Praise for M. T0028608

"This powerful book will revolutionize the way you think about diabetes. Written by two guys with type 1 diabetes at the forefront of the diabetes revolution, Cyrus and Robby have created a roadmap to understand the physiology of insulin resistance and give you the tools to reverse it using powerful scientific evidence."

—Michael Greger, MD, FACC, *New York Times* bestselling author of *How Not to Diet*

"When you are a type 2 diabetic, my message is don't control it—instead, get rid of it. *Mastering Diabetes* is a masterpiece with critical information that every diabetic should know. Knowledge is power. Why be a diabetic when you can recover?"

—Joel Fuhrman, MD, *New York Times* bestselling author of *The End of Diabetes*

"Cyrus and Robby's work is methodically researched, brilliantly written, and substantiated by hundreds of scientific studies. Autoimmune diseases can be successfully treated with a plant-based diet. I see it every day in my work with inflammatory bowel disease patients, and now Cyrus and Robby have shown us the incredible results of eating this way to master all forms of diabetes."

—Robynne Chutkan, MD, author of *The Microbiome Solution*

"As a physician, I am under tremendous pressures and time constraints, so it is imperative that I have excellent resources at hand to refer my patients to. *Mastering Diabetes* is my go-to resource for my diabetic patients. Robby and Cyrus have done a phenomenal job putting this book together so that everyone can benefit from their years of personal and coaching experience. I wish every physician knew as much about diabetes and could communicate it to their patients as well as Robby and Cyrus do."

—Laurie L. Marbas, MD, MBA

"*Mastering Diabetes* is a landmark book that shows how common beliefs about carbohydrates and diabetes are exacerbating a tragic epidemic. The knowledge and advice on these pages will improve millions of lives and provide a clear scientific model that can end diabetes as we know it."

—Brian Wendel, founder and creator of Forks Over Knives

"In the world of ultra-processed convenience foods, it's a struggle for many people to eat naturally, especially for people at risk for all forms of diabetes. This book will not only teach you the fascinating biology of diabetes, it lays out a daringly simple approach to eating whole foods that's actually the most powerful form of medicine ever discovered. If you're at risk or living with diabetes, read this book—it will completely change your view of diabetes and help you live with exceptional health for many years to come."

—John Mackey, cofounder and CEO of Whole Foods Market

# MASTERING DIABETES

The Revolutionary Method to Reverse
Insulin Resistance *Permanently* in Type 1, Type 1.5,
Type 2, Prediabetes, and Gestational Diabetes

Cyrus Khambatta, PhD,
and Robby Barbaro, MPH

*with Rachel Holtzman*

*Foreword by Neal Barnard, MD*

*Illustrations by Samantha Stutzman*

AVERY
an imprint of Penguin Random House
New York

AVERY

an imprint of Penguin Random House LLC
penguinrandomhouse.com

First trade paperback edition 2022
Copyright © 2020 by Cyrus Khambatta and Robby Barbaro

Most Avery books are available at special quantity discounts for bulk purchase for sales promotions, premiums, fund-raising, and educational needs. Special books or book excerpts also can be created to fit specific needs. For details, write SpecialMarkets@penguinrandomhouse.com.

ISBN 9780593189993 (hardcover)
ISBN 9780525540045 (e-book)
ISBN 9780593542040 (paperback)

Printed in the United States of America
4th Printing

Book design by Patrice Sheridan

Neither the publisher nor the author is engaged in rendering professional advice or services to the individual reader. The ideas, procedures, and suggestions contained in this book are not intended as a substitute for consulting with your physician. All matters regarding your health require medical supervision. Neither the author nor the publisher shall be liable or responsible for any loss or damage allegedly arising from any information or suggestion in this book.

This book is dedicated to those willing to challenge the status quo and to those willing to reevaluate outdated and incomplete scientific principles.

# Contents

# Foreword

My father arrived home from work every night around six o'clock. He set his heavy medical bag next to the door and plunked down in a living room chair to read the newspaper until dinnertime. He was the diabetes expert for Fargo, North Dakota. Patients from eastern North Dakota and western Minnesota came to see him to find out how they were doing and to regulate their insulin doses. Not once did he come home proclaiming that a patient had been cured. He never even mentioned that a patient with diabetes got better. His goals were much more modest. He worked only to slow the inevitable complications of the disease.

For many people with diabetes, that is about as good as it gets, even today. Diagnosed with type 2 diabetes, they are advised to make a few perfunctory diet changes and to take a gradually escalating regimen of medications. Drugs for diabetes. Drugs for cholesterol. Drugs for blood pressure. And the disease never goes away and never really gets better. People with type 1 diabetes manage the disease as best they can, hoping to stave off complications. Women with gestational diabetes assume the disease will recur with each pregnancy.

If that has been your experience, you are about to enter a completely new world. It is time to *master* diabetes. For some people, that may even mean getting rid of it.

The first clues that diabetes could be tamed came from observations in countries that changed their diets. In Japan in the 1980s, for example, the fast-food invasion meant that chicken wings, burgers, and milkshakes replaced the traditional rice-based diet. In the process, diabetes rates soared. Similarly, as America's appetite for meat and cheese grew decade after decade, so did the prevalence of type 2 diabetes. That led to the question, what if we do exactly the opposite? What if we throw out these unhealthy foods and move to a more plant-based diet?

Our research team, funded by the National Institutes of Health, did just that. In a group of adults with type 2 diabetes, we randomly assigned half to a conventional "diabetes diet" that called for reducing calories and keeping carbohydrates fairly steady from day to day. The other participants began a totally new diet, throwing out meat, cheese, and other animal products altogether and minimizing oils. Rather than restricting fruits, as many people with diabetes have been told to do, they had all the fruit they wanted. And they ate vegetables, beans, whole grains, and all the foods these ingredients turn into: vegetable stews, lentil soup, bean burritos, angel hair pasta topped with artichoke hearts and grilled mushrooms, vegan lasagna, curries, vegetable sushi, and countless others, without counting calories or carbohydrates.

In the process, their laboratory tests showed surprising results. In 2006, the American Diabetes Association published our first findings: The plant-based diet was three times more effective at improving blood glucose control compared with the conventional diet. Three years later, we published our longer-term findings in the *American Journal of Clinical Nutrition*, confirming that the benefits last. Many other research teams have studied similar diets, consistently finding weight loss and improved cholesterol levels and blood pressure. Perhaps surprisingly, it has turned out to be rather easy. Yes, our research participants do have to learn some new tastes and unlearn others. But unlike every other diet they have been on, there is no hunger—they are free to eat as much as they want. There is no roller coaster ride of weight loss followed by weight gain. And they never have to fear carbohydrates as many people do. They are free to explore a new world of delicious foods.

We have also put the diet to work for people with long-standing diabetes, whose disease has led to painful neuropathy in their feet or hands. And despite their long history with the disease, they, too, improve to a surprising degree.

Meanwhile, our colleagues at Yale University have looked inside the human body to understand what is actually happening during a diet change. Using magnetic resonance spectroscopy, they have found that fats from the foods we eat accumulate inside muscle and liver cells. As these fats build up, they interfere with insulin function, causing a condition called *insulin resistance* and setting the stage for type 2 diabetes. A low-fat plant-based diet, of course, has no animal fat and very little vegetable fat. So it helps that built-up fat to dissipate, allowing insulin function to be restored to a great degree.

Many people have put this approach to work for type 1 diabetes, too, finding that it greatly improves their glucose control, slashes their insulin requirements, and helps them feel better overall. Researchers are also investigating ways of preventing type 1 diabetes, finding that breast-feeding (especially avoiding exposure to cow's milk proteins) may reduce the chances of sparking the autoimmune reaction that destroys the insulin-producing beta cells of the pancreas. While that research is by no means finished, there is every reason to take advantage of the power of a plant-based diet.

*Mastering Diabetes* puts this power in your hands. Cyrus and Robby know diabetes inside and out, having dealt with it personally and having thoroughly researched the published literature. They are experts, and they will guide you step by step. Soon, you will have the confidence of knowing you are on the right path. You will see the results in how you feel, and you will confirm these benefits in your laboratory tests.

Let me encourage you to read this book from cover to cover, to put its power to work, and to share it with others who could benefit from this life-changing new approach.

Neal D. Barnard, MD, FACC
President, Physicians Committee for Responsible Medicine
Adjunct Associate Professor of Medicine, George Washington
University School of Medicine and Health Sciences
Washington, DC

In the process of writing this book, we read thousands of scientific papers and referenced more than 800 peer-reviewed articles. Even though there are too many references to print in this book, we are passionate about empowering you to make informed decisions for your health. Visit www.mastering diabetes.org/bookinfo to explore every scientific reference in this book.

# Mastering Diabetes

# Chapter 1

# This Book Can Save Your Life

As you're probably aware, diabetes is currently one of the fastest-growing chronic diseases in the United States and around the world. It has officially been classified as a pandemic by the Centers for Disease Control and Prevention (CDC), which estimates that more than 29 million people in the United States are living with type 1 and type 2 diabetes and that a staggering 86 million more have prediabetes. In 2017, the total cost of diagnosed diabetes on the American healthcare system was $327 billion, and is expected to grow to $490 billion by 2030. By 2050, experts estimate that diagnosed diabetes will affect 33 percent of the US population—*that's 1 in every 3 people.*

To make matters even more real, people with diabetes incur an average of $13,700 of medical expenses per year—2.3 times as much as nondiabetic individuals. Receiving the diagnosis of diabetes dramatically increases your risk for the development of many chronic diseases, making you more likely to be absent from work, less productive at your job, and at risk for premature death.

If you've been diagnosed with any form of diabetes, it may seem like the odds are against you. If you're losing energy, gaining weight, facing rising medical expenses, or worried that your life may be cut short, it may be time to put the right lifestyle habits into place and avoid the slow-moving disaster that diabetes often creates.

That's exactly why we wrote this book.

Even though the statistics are scary, the truth is that the solution to diabetes is actually more readily available than you may think. In this book, we'll explain how people living with all forms of diabetes can optimize their diet and exercise habits to feel great, look amazing, and minimize the risk of long-term complications, including conditions like coronary artery disease, atherosclerosis, cancer, high cholesterol, high blood pressure, obesity, peripheral neuropathy, retinopathy, Alzheimer's disease, chronic kidney disease, and fatty liver disease.

Many people are skeptical about the scientific research in support of low-fat plant-based whole-food nutrition, and often claim that the Mastering Diabetes Method has no scientific basis. In the process of writing this book, we read thousands of scientific papers covering a wide range of topics (including low-carbohydrate nutrition) and were amazed at just how much research exists in support of a low-fat plant-based whole-food diet. This book references more than 800 scientific articles, which is too many to print in the book itself. We are passionate about empowering you to make informed decisions for your health, so please visit www.masteringdiabetes.org/bookinfo to explore every scientific reference in this book.

If you're ready to eat delicious meals made from ingredients that people living with diabetes have been told to limit or avoid for years, this is your opportunity. If you're excited to eat carbohydrate-rich foods like bananas, mangoes, potatoes, squash, corn, beans, lentils, quinoa, and rice, and lose weight, reduce your blood glucose, and minimize or eliminate your need for oral medications and insulin, then you're going to love learning how simple changes to your diet can fully transform your health from the inside out.

If you're living with prediabetes or non-insulin-dependent type 2 diabetes, we'll teach you how to completely reverse both conditions using your food as medicine. For those living with insulin-dependent diabetes, including type 1 diabetes, type 1.5 diabetes, or insulin-dependent type 2 diabetes, we'll teach you how to maximize your insulin sensitivity and make your blood glucose significantly easier to control while reducing your overall need for basal and bolus insulin. Regardless of the type of diabetes you may be living with, the system outlined in this book will dramatically reduce your risk for diabetes complications, help you achieve your ideal body weight, increase your mental clarity, and dramatically increase your energy levels.

If you enjoy eating, then you'll love this book. Why? Because we'll spend the majority of our time focusing on food, then venture into the world of intermittent fasting and exercise, so that you have a full picture of why each puzzle piece helps reverse insulin resistance and how to put the puzzle pieces together in your busy life.

We know this might sound crazy, but stick with us—it's going to be a fun ride. You're about to get a full picture of how to maximize your total body health, and get the nitty-gritty details about the most powerful insulin-sensitizing method ever developed. We'll address the incredible confusion that exists in the world of diabetes head on and provide you with a complete understanding of the long-term dangers of eating a low-carbohydrate or ketogenic diet. You'll learn why low-carbohydrate diets actually *increase* insulin resistance and dramatically increase your risk for many chronic diseases in the long term.

We wrote this book not only to provide you with the evidence-based science of insulin resistance but also to give you a detailed and straightforward how-to guide that we know works from extensive personal experience and from helping thousands of people with all forms of diabetes maximize their insulin sensitivity.

We wrote this book because we want you to know that you are in full control of your diabetes destiny. We want you to know that you can reverse insulin resistance by following the Mastering Diabetes Method, which will in turn drop your risk for the development of diabetes complications both now and in the future. The exact foods that have been demonized for almost a hundred years are actually the solution, and we'll show you exactly why.

## A Note to the Reader

The information contained in this book will educate you about how to reverse insulin resistance permanently. Do not underestimate the effectiveness of this program. Because this information is so effective, you must implement these changes with the help, support, knowledge, and guidance of your physician. Many people living with diabetes around the world have found that the Mastering Diabetes Method results in a strong reduction in their requirement for oral medication, insulin, or both. Failure to reduce your medications appropriately may result in life-threatening hypoglycemia and even death.

Many physicians are unaware of the power of low-fat plant-based whole-food nutrition and may be hesitant to reduce your medication dosages sufficiently. Because of this, it is important for you to monitor your blood glucose very carefully as you change your diet step by step. If you are currently taking oral medications for high blood pressure or high cholesterol, the Mastering Diabetes Method is also very likely to lower your blood pressure and cholesterol levels significantly. Work closely with your physician to prevent dangerous and life-threatening situations that could arise from not reducing your oral medication and insulin use quickly when participating in this program.

## This Book Can Save Your Life

How do we know? Because we have been living with type 1 diabetes ourselves for a combined total of more than thirty-six years. Because we have extensively read almost a hundred years of evidence-based scientific research. Because our colleagues are healthcare professionals who have observed remarkable and repeatable results in thousands of patients for decades.

And what's more, we've developed an online coaching program for people with all forms of diabetes that is like no other program currently on the market. Not only does it work incredibly well (we and our clients test-drive it every single day), but it also addresses all the day-in-the-life questions, concerns, and frustrations that affect those of us living with diabetes.

For more than four years, our Mastering Diabetes Coaching Program has helped people with all forms of diabetes reduce or eliminate diabetes medications while increasing their consumption of carbohydrate-rich whole foods. Most people living with prediabetes and type 2 diabetes have been able to completely reverse diabetes, discontinue the use of oral medications and insulin, and drop their A1c to 5.6% or less. Those living with insulin-dependent diabetes often experience a 10 to 60 percent reduction in both basal and bolus insulin use, with more stable and predictable blood glucose values, and an A1c value between 5.5% and 6.5%. In addition, thousands of clients have been able to lose weight; dramatically lower their cholesterol, blood pressure, and triglycerides; improve their digestive function; and live without the fear of future complications.

Our clients come to us because they're disappointed (and sometimes outraged) by the advice they have received in the past, which may have seemed attractive and logical at the time. They enlist our help because they are frustrated with a decreasing quality of life and an increasing need for oral medications and insulin. They're gaining weight, have unpredictable blood glucose, and are constipated, inflamed, and exhausted. We hear them. The truth is, *we were them.*

## A New Approach to Understanding—and Mastering—Diabetes

We were both diagnosed with type 1 diabetes early in life—Robby as a preteen and Cyrus in his early twenties—and as outgoing, athletic, adventurous, motivated guys, we didn't want to put our lives on hold. But after following the popular medically orthodox low-carbohydrate, high-fat, high-protein diet to help manage our blood glucose, we were far from being in the driver's seat of our metabolic health. Instead of making our blood glucose more controllable and increasing our insulin sensitivity, the nutritional steps we followed had exactly the opposite effect. It seemed that no matter how "perfectly" we ate, our insulin sensitivity decreased and our physical and emotional health suffered immensely because of it.

Even though we didn't know each other at the time, we each made the decision to reexamine the nutritional advice given to us by the conventional medical system. We started by looking to "alternative" diet philosophies for guidance, including vegetarian, vegan, raw vegan, and the Weston A. Price Foundation diet. Amazingly, our two different tracks led us to the same conclusion:

**A low-fat plant-based whole-food lifestyle is the most effective way to gain insulin sensitivity using your food as medicine.**

Even though this may seem counterintuitive at first, this form of nutrition is extremely powerful at reversing insulin resistance because carbohydrate-rich whole foods require large amounts of insulin *if and only if the total amount of fat in your diet is also high,* as you will learn about in detail in chapter 3. But when you eat a low-fat plant-based whole-food diet and reduce your intake of fat- and protein-rich foods, you gain insulin sensitivity very quickly, which in turn drops your need for oral medications and insulin in the short and long term.

Within days of changing our diets, we both observed that our insulin sensitivity increased dramatically. In addition, our energy levels increased, and our blood glucose became much easier to control. After only a few months of eating this way, Cyrus saw his total insulin use drop by 40 percent and Robby saw his insulin sensitivity improve by 600 percent. To put it in perspective: The average adult with type 1 diabetes injects approximately 0.5 to 1.0 units of insulin per kilogram of body weight per day. Following the Mastering Diabetes Method, those living with type 1 diabetes inject as little as 0.35 units of insulin per kilogram body weight per day, and experience dramatically improved blood glucose values, while increasing carbohydrate intake as much as twenty-fold. When we transitioned to eating more plants, we began eating more fruits and vegetables than ever before—including many foods that previously had been forbidden on a low-carbohydrate diet. *And despite this counterintuitive approach, we both felt better than ever—even better than before we were diagnosed.*

This radical shift in our own personal diets sparked an adventure to learn as much as possible about nutrition-driven wellness. It's what originally led Robby to help build the revolutionary Forks Over Knives empire and earn a master's degree in public health. It's also what inspired Cyrus to leave his job at the NASA Ames Research Center as a Stanford University–educated mechanical engineer to earn a PhD in nutritional biochemistry at the University of California, Berkeley. But the real magic was in realizing that we could take our unique insights, knowledge, and experience as people with diabetes and turn it into usable, relatable, and *effective* advice for other people living with all forms of diabetes, including type 1 diabetes, type 1.5 diabetes, type 2 diabetes, prediabetes, and gestational diabetes. That's the ethos behind our coaching program, and it's what lies at the foundation of this book.

Over time, we have fine-tuned the Mastering Diabetes Method into something that is truly unique. It encompasses the following four components:

**Component 1: Low-Fat Plant-Based Whole-Food Nutrition.** We encourage carbohydrate-rich whole foods, including fruits, starchy vegetables, legumes, and intact whole grains. As you will learn in this book, carbohydrate-rich food is not the enemy when you are living with diabetes, and we'll provide you with the scientific rationale as to why eating fruit and starchy foods is actually an integral part of reversing insulin resistance and maximizing your longevity.

**Component 2: Intermittent Fasting.** Not eating is one of the most powerful ways to improve your insulin sensitivity, improve your cardiovascular health, lose weight, and actually *increase* your lifespan. You'll learn about various intermittent fasting routines and ways to successfully integrate this time-tested and proven practice into your busy lifestyle.

**Component 3: Daily Movement.** Your body is designed for physical activity, and when you make daily movement a part of your lifestyle, you're likely to dramatically improve your insulin sensitivity, your energy levels, and your mood. We'll teach you how to move your body, how often to move your body, and how to combine movement with a low-fat plant-based whole-food diet for maximum effect.

**Component 4: Decision Trees.** We have created a specific tool that helps you address hour-by-hour decisions, look for patterns, and establish cause-and-effect relationships between your lifestyle choices and your blood glucose profile. The process of filling out decision trees helps you troubleshoot confusing everyday scenarios relating to oral medication use, insulin use, and blood glucose management. In addition, decision trees can help you address little-picture scenarios like managing your blood glucose before, during, and after exercise; safely reducing your use of oral medications and insulin as your insulin sensitivity significantly increases; understanding why your fasting glucose might be higher than your post-meal glucose at times; dealing with post-meal blood glucose spikes and dips; and timing your insulin use to properly control your blood glucose after meals.

Furthermore, you'll learn how to use and interpret important diabetes blood tests and how to incorporate various medicinal plants as alternatives to pharmaceutical medications. We'll also answer such questions as: *Should I exercise before or after a meal? Why does my blood glucose increase when I eat certain foods?* and *Do fruits really metabolize to sugar?*

One aspect of the Mastering Diabetes Method that is very important to understand is that we welcome people with all forms of diabetes including type 1 diabetes, type 1.5 diabetes, type 2 diabetes, prediabetes, and gestational diabetes, because our collective struggles controlling blood glucose all originate from the same underlying condition: insulin resistance.

Even though we are diabetes experts, our understanding of diabetes does not originate from a traditional medical background and instead comes from personal experience, a PhD in nutritional biochemistry, a rigorous analysis of almost a hundred years of evidence-based scientific research, decades of repeatable results from our colleagues, our in-person retreats, and our work with thousands of people via our online coaching program. Unlike any other program or book currently on the market for diabetes, *Mastering Diabetes* is written by two experts who have proven firsthand that our prescription works by helping more than 3,000 people around the world adopt lifestyle changes that transform their metabolic health from the inside out. This program is based on thirty-six years of combined personal experience living with type 1 diabetes and twenty-nine years of combined experience following the Mastering Diabetes Method.

Even though we're not MDs, we are well versed in the evidence-based research of nutritional biochemistry and use rigorous scientific evidence as the basis for our recommendations. Because we put this data to the test every single day in our own lives, we are able to translate complex scientific concepts into easy-to-understand principles. Many people tell us that watching a few of our videos or webinars—like the ones that debunk the misleading science of low-carbohydrate and ketogenic diets, reveal the true causes of high cholesterol, or demonstrate why increasing your protein intake can help you lose weight but increases your long-term disease risk—has taught them more about the biological details of living with diabetes than their doctor ever has. Evidence-based science (not pop science) is the foundation of our platform, and we make it a point to translate complicated biological phenomena into easy-to-understand topics so that you can understand *how* and *why* specific foods can transform your health from the inside out, and *how* and *why* other foods can increase your chronic disease risk.

Last but not least, we'll plug you into a community. We've honed and strengthened the Mastering Diabetes Coaching Program based on the feedback from thousands of clients who follow it every day, and the most important thing we've found is that our clients do best when surrounded and supported by other people going through the same experience. Success is truly contagious! Too often, when you read a book or try a new program to improve your diabetes health, you're a solo rider. The Mastering Diabetes Coaching Program is designed to put an end to that isolating feeling that comes from attempting to manage diabetes on your own. To help you plug into our support system, we have created a private online community that we monitor 24/7 to give real-time responses to our clients. We also host regular video conferences where community members can bring questions and concerns and interact directly with our highly educated and experienced coaching staff.

What began years ago as a cautiously optimistic plan originally using ourselves as test subjects—bolstered, of course, by sound research—has since blossomed into a life-changing program that has received the praise and support of well-regarded experts and friends including Dean Ornish, MD; Michael Greger, MD; Neal Barnard, MD; John McDougall, MD; Garth Davis, MD; Joel Kahn, MD; Caldwell Esselstyn, MD; Brenda Davis, RD; Michelle McMacken, MD; Dean and Ayesha Sherzai, MD; Rip Esselstyn; Danielle Belardo, MD; Robert Ostfeld, MD; Ocean Robbins; and many more. It's a scientific method that has transformed the lives of the thousands of individuals who have already followed our program and will do so for you, too. If you stay faithful to the steps and insights outlined in this book, you are likely to experience the same results as our clients. You'll lose the weight that you never thought you'd be able to lose, you'll achieve the best A1c values you've ever experienced, you'll lower your total and LDL cholesterol, you'll reduce your blood pressure, you'll reduce your need for oral medications and insulin, and most importantly, *you'll significantly decrease or completely reverse insulin resistance now and for the rest of your life.*

The most important thing that you can take away from this book is that the Mastering Diabetes Method is a time-tested and proven system that is designed to teach you how to control your blood glucose with precision and maximize your overall metabolic health for the rest of your life. While many diabetes books teach you how to improve the numbers on your blood glucose meter, we have worked tirelessly to ensure that the recommendations set forth in this book dramatically improve your diabetes health both in the short and long terms and give you the highest chance of preventing and reversing many chronic diseases that often travel together with insulin resistance.

> *I have had diabetes for 31 years, and after 4 months in the Mastering Diabetes Coaching Program I lost 23 pounds and got off all my cholesterol medication. Anyone who is new to this approach, just stick with it—it's incredibly rewarding.*
>
> —John L., type 1 diabetes

> *In less than one month, I stopped taking 2,000 mg of metformin every day. In 4 months, I lost 45 pounds and dropped my blood pressure and cholesterol medication completely. I have lots of energy and think clearly now.*
>
> —Gerry B., reversed type 2 diabetes

> *I just got my labs back and I did it! I reversed type 2 diabetes and high blood pressure with a whole-food plant-based diet with your help. I'm on cloud nine right now basically crying with joy. Thank you, Robby and Cyrus, for helping me change my life.*
>
> —Cheryl K., reversed type 2 diabetes

*When I first started in the Mastering Diabetes group 8 months ago,*
*I was a prediabetic and very overweight. Since adopting this program,*
*I have lost more than 70 pounds, and prediabetes just went away. The*
*Mastering Diabetes plan is the best plan for achieving lasting health,*
*even if you don't have diabetes. We only live once, and I personally*
*believe we are all in this together.*

—John D., reversed prediabetes

*I started at 285 pounds and I am now down to 183 pounds. My A1c*
*dropped from 11.6% to 5.6%. My fasting blood sugars are between 88*
*and 93 every day. I am eternally grateful for the Mastering Diabetes*
*Coaching Program.*

—Stefanie S., reversed type 2 diabetes

When Cyrus first started his doctorate in nutritional biochemistry, he had a difficult time understanding why insulin resistance was such a problem. Only after thousands of hours of research did the answer to this question become extremely clear. Insulin resistance is a major condition that underlies many chronic metabolic diseases, including (but not limited to) type 1 diabetes, type 1.5 diabetes, type 2 diabetes, prediabetes, gestational diabetes, coronary artery disease, atherosclerosis, cancer, high cholesterol, high blood pressure, obesity, polycystic ovary syndrome (PCOS), peripheral neuropathy, retinopathy, Alzheimer's disease, chronic kidney disease, and fatty liver disease.

Think of insulin resistance as the central culprit that elevates your risk for most chronic diseases and as the root condition that accelerates the development of cardiovascular disease, cancer, type 2 diabetes, and obesity—our planet's leading causes of death. More than any other condition, insulin resistance is the strongest predictor of chronic disease, and recent research suggests that 65 percent of all people living with type 1 diabetes for more than 20 years will die of cardiovascular disease and that more than 50 percent of people living with type 1 diabetes for more than 30 years will die of kidney failure. And unfortunately, achieving tight blood glucose control without reversing insulin resistance **is not enough to minimize your risk for future diabetes complications,** as you will learn in detail in chapter 7.

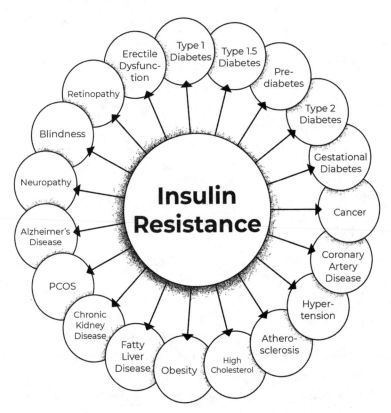

Insulin resistance influences your risk for the development of a number of chronic health conditions in addition to diabetes.

The good news is that insulin resistance is often detectable up to twenty years before the symptoms of diabetes and heart disease become noticeable, which means that controlling and reversing insulin resistance today can prevent the onset of many chronic metabolic diseases in the future.

## How Many Types of Diabetes Are There?

**Even though most people** have heard of type 1 and type 2 diabetes, it turns out that there are many types of diabetes—and that they can all be improved using the Mastering Diabetes Method. That's because there are many reasons why your blood glucose can increase, and taking the time to understand which specific tissues in your body are affected is your key to understanding which type of diabetes you are living with. Throughout this book, we'll refer to various types of diabetes, but before we go any further, let's get clear about the differences between each type.

- **Type 1 diabetes** is commonly referred to as *juvenile onset diabetes* because it has traditionally affected young children and adolescents. It is an autoimmune condition that can completely destroy insulin-producing beta cells in your pancreas, dramatically decreasing *endogenous* (self-made) *insulin* production, while increasing the need for *exogenous insulin* (insulin injected through a syringe, pen, or insulin pump). When you are living with type 1 diabetes, the goals of following the Mastering Diabetes Method include increasing your carbohydrate-to-insulin ratio; maximizing your insulin sensitivity; making your blood glucose extremely predictable; preventing common complications such as heart disease, neuropathy, retinopathy, and kidney disease; reaching your ideal body weight; and dramatically increasing your energy levels.

- **Type 1.5 diabetes,** or latent autoimmune diabetes in adults (LADA), is also an autoimmune version of diabetes that destroys insulin-producing beta cells. Unlike type 1 diabetes, however, type 1.5 diabetes affects people over the age of 30 and is a slower-progressing autoimmune reaction that gradually destroys beta cells and decreases endogenous insulin production, often over the course of five to ten years. Think of type 1.5 diabetes as an adult-onset, slow-progressing version of type 1 diabetes that is often misdiagnosed as type 2 diabetes. As is true with type 1 diabetes, when you are living with type 1.5 diabetes, the goals of following the Mastering Diabetes Method are to preserve beta cell function for as long as possible; increase your carbohydrate-to-insulin ratio; maximize your insulin sensitivity; make your blood glucose extremely predictable; prevent common complications such as heart disease, neuropathy, retinopathy, and kidney disease; reach your ideal body weight; and dramatically increase your energy levels.

- **Prediabetes** is a condition that precedes type 2 diabetes and is diagnosed when your fasting blood glucose is between 100 and 125 mg/dL, or when your A1c value is between 5.7% and 6.4%. Prediabetes occurs when your muscles and liver have become resistant to the effects of insulin, resulting in a minor traffic jam of both glucose and insulin in your blood that slightly elevates your fasting blood glucose. Think of prediabetes as a warning sign that type 2 diabetes is fast approaching. The goal of following the Mastering Diabetes Method living with prediabetes is to eliminate insulin resistance and avoid the transition to type 2 diabetes altogether.

- **Type 2 diabetes (non-insulin-dependent)** occurs when your fasting blood glucose increases beyond 125 mg/dL or when your A1c level is 6.5% or greater, yet you are still producing sufficient quantities of endogenous insulin. A type 2 diabetes diagnosis follows when prediabetes progresses beyond mild insulin resistance, often resulting in an increased risk for high blood pressure, high cholesterol, atherosclerosis, weight gain, fatty liver disease, chronic kidney disease, and low energy. The goals of following the Mastering Diabetes Method living with non-insulin-dependent type 2 diabetes are to maximize your insulin sensitivity until you no longer require diabetes medications, drop your A1c to 5.6% or below, and remove type 2 diabetes from your health record. If you have been diagnosed with type 2 diabetes, eating to reverse insulin resistance is your ticket to becoming nondiabetic.

- **Type 2 diabetes (insulin-dependent)** occurs when your fasting blood glucose increases beyond 125 mg/dL or when your A1c level is 6.5% or greater, and you are not producing sufficient quantities of endogenous insulin. Insulin-dependent type 2 diabetes occurs when beta cells have overproduced insulin for a long period of time, resulting in an inability to produce sufficient insulin. In this situation, managing your blood glucose with precision can be accomplished only by using your diet in combination with insulin and/or oral medications. As is true in type 1 and type 1.5 diabetes, the goals of following the Mastering Diabetes Method living with insulin-dependent type 2 diabetes are to maximize your insulin sensitivity; make your blood glucose extremely predictable; minimize or eliminate oral diabetes medications; prevent common complications such as heart disease, neuropathy, retinopathy, and kidney disease; reach your ideal body weight; and dramatically increase your energy levels.

- **Gestational diabetes** is a version of diabetes that affects pregnant women and usually disappears after giving birth. Gestational diabetes can occur at any stage of pregnancy, but it is more common in the second half, when a woman fails a diagnostic screening known as a *glucose tolerance test*. Much like prediabetes and type 2 diabetes, gestational diabetes can result when a pregnant woman develops insulin resistance, and can be managed, prevented, and even reversed using the Mastering Diabetes Method. Even though gestational diabetes often disappears after birth, it's still important to address it during pregnancy because it can increase the risk for premature birth, preeclampsia (high blood pressure), and stillbirth, and can dramatically increase the risk for developing type 2 diabetes in the months and years after pregnancy.

# The Mastering Diabetes Method

Like our coaching program, this book is designed to help you create a long-term and sustainable lifestyle that is very effective at decreasing or eliminating your biological need for oral medications and insulin while increasing your intake of carbohydrate-rich foods. Using evidence-based research and making the information easily understandable for anyone who isn't a scientist, we'll help you understand why you'll benefit from changing the way you eat and how to do it successfully *and* safely. All of the expertise, planning, strategies, tips, tools, and tricks that we've acquired living this very same lifestyle will be there for the taking, just as they are for our coaching clients. And by following this step-by-step process, you'll be setting yourself up for success more effectively than any other program that promises a "quick fix."

Ultimately, at the foundation of this process is what we have personally experienced to be true—your diabetes health is only as good as your daily habits. If you have taken the time to create strong, effective, and reliable habits that improve your blood glucose control and metabolic health, then you're likely to reap the rewards of this lifestyle for a long time. If instead you speed through making lifestyle changes and don't take the time to create a collection of long-lasting habits, then you're likely to revert back to your old habits when confronted with challenging situations.

Understanding exactly what components of your diet affect your blood glucose is more powerful than any medication you can buy, and it can save you thousands of dollars on test strips, oral medications, and insulin every year. In addition, you'll learn exactly which foods will help your body repair long-standing metabolic damage, how to easily integrate them into your daily life, and how to maximize these effects with other highly effective lifestyle changes, including intermittent fasting and exercise. And if you choose to join our online coaching program, we'll connect you with an online community so that you have plenty of support, and we'll include a number of case studies throughout the book so you can learn from others about how to apply these teachings in real life. So settle in, peel yourself a mango, and let's get started.

To view the 25+ scientific references cited in this chapter, please visit us online at www.masteringdiabetes.org/bookinfo.

# Chapter 2

# The Mastering Diabetes Approach

**Reversing Type 2 Diabetes and Achieving a Nondiabetic A1c: Tami's Story**

As a child and teenager, Tami was very active in sports, but by the time she was 19, she had undergone two surgeries on the same knee. Over the course of the next thirty years, she wore out her other knee, destroyed the arches in both feet, and developed chronic hip pain. As a result of these injuries, Tami became inactive and steadily gained weight. She began to lose hope that she could ever be a normal weight again, and as she witnessed family members struggle with heart disease and cancer, she was scared that she was next in line.

When Tami was 51, she got a blood test at a wellness fair. She found out that her A1c and lipids were elevated, and after further investigation, she was diagnosed with not just one, but a collection of chronic diseases including type 2 diabetes, high cholesterol, obesity, fatty liver disease, and vitamin D deficiency. She was shocked and angry at herself for allowing her health to deteriorate to this point, but she was also determined to figure out the root cause. When one of her doctors told her that insulin resistance was the culprit in all of these conditions, she began researching this idea online and found a community of people claiming that they could "reverse insulin resistance and lower their A1c using their diet," in the Mastering Diabetes Coaching Program.

Meanwhile, Tami's A1c had reached 7.1%, her total cholesterol was 266 mg/dL, and her triglycerides had climbed to 194 mg/dL. Her doctor prescribed her 2,000 mg of metformin per day, and she used that to manage her blood glucose, given a lack of other effective options. Despite this, she was determined to reverse insulin resistance and reduce her A1c (as she had read about online). Motivated by the opportunity to transform her health from the inside out without the use of pharmaceutical medications, she decided to join the Mastering Diabetes Coaching Program.

During the first few weeks of the program, she resisted the idea of changing her eating habits because she found it challenging to give up the foods that she had eaten her whole life. But once she gained momentum and began making the recommended changes, Tami began losing weight, gaining energy, and reducing her fasting blood glucose. As the weight came off, she began exercising more frequently and experienced less joint pain than she had over the previous thirty years.

Four and a half months after applying the Mastering Diabetes Method, Tami's A1c dropped to 5.3%, she had discontinued diabetes medications, her fasting glucose had normalized, her chronic cough was gone, her plantar fasciitis went away, her chronic allergies had disappeared, and she no longer experienced acid reflux. She had lost 34 pounds, and you can now find her back in motion doing the activities she loves, including riding her bike or hiking in the hills—without pain or inflammation in her knees, feet, or hips. In addition, she absolutely loves the wide variety of fresh whole foods that maximize her insulin sensitivity, and she shares her delicious meals with her family and friends. She enjoys her lifestyle so much that she has started her own online community to inspire others to do the same for their health.

---

You may have picked up this book for many reasons—maybe you're struggling with living with type 1 diabetes, type 1.5 diabetes, type 2 diabetes, prediabetes, gestational diabetes, polycystic ovary syndrome (PCOS), obesity, high blood pressure, high cholesterol, fatty liver disease, or chronic kidney disease. Maybe you're an athlete looking to improve your athletic performance and recovery, or you're seeking more energy or sharper mental clarity. Maybe you're reading this book to help a loved one improve his or her overall health. The good news is that no matter what brought you here, you're here! Which means we can get started unpacking our method, which is specifically designed to combat the root cause of all blood glucose variability: insulin resistance. By addressing insulin resistance directly, you will learn how to stop *managing the symptoms* of blood glucose fluctuations and instead *reverse the cause* of unmanageable blood glucose once and for all. This book is divided into five steps.

## Step 1: Making a Plan to Succeed

More than anything else, we want you to *succeed* in the long run. That's why it's just as important to understand both the *how* and the *why*. We'll talk about what insulin resistance is (complete with handy visuals for understanding how this complex issue works) and what really causes it (it may not be what you think). Then we'll discuss why slow change is helpful for both your body *and* for long-term success, why consistency is your new best friend, and how you can set realistic and achievable goals. For those living with insulin-dependent diabetes, we'll describe how to adjust your insulin dosing strategy as your insulin needs drop significantly. For those living with non-insulin-dependent diabetes, we'll explain which diabetes medications are safest to reduce first and what you can expect as your need for medications is reduced or completely eliminated.

Then it's on to the *what*, as in *what do I eat?* In chapter 8 we'll give you all the concrete answers about *what* to eat, *what* to minimize or eliminate, *how much* to eat, *when* to eat, and *how* to make your new lifestyle sustainable in the long term. Our goal in this section is to help you feel as confident as possible in your new way of eating. To make the Mastering Diabetes Method as simple as possible to follow, we've categorized foods as **green light foods** (fruits, starchy vegetables, legumes, intact whole grains, non-starchy vegetables, leafy greens, herbs and spices), **yellow light foods** (fatty plants like avocados, olives, coconuts, nuts including peanuts, seeds, edamame, and pasta alternatives), and **red light foods** (red meat, white meat, fish, dairy products, eggs, refined grains and processed foods, vegetable oils, and refined sugars). Green light foods are those that actually *improve* your insulin sensitivity and can be enjoyed in abundance, yellow light foods are okay to include in your diet occasionally (i.e., they are not to be eaten in unlimited quantities), and red light foods are those that actually *create* insulin resistance and should be minimized or completely avoided for best results.

The most common complaint about eating a low-fat plant-based whole-food diet (and the reason why most people abandon plant-based diets in general) is *not understanding how to eat enough calories.* People often report that they have low energy or are losing weight too rapidly—and we'll address all of these concerns by showing you how to eat foods with the optimal calorie density to keep you satisfied as you transition to a plant-based diet.

## Step 2: Changing Your Diet One Meal at a Time

We have found that our clients who have the most success making the transition to the Mastering Diabetes Method are the ones who change their diets *one meal at a time,* so we'll spend the next part of the program focusing on doing just that:

- **Breakfast:** The obvious place to start. We'll describe how to shift from the typical high-protein, high-fat meal (including eggs, bacon, avocados, sausage) that leaves most people feeling sluggish to eating a high-carbohydrate breakfast that not only energizes you for the day but also keeps your blood glucose very well controlled.
- **Lunch:** Here's where we'll teach you how to eat a calorie-dense plant-based meal to fuel you when you're most cognitively and physically active and to keep you going strong all afternoon. We'll make the case for adding starches to your day (long thought to be the "bad guys" of nutrition) and explain how adding foods like

legumes and intact whole grains to your diet will help keep you fueled and feeling full while providing a generous serving of fiber to feed trillions of bacteria in your gut microbiome.

- **Dinner:** Reexamining this meal is sometimes difficult because it's usually the most social meal of the day, and many people are accustomed to eating a large meal centered around a piece of meat. To us, the perfect dinner is one that's centered around green leafy vegetables (like spinach, arugula, kale, lettuce, and cabbage), non-starchy vegetables (like tomatoes, cucumbers, zucchini, carrots, okra, cauliflower, and onions), and mushrooms, but also includes fruit, starchy vegetables, legumes, or intact whole grains. Since it's the last meal of the day, we focus on eating a generous serving of foods with a lower calorie density that are high in vitamins, minerals, fiber, water, antioxidants, and phytochemicals—all the behind-the-scenes players necessary for maximizing your metabolic health while you sleep. In addition to explaining the science behind the ideal macronutrient target for your overall diet, we'll provide simple and delicious recipes that offer general guidance and room for improvisation depending on what you like to eat or what you have on hand in your kitchen.

# Step 3: Using Intermittent Fasting for Maximum Insulin Sensitivity and Weight Loss

Here we'll explore a wildly popular and extremely effective technique called intermittent fasting, which involves changing the timing of your food intake to significantly increase your insulin sensitivity. Intermittent fasting is one of the most effective ways to liberate stored fat, including fat that is tucked away in your muscles and liver that inhibits the action of insulin. Over eighty-five years of research has documented amazing benefits of both calorie restriction and intermittent fasting for preventing and delaying the onset of heart disease, diabetes, hypertension, and cancer, and reducing important biomarkers like blood pressure, LDL cholesterol (the bad cholesterol), and triglycerides.

Specifically with regard to diabetes, performing regular intermittent fasts often leads to:

- Reduced fasting blood glucose
- Reduced post-meal blood glucose
- Reduced blood glucose variability
- Increased insulin sensitivity
- A way to test your basal rate for those living with insulin-dependent diabetes

Calorie restriction is in fact the only known way to increase longevity. We will walk you through the differences between calorie restriction and intermittent fasting, and teach you how and when to safely perform an intermittent fast, whether it's performed by skipping one meal every day or choosing one day of the week to let your digestive system fully rest.

## Step 4: Exercising to Reverse Insulin Resistance

We don't talk about exercise right away for one simple reason: It's not required to begin experiencing improved blood glucose control. However, we are firm believers that regular exercise (in combination with other important aspects of the Mastering Diabetes Method) is the holy grail of insulin sensitivity. Because it's easy to make excuses and prioritize other things in place of exercise, we'll help you to define what activities you enjoy doing (and what you don't enjoy doing), and then help you commit to a routine in writing.

Ultimately, the best exercise routine is the one you'll actually do. The second best exercise routine—in terms of its effectiveness on insulin sensitivity—is one that includes resistance training, and we'll give you ways to integrate this into your exercise regimen. Performing a minimum of three hours of exercise per week divided into five or six sessions spread over a seven-day period will keep your insulin sensitivity high at all times. This approach is much more effective than spending longer periods of time exercising a few days a week, which temporarily boosts your insulin sensitivity for only a few days at a time while you become less insulin sensitive on your rest days. We'll also discuss simple ways to manage your blood glucose and insulin needs before, during, and after exercise to minimize your risk for high or low blood glucose, all while maximizing your athletic recovery.

## Step 5: Mastering Your Lifestyle

In the latter part of this book, we'll discuss specific lifestyle strategies that will help you integrate the Mastering Diabetes Method into your life and create a sustainable regimen that you can stick to in the long term. We'll help you preemptively troubleshoot tricky situations, such as eating at a restaurant or at someone's house.

We understand that modifying your lifestyle can be difficult because even small changes can disrupt the way you live your life. Especially as you age, your desire to modify your habits tends to decrease significantly. The Mastering Diabetes Method is designed with a long-term vision in mind so that none of the changes feel overwhelming—and yet our step-by-step nutrition, fitness, and lifestyle recommendations are designed to add new tools to your "insulin sensitivity toolbox" to significantly reduce your long-term disease risk.

## One Size Fits . . . No One

If you are like many of our clients, you may have tried many diets over the years. Perhaps some of these diets helped you lose weight and gain energy, while some of them caused you to gain weight and lose energy. In an effort to regain control of your health, you may have spent countless hours reading books, surfing the internet, watching videos on YouTube, or participating in Facebook discussions to learn how to feel better. Over the course of time you may have lost your enthusiasm for living an active life, managing your blood glucose, or taking the medicine prescribed by your doctor. Many of our clients tell us that they have stopped taking their medication out of frustration.

If you've ever experienced any of these problems, join the club. We've been there. We know what it's like to feel sick and tired of it all. Luckily, the Mastering Diabetes Method has completely transformed the two of us from the ground up—mind, body, and spirit. Gone are the days when lethargy kept us in bed until noon, when we couldn't exercise because our joints and muscles hurt, when checking our blood glucose was a terrifying and annoying guessing game, and when going to the doctor's office to get an A1c test felt like judgment day.

The real power of the Mastering Diabetes Method is that you have the ability to customize it to your unique preferences. As you learn the fundamentals about how to change the foods you eat, when to not eat, what type of exercise to perform, when to exercise, and how to handle stressful situations, you will have the ability to adapt this program to *your* life. One of the most important lessons we've learned as coaches is that there is no one-size-fits-all approach to health. Therefore we strongly encourage you to tailor this program to you, your family, your friends, and your career so that it becomes part of your life in the long term and keeps you free of insulin resistance for the rest of your life.

## Meet Your Coaches

### Cyrus: The PhD "Super Nerd College Professor"

I was diagnosed with type 1 diabetes at the age of 22, during my senior year of college at Stanford University. Plagued with excessive thirst and low energy, I spent a few days trying to study for finals even though I could barely muster the energy to stay awake. I remember feeling drained and assumed that it was because I was studying around the clock. For a few days, I urinated between seventeen and twenty times per day, and yet no matter how much water I drank, my thirst increased. After two days of frustration, I picked up the phone to call my sister Shanaz Khambatta—a family practice doctor of osteopathy—who instructed me to go to the campus health center immediately. I asked her why, and she responded with "Your symptoms are telling me that you have type 1 diabetes. I'll explain later. For now, just go to the health center. And, Cyrus, please go quickly."

I took her advice and checked myself into the campus health center within thirty minutes. I was immediately seen by a nurse, who discovered that my blood glucose was over 600—six times higher than normal. I was rushed to the emergency room, where I was hooked up to monitors, intravenous saline, and intravenous insulin. Over the next twenty-four hours, a team of doctors asked me detailed questions about my health history and lifestyle, then officially diagnosed me with insulin-dependent type 1 diabetes.

Even though type 1 diabetes is one of the most common autoimmune diseases in children, affecting approximately 100,000 people in the United States every year, this diagnosis seemed very atypical. Why? Because in the six months prior to this diagnosis, I had developed two other autoimmune conditions—Hashimoto's thyroiditis (autoimmune hypothyroidism) and alopecia universalis (total body hair loss)—making type 1 diabetes the *third* autoimmune condition that I developed within six months. My doctors diagnosed me with a *polyglandular autoimmune syndrome*—a term used to describe a collection of autoimmune conditions with no known cause. My doctors had never before cared for a patient with a polyglandular autoimmune condition, and as a 22-year-old, I was terrified that my health was deteriorating rapidly, even though I thought I lived a healthy lifestyle.

My family came to my hospital room, and we all tried to make sense of this situation together. We were confused and had more questions than we were willing to admit. The next day I was discharged from the hospital with a blood glucose meter, test strips, a prescription for basal and bolus insulin, a box of syringes, a carbohydrate counting guide, and a somewhat cryptic piece of paper with discharge information about how to return to a normal life. In slightly over twenty-four hours, I went from being a normal happy-go-lucky college senior to a medical patient with multiple autoimmune diseases, now in charge of controlling my blood glucose using my lifestyle and insulin. Even though I did my best to remain calm and practical, I returned to my dorm room terrified that something was very wrong with me. I felt extremely alone and victimized, and I didn't know a single other person living with type 1 diabetes that I could contact for guidance, support, or a simple hug.

Controlling my blood glucose was considerably more difficult than I had anticipated. I knew that type 1 diabetes was a life-threatening condition that demanded my full attention, and that if I didn't take it seriously, I ran the risk of overdosing on insulin and seriously harming myself. I needed answers, and the only answer that I consistently read was "eat a low-carbohydrate diet, because your body can't metabolize carbohydrates anymore." No matter how diligently I controlled my diet and exercise patterns, maintaining my blood glucose within a "normal" range took most of my mental, emotional, and physical energy. I felt vulnerable, weak, confused, and I grew increasingly angered because there weren't many answers. Often when I asked a troubleshooting question, I was given the same response: "Everyone's different."

In the quest to gain more energy, control my blood glucose, and return to being "normal," I desperately listened to the advice of my doctor and nutritionist, both of whom gave me the same advice that they extended to all people newly diagnosed with diabetes: "Restrict your carbohydrate intake and eat foods high in fat and protein." Their advice seemed reasonable, so I followed their recommendations to the best of my ability.

About nine months into living with diabetes, one day I returned home from work excited to eat a hard-earned dinner. I remember that my body felt overly stiff. My muscles felt unusually sore. True, I was recovering from a soccer game that I had played three days earlier, but the soreness seemed to be getting worse with time. My hamstrings were tight, my back was rigid, and I was extremely tired. I checked my blood glucose, and it was *three times* higher than it should have been, despite eating a low-carbohydrate diet and moving my body the way I was told.

I felt out of shape, excessively tired, and downright confused—I was a 23-year-old living in what felt like the body of a 90-year-old. I had just graduated with a degree in mechanical engineering—a rigorous science that teaches you how to control complex mechanical and electrical systems with exquisite detail—and the irony is that despite my academic training, diabetes was a system that I simply couldn't figure out. No matter how hard I tried, no matter how many variables I worked to control, no matter how systematic I was about documenting my daily activities, my blood glucose meter acted like a random number generator, which frustrated me beyond belief.

In that moment of pure frustration I decided that it was time to take matters into my own hands and begin experimenting with the food I put in my mouth. I heard a voice in my head that said, "Cyrus, you're 23 years old, but you never learned how to eat. Learn how to eat and it will change your life." The next day I began looking for answers about food with a newfound enthusiasm that I had never experienced before. I searched for information wherever I could find it—on the internet, at the bookstore, in recipe books, at scientific lectures—and noticed that practically every avenue I opened pointed me toward this thing called plant-based nutrition, of which I knew absolutely nothing.

For the first time in my life, I opened my mind to the idea of becoming a plant-based eater, even though I used to be *that guy* who ridiculed vegetarians and vegans in my teenage years, including my middle sister, Persis, who adamantly tried to be a vegetarian from the time she was in middle school. When I would overhear people ordering a salad at a restaurant or watch as friends did the same, I would think to myself, *I'm sorry that you can't eat real food. I wish things were better for you.* At the time, I didn't know any better. I was ignorant about why people chose to eat a plant-based diet, and charged through life with a typical protein-centric view of nutrition, arguing that I had to eat meat at least twice a day in order to fuel my body properly so that I could play high-intensity sports. It seemed logical at the time, but in reality I had absolutely no idea what I was talking about. I told myself exactly what I wanted to hear—that eating more meat and dairy products was the secret to excellent athletic health.

But being diagnosed with type 1 diabetes was a wake-up call, to say the least. I began consulting with "alternative" medical professionals and read books by doctors who had outside-of-the-box solutions to common health conditions that couldn't be solved by modern medicine. I began eating a more plant-based diet by replacing foods like steak, eggs, cheese, meat loaf, chicken, and turkey burgers with foods like tomatoes, carrots, eggplant, peanut butter, and mushrooms. I thought I felt better. But I still couldn't control my blood glucose with precision and knew that there was a whole world of nutrition and human biology about which I didn't understand anything technical.

After a few months of eating more plants, I traveled to Texas with my mother to consult with a physician who had come highly recommended to me from a trusted friend. While we were waiting for the appointment to begin, my mother and I sat in his office preparing to ask him a laundry list of questions we had written over the course of many weeks. My eyes scanned his bookshelf from top to bottom, which contained hundreds of textbooks, manuals, journals, and technical information. I thought to myself, *This guy must be really smart. I'm excited about what we're about to learn.* As my eyes scanned toward the bottom of his bookshelf, one book jumped out at me as if it were trying to speak to me. The book appeared to be about 500 pages thick, it had a blue binding, and it had the word *biochemistry* printed prominently on the spine. I stared at that book for about thirty seconds and was filled with an overwhelmingly inspiring feeling that washed over my body from head to toe. I got goose bumps. My eyes grew wide. My gaze grew deeper. I read the word *biochemistry* over and over, and knew instinctively that biochemistry was the very subject that I had been searching for from the moment I was a young kid asking myself questions like "Why am I eating this food—is it actually good for my body?" and "How does my body actually process this stuff I'm eating?"

The truth is that while at that very moment I didn't know anything about the details of biochemistry, I was overcome with a strong sensation that biochemistry could be the gateway to helping me answer a collection of challenging questions I had asked since childhood. More important, I was overcome with a sense of hope that biochemistry would help me answer the ever-increasing list of detailed and technical questions about type 1 diabetes.

When I returned home, I mustered the courage to radically transform my diet from the ground up. I sought out the guidance of Doug Graham, DC, a nutrition coach with many years of experience working with people with diabetes and with athletes, who instructed me to do the opposite of what I had been advised by my medical team. I began eating large quantities of fresh fruits and vegetables and stopped eating meat, dairy, fish, poultry, and eggs entirely. I was excited to experience positive change but was quite nervous that eating more fruit-based carbohydrate energy would increase my insulin use considerably.

In the first week of eating a strictly plant-based diet, my insulin requirements dropped by approximately 35 percent, my energy levels increased, and my blood glucose became significantly more predictable. After performing a few back-of-the-envelope calculations, I determined that my carboyhdrate intake had increased almost sixfold, from about 75 grams per day to about 500 grams per day. That meant that I was eating significantly more carbohydrate energy using *less* insulin, which went against everything that I had been told since day one. This made no sense at all.

When I began eating more carbohydrate-rich foods, I found that my biological requirement for insulin dropped significantly and quickly, and naturally this piqued my intellectual curiosity. I became increasingly convinced that the carbohydrate-phobic view of diabetes was either incomplete or flawed at its core—I just didn't yet have the scientific knowledge to explain why. Fascinated by the exciting "n-of-1" scientific experiment under way in my own body, I enrolled in graduate classes at the University of Hawaii and began feverishly studying human biology, chemistry, organic chemistry, anatomy, physiology, and nutritional biochemistry with a newfound excitement that motivated me to learn everything I could possibly get my hands on. I considered myself extremely fortunate to be able to study the subject that would enable me to articulate the details of the exciting (and finally *controllable*) biological experiment under way in my own body.

After a few years of coursework, I applied to PhD programs around the country and enrolled in a program to study nutritional biochemistry at the University of California at Berkeley to investigate the nutritional causes and effects of diabetes. It was at UC Berkeley that I dove deep into the biological phenomenon known as insulin resistance, a highly misunderstood and intricate condition present in people with and without diabetes that helps to explain the ins and outs of blood glucose management as well as chronic disease as a whole. I learned that simple nutrition strategies that reliably reverse insulin resistance apply to *all* individuals living with diabetes, including those with type 1 diabetes, type 1.5 diabetes, type 2 diabetes, prediabetes, and gestational diabetes. Over the course of five years I taught classes on topics ranging from nutrient metabolism to disease prevention, and in the process I became a published author in peer-reviewed scientific journals. I wrote a dissertation on the effect of calorie restriction on mitochondrial health and insulin sensitivity, and we'll explore many of these concepts in the following chapters as it pertains to reversing insulin resistance.

What I love the most—aside from the rigorous science—is translating complex scientific information into bite-sized chunks that save you the time and effort of having to seek out reliable and credible information for yourself. My mission is to educate, inspire, and motivate people living with all forms of diabetes and to turn an otherwise grim diagnosis into a rewarding experience that can transform your life from the inside out. I strive to teach people with diabetes that the "tunnel vision" view of controlling your blood glucose using a low-carbohydrate diet is a dangerous game that can cause your overall metabolic health to deteriorate rapidly and decrease the number (and quality) of days you live on this planet. I love giving people with diabetes the education that is both immensely helpful at the time of their diagnosis and **required** to take full control of their metabolic health by using food as medicine.

But most important, I want you to understand that diabetes is the **best** thing that ever happened to me, because it opened my eyes to a world of evidence-based nutrition that has transformed not only my life but the lives of thousands of people around the world. Type 1 diabetes was the gateway to discovering this information, and without this diagnosis I might have never found it.

## Robby: The Seeker

On January 26, 2000, when I was 12 years old, I was diagnosed with type 1 diabetes. Steven, my middle brother, had been diagnosed nine years prior, so I was familiar with the symptoms and the daily maintenance required to live a normal life. I said to my mom, "I think I have diabetes, just like Steven," and she responded by saying, "Don't be silly, Robby." Even though I listened to my mom, my symptoms persisted. I was incredibly thirsty and urinated very frequently. A few weeks later, my parents had left our home in St. Cloud, Minnesota, to visit my grandparents in Florida and prepare for our upcoming move. My mom called to check in, and I told her that I had difficulty sleeping the night before and that my legs were cramping—two more symptoms that convinced me that I was developing type 1 diabetes. At this point she became concerned, so she instructed me to go upstairs and use Steven's blood glucose meter. He helped me prick my finger, and a few seconds later, I saw my blood glucose for the first time: it was over 400 mg/dL—more than four times higher than normal.

As we drove to our family doctor, I didn't fully realize what was happening to me. Even though my brother Steven had type 1 diabetes, I was too young to fully understand the gravity of the situation. As soon as my doctor delivered the news that I did in fact have type 1 diabetes, Steven began crying, saying, "I'm so sorry that you have to deal with the same thing that I have to." Upon hearing this news, my parents flew back to Minnesota immediately, and as I was lying in the hospital bed with intravenous saline and insulin, my dad reassured me that type 1 diabetes is merely an "inconvenience" and that I would still be able to do whatever I wanted. To this day, those words are still in the forefront of my mind and are a daily reminder that I choose not to let type 1 diabetes get in the way of achieving my dreams in life. In fact, type 1 diabetes has given me a newfound mission, which has filled my life with growth opportunities, community, purpose, and joy.

I'm a type A personality, and because of that I took my diagnosis very seriously from day one, managing my blood glucose to the best of my ability. As a child, I played tennis competitively and worked hard to become one of the top-ranked tennis players in the Midwest Region between the ages of 10 and 14. I grew up with the typical athlete's mindset that "I could eat whatever I wanted, because I was getting plenty of physical activity."

It wasn't until after my diagnosis with type 1 diabetes at age 12 that I became interested in living a healthy life and paying attention to what I ate. Because I was new to this idea and quite young, I didn't exactly know where to begin, so I started by taking daily supplements that my dad sold at the time. By the time I was 14, I had eliminated virtually all junk food from my diet, avoided food additives like MSG, and made an effort to eat as much unprocessed food as possible.

Despite eating a cleaner diet, I suffered from allergies every year, even though I routinely took medications like Claritin-D and Nasonex. I also suffered from plantar fasciitis, a frustrating condition that made the soles of my feet tight and painful, and I wore big blue boots at night for passive stretching. Throughout high school, I battled with cystic acne. I tried to treat acne with everything I could get my hands on, from creams to oral pills to microdermabrasion to laser treatments and eventually Accutane—the medication doctors prescribe only if nothing else has worked. Accutane is known for severe side effects, including depression and suicide, so I was hesitant to take it but felt like I didn't have a choice.

While in high school, I stumbled across a book that changed my life forever called *Natural Cures "They" Don't Want You to Know About* by Kevin Trudeau. I remember walking away with the belief that I can and will reverse type 1 diabetes, and that one day I will no longer need insulin to manage my blood glucose. It was the beginning of a series of desires to solve the mystery of type 1 diabetes, to learn about autoimmunity, to learn how stem cells could lead to new beta cell growth, and to try anything in my power to reverse type 1 diabetes in my own body. (Kevin Trudeau has since been imprisoned for misleading health claims and fraudulent advice. We do not condone his advice; it was merely a book that planted a seed to learn more about evidence-based lifestyle change.)

I began visiting a naturopathic doctor in Tampa, Florida, on a regular basis, who used electrodermal testing to identify foods that were both compatible and incompatible with my body. After every visit, I left her office with many supplements and a long list of approved foods and guidelines that said things like "Eat chicken but not beef and eat bread made from millet but not spelt." I followed her advice, and soon became the weird one at the high school lunch table.

Next, I came across the Weston A. Price Foundation and became convinced that it was smarter to drink raw milk instead of pasteurized milk and eat grass-fed beef instead of factory-farmed beef. Even though nothing dramatic happened to my health or diabetes management, I continued to follow this advice through high school because I felt like I was doing the right things to improve my well-being.

When I began college at the University of Florida, I continued to experiment with anything I could get my hands on. Fueled by the desire to stimulate my own insulin production once again, I maintained an open mind about new and exciting opportunities to become healthier. One day I flew to San Jose, California, and met with an underground Chinese medicine man who I had heard was extremely talented. He made me a tea and instructed me to take it every day. The problem was that the tea smelled and tasted *terrible*. In fact, it smelled so bad that in order to prevent my roommates in college from kicking me out of our dorm room, I brewed it outside on the sidewalk using an electric hot plate.

Later, while taking a break from college essays, I was on a website forum explaining to others why it was important to drink raw milk for optimal health. The members of the board were very kind and shared health resources to help me understand a different perspective, and also suggested that I watch an animal-rights movie called *Earthlings* to learn more details about where milk comes from. I watched the film and was blown away by the shocking imagery. Even though I was quite educated and attended a well-respected university, I couldn't believe that I didn't understand how my food got on my plate. This opened my mind greatly, so I returned to the forum and absorbed their nutritional resources with a new level of openness.

This led me into the world of raw food, where I came across a doctor named Gabriel Cousens, MD. He recommends eating a plant-based ketogenic diet including only raw food that was very low in carbohydrate energy, high in fat, and included plenty of greens. At this point in my dietary journey, I ate approximately 30 grams of carbohydrate energy per day and my total insulin use dropped to about 10 units per day. This was the least amount of insulin I had ever used.

The problem was that even though my blood glucose control was excellent and my insulin use was very low, I felt terrible. I suffered from extremely low energy, and I blacked out several times on my college campus. Naturally this scared me and made me realize that even if I could drop my insulin use and stabilize my blood glucose in the short term, I still hadn't found a dietary approach that could ensure my long-term health and keep me feeling energetic, alert, and vibrant for many years to come.

At this point I was lost and confused. I went back to the naturopath I worked with in high school to see if she could help, and she recommended that I try chelation therapy to eliminate heavy metals. This process was quite expensive and required driving several hours on a regular basis, and just as I was about to commit, I heard a podcast that changed the course of my life forever.

On this podcast, I learned about the work of Douglas Graham, DC, an educator who helps people adopt a raw low-fat plant-based high-carbohydrate diet. He talked about the health benefits of eating fruit and explained how the human body is capable of reversing many chronic diseases when fueled properly. He released a book called *The 80/10/10 Diet* in 2006, and as soon as it became available, I read it all in one sitting. Cyrus was one of the testimonials profiled in the book, and his story was incredible! I subsequently found an article about Cyrus online that further documented his athletic endeavors and insulin sensitivity and showed off his impressive physique. What Dr. Graham wrote in his book resonated with me like nothing I had ever read before.

I began a ninety-day email coaching program with Dr. Graham, who taught me the fundamental principles, explaining why a low-fat diet high in fruit was not only great for my blood glucose control but also great for my overall health. I began adding more fruits to my diet, including bananas, mangoes, cantaloupe, papayas, grapes, oranges, persimmons, and dates. Even with all the education and reassurance from Dr. Graham, I anticipated that my insulin use would skyrocket given the carbohydrate content of fresh fruit, but what I finally began to realize was that tracking *only* my insulin use was only half of the insulin sensitivity equation. Following Dr. Graham's advice, I tracked both my carbohydrate and insulin use, and watched as my 24-hour carbohydrate-to-insulin ratio increased from 3:1 on a high-fat plant-based diet to 22:1 on a low-fat plant-based diet. To this day, I think that signing up for his coaching program was one of the best decisions I have ever made.

For the first time since being diagnosed with type 1 diabetes, I began to feel amazing and had a newfound optimism for life. My purpose had never been clearer. I started to learn about the world of low-fat plant-based whole-food nutrition, and began making videos about peer-reviewed journal articles that confirmed the results I experienced in my own body. The beauty is that this research had been published in the world's most respected scientific journals dating back to the early 1900s. It had been there the whole time, but I just didn't know where to look. I was shocked to see that more people did not know about this proven approach to reversing insulin resistance, and thus began my mission to share this information with anyone who would listen.

While in college I started a nonprofit organization to spread the message about a low-fat plant-based whole-food lifestyle. Part of the content on my website were details about my experience living with type 1 diabetes and eating "buckets" of fruit each day. For 365 consecutive days, I documented all of the food that went in my body (including pictures of every meal and every snack), including every blood glucose reading, every insulin injection, and the corresponding nutritional data. To this day, documenting these details consistently is one of my proudest accomplishments, and serves as a precursor to the all-important decision tree you'll learn about later.

When I graduated from college, I began working as operations manager for Forks Over Knives in the prescreening phase. While working at Forks Over Knives for six years, I connected with plant-based doctors and researchers and deepened my understanding of the vast array of scientific and clinical evidence that shows why each aspect of the Mastering Diabetes Method works well to improve both short-term and long-term health. I thoroughly enjoyed my time at Forks Over Knives and was honored to be part of a company that was impacting thousands of lives across the planet every day.

In 2016, I left my position at Forks Over Knives to create the very thing that did not exist for those living with diabetes—an evidence-based program to help people with diabetes transition to a lifestyle scientifically proven to improve short-term health and maximize longevity, operated by people living with diabetes. Cyrus and I created Mastering Diabetes to educate and inspire millions of people around the world about the truth behind evidence-based nutrition, and it is without doubt the most rewarding thing I've ever created.

I decided to attend graduate school and earn a master's in public health so I could further my knowledge of conducting and analyzing peer-reviewed research. My graduate education has deepened my understanding of the diabetes crisis and further ingrained my desire to help distribute credible information to the public about diabetes. In addition, it has helped strengthen my desire to create resources so that people can transition to a healthier lifestyle no matter their race or economic status.

Since December of 2006, I have diligently followed a low-fat plant-based whole-food diet, and I am able to control my blood glucose with precision. I eat approximately 750 grams of carbohydrates per day, the majority of which comes from fruit. To put that in perspective: I'm buying enough fruit at the Santa Monica Farmers Market or Los Angeles Wholesale Produce Market per week to fill a seven-shelf baker's rack and fridge every week. There's always an abundance of mangoes, papayas, berries, bananas, various citrus fruits, peppers, lettuces, greens, zucchinis, and tomatoes as well as exotic fruits like jackfruit. And I'm eating these foods using about 34 units of insulin per day, a physiologically normal amount of insulin that my pancreas would produce if I were nondiabetic. Since I adopted this lifestyle, my A1c values have ranged between 5.3% and 6.6%, I don't take any oral medications, I have abundant energy, my acne has cleared up, and both allergies and plantar fasciitis are things of the past.

I'm grateful that you are taking the time to read this book. Unfortunately, I don't have the answer for reversing type 1 diabetes yet, but I can promise you that the information in this book is the key to living a long, healthy, complication-free life for those living with insulin-dependent diabetes. This book will show you how to control your blood glucose with precision, get your best A1c values today and in the future, and dramatically reduce your risk for coronary artery disease, cancer, retinopathy, Alzheimer's disease, chronic kidney disease, fatty liver disease, and more. If you are living with non-insulin-dependent diabetes, this book will give you the knowledge to make diabetes (and associated complications) a thing of the past.

# Diabetes Is You. You Are Diabetes.

If you spend time around people living with diabetes, one of the first things that you may notice is the choice of words that many use when talking about their health. It is not uncommon to hear people using combative and aggressive language that personifies diabetes as an evil villain who has hijacked their body. Often those living with diabetes refer to their condition as a *monster,* and talk about *beating, crushing, defeating, outsmarting, killing, conquering,* and *overpowering* this invisible enemy. This phraseology is plastered around many prominent diabetes blogs, and it runs rampant across social media platforms. A simple search on Twitter or Instagram reveals common hashtags used in diabetes-related conversations, including #diabetessucks, #diabetesprobs, #thestruggleisreal, and #curediabetes.

But here's the thing: Diabetes is not a monster. Diabetes is not a villain. Treating diabetes as an enemy reinforces a combative relationship that only serves to fuel its inflammatory nature. The angrier you become when living with diabetes, the more likely your biological machine will increase its production of stress hormones, fueling unwanted blood glucose fluctuations that only increase your level of anger.

The truth is that diabetes is not a villain, nor is it even a separate entity from you. *Diabetes is you, and you are diabetes.* Embracing this "demon" as a part of you is one of the most powerful early steps you can take in managing your relationship together. When you embrace diabetes as a part of your physical, emotional, and spiritual being, you'll feel empowered and at peace, and you'll maximize your chances of taking full control of your health. So let's embrace diabetes for what it is, and dive right into understanding the causes of insulin resistance.

# Chapter 3

# What *Really* Causes Insulin Resistance?

## The Diabetes Lightbulb: Joaquin

During a routine doctor's visit in May of 2017, Joaquin was diagnosed with type 2 diabetes when a blood test revealed that his A1c was 7.1%. In the months prior, he had been experiencing severe headaches, nasal congestion, and nerve tingling in his toes, and after receiving this diagnosis, he realized that these symptoms were all connected.

He began searching online for information about type 2 diabetes and learned that the condition is caused by insulin resistance. After watching a video presentation given by Cyrus at the Torrance Memorial Medical Center, Joaquin immediately signed up to participate in the next Mastering Diabetes retreat, excited to eat large quantities of his favorite foods—mangoes, potatoes, rice, and beans. At the retreat, Joaquin began exercising every day, and when he returned home, he continued to exercise without equipment, using only his body weight as resistance. He learned as much as he could about the underlying causes of insulin resistance and considered himself very knowledgeable about why the Mastering Diabetes Method is an incredibly effective solution to reverse insulin resistance and maximize his long-term health.

In three months, Joaquin lost 35 pounds. And he no longer experienced daily headaches, nasal congestion, or tingling in his toes. His fasting blood glucose dropped below 100 mg/dL within the first week of following the Mastering Diabetes Method, and his energy levels began increasing quickly. For the first few months, he checked his blood glucose multiple times a day to confirm that type 2 diabetes was fading into the background, and after three months he stopped entirely. In six months, his A1c dropped from 7.1% to 5.6%, and Joaquin is now free of diabetes altogether. He calls this lifestyle a no-brainer and has successfully helped many family members and friends transition to the same lifestyle. "Don't overcomplicate this lifestyle," he says. "After one month you're going to thank yourself and see that it's well worth it."

---

There are countless misconceptions about what causes diabetes, and in today's internet-dominant era, it's becoming increasingly difficult to separate scientific truth from theory and opinion. Regardless of your understanding of diabetes physiology, we encourage you to keep an open mind when reading these next chapters. Some of these concepts might be difficult for you to wrap your head around at first, and you might even feel overwhelmed by the information in this book because it directly conflicts with what you have been taught in the past. And if that's the case, you'll feel exactly how we felt when we first learned it. Don't worry, the information in this chapter may seem counterintuitive, but rest assured that it's biologically accurate.

Without doubt, our most ardent followers are those who have struggled with the concept of low-fat plant-based whole-food nutrition from the beginning of their journey because it was so different from what their doctors recommended and from what they previously believed to be the truth. We remember feeling very apprehensive ourselves when we learned about the root causes of insulin resistance. But once we started to experience improved insulin sensitivity, there was no denying the power of this "unconventional" approach to nutrition.

We understand that changing old patterns can be very difficult, especially when it comes to your health. That's another reason why we strongly encourage you to understand the fundamental science of insulin resistance before making long-term lifestyle changes. As is true for many of our clients, understanding the science-based relationship between your blood glucose, your weight, your energy, and your level of insulin resistance is the key to implementing the Mastering Diabetes Method—and to seeing quick and long-lasting results. And that all starts with recognizing that what you may have learned about diabetes up to this point may in fact be leading you down the wrong path.

## Your Doctor Didn't Learn
## Nutrition in Medical School

There is no arguing the fact that the overwhelming majority of doctors around the world are extremely well intentioned and have a genuine desire to improve the quality of life of their patients. The fundamental problem is that doctors have been trained in a system that is designed to treat symptoms using pharmaceutical and surgical intervention instead of addressing the root cause of chronic disease. In the same way that a carpenter selects the right tool for the job, a doctor selects the right tool for a given medical condition. The problem is that the main tools that doctors are trained to use are pharmaceutical medications, not food. The result is that doctors treat diabetes and its complications using medications rather than evidence-based nutrition.

It's not your doctor's fault. Medical schools barely scratch the surface when it comes to providing nutrition-related education. A 2010 survey revealed that only 25 percent of medical schools in the United States require their students to take a nutrition course as part of their medical curriculum, resulting in an average of less than 20 hours of nutrition education total, as compared to more than 10,000 hours of medical and clinical education. Even worse, less than 30 percent of the schools met the minimum requirement of 25 hours of nutrition education, a standard set by the National Academy of Sciences.

Given that nutrition education is only a minor focus in medical schools, it is unrealistic to believe that physicians can effectively recognize or treat the root causes of insulin resistance, obesity, diabetes, and cardiovascular disease through diet. More specifically, physicians are not trained on the power and efficacy of a *low-fat diet* in reversing insulin resistance and improving insulin sensitivity, and are just as susceptible to fad diets and catchy marketing as is the general public. As a result, people living with prediabetes and type 2 diabetes are rarely presented with evidence-based information, and instead are encouraged to focus only on short-term methods to control their blood glucose using either a low-carbohydrate diet or a very low-carbohydrate ketogenic diet. Because doctors are insufficiently educated about nutrition in medical school, we believe that the solution to reversing insulin resistance lies in **your** hands.

## The Carbohydrate-Centric Diabetes Model

If you're like most people with diabetes or prediabetes, you may have been encouraged to eat a low-carbohydrate diet to control your blood glucose, or you may have been told that carbohydrate-rich foods will increase your risk for diabetes complications and worsen your long-term health. Whether you open *The New York Times,* scan the bookshelves at your local bookstore, or search online for diabetes-related advice, the prevailing wisdom in the world of diabetes nutrition is that a low-carbohydrate diet is the safest and most effective way to control your blood glucose and will help you lose weight, reduce your fasting blood glucose, drop your A1c, lower your cholesterol, and reduce your blood pressure. Even at scientific conferences you'll see some of the most accomplished professors pointing a finger at foods like bananas and rice, showing detailed scientific evidence that all foods containing carbohydrates act the same way in your body, causing uncontrollable blood glucose fluctuations that then lead to increased appetite, weight gain, and obesity.

The carbohydrate-centric diabetes model states that when you eat any foods containing a sufficient quantity of carbohydrate energy (regardless of whether they are processed or whole foods), the carbohydrate energy turns into "sugar." In turn, these "sugar" molecules rapidly increase your blood glucose, which then triggers your pancreas to secrete large amounts of insulin. As a result of large surges of insulin in your blood, tissues downregulate their insulin receptors, which creates a state of insulin resistance in which "sugar" can't get out of your blood. In addition, since insulin is your "fat-storage hormone," large insulin spikes increase the amount of fat you store. Your liver then converts large amounts of "sugar" to fat, and this causes you to gain weight, which in turn makes you more insulin resistant. The model looks like the illustration on the next page.

In effect, *the carbohydrate-centric diabetes model says that excess insulin causes insulin resistance.* It points a finger at insulin as being the cause of insulin resistance, arguing that insulin is your "fat-storage hormone" and that it is responsible for unwanted weight gain. According to this model, the solution to diabetes is to eat foods that minimize or eliminate your need for insulin, which includes foods that are low in carbohydrate energy, high in fat, and high in protein. Following this logic, carbohydrate-rich foods are to blame for high insulin levels, and high insulin levels are to blame for insulin resistance and weight gain.

In the subsequent chapters of this book, we will demonstrate with overwhelming evidence that the carbohydrate-centric model of diabetes is more than just wrong; it is an overly simplified attempt at explaining diabetes using a single variable. It is a great example of flawed logic that focuses on only one component of your diet (carbohydrates) and teaches you how to eat foods high in fat and protein to minimize your insulin needs in the short term, with no regard for almost a hundred years of scientific evidence that demonstrates the long-term chronic disease risks of eating foods high in fat and protein.

The reason why millions of people around the world believe that the carbohydrate-centric diabetes model is correct is because carbohydrate-rich foods will spike your blood glucose *if and only if your baseline level of insulin resistance is high to begin with.* As you will learn in the subsequent chapters, insulin resistance makes it extremely challenging to eat carbohydrate-rich foods without experiencing high blood glucose, which means that if you are already insulin resistant, then you are likely to experience high blood glucose any time you eat carbohydrate-rich foods. So the question then becomes . . . *is insulin resistance actually caused by something other than insulin?*

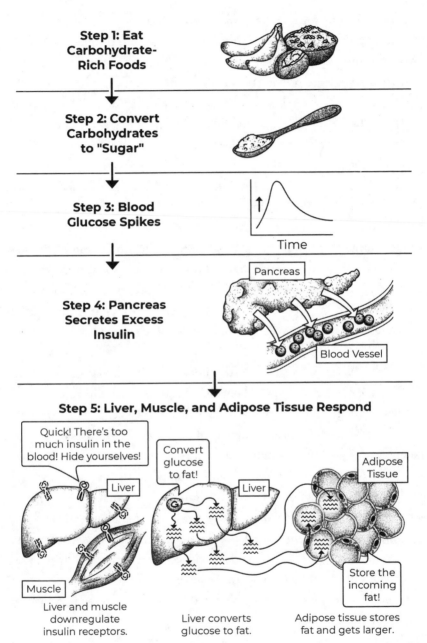

The carbohydrate-centric diabetes model argues that carbohydrates turn into sugar, which then spikes your blood glucose and triggers the production of large amounts of insulin. As a result, your muscle, liver, and adipose tissue become resistant to insulin, in an effort to protect themselves against excess insulin.

The truth is that insulin resistance is not caused by insulin at all—it's caused by something entirely different that creates the *symptom* of excess insulin in your blood. Pointing a finger at insulin as the cause of insulin resistance is akin to pointing a finger at a sore throat as the cause of the common cold. You probably know that a sore throat is not the *cause* of a common cold; it is simply one of many *symptoms* that can make your life temporarily uncomfortable. Sure, treating the symptoms of your cold will help you feel better in the short term, but it does nothing to improve your immunity in the long term. In the same way, treating the symptom of insulin resistance (high blood glucose and excess insulin) rather than treating the cause (a high-fat diet causing insulin resistance) works in the short term but fails to minimize your risk for many chronic diseases and worsening diabetes health in the long term.

In this book you'll learn the exact method for eating significantly larger quantities of carbohydrate-rich foods by first increasing your *carbohydrate tolerance.* By doing so, you're also likely to experience normal blood glucose, reach your ideal weight, lower your cholesterol, normalize your blood pressure, prevent and reverse heart disease, and much, much more. As long as you are living with insulin resistance, your ability to metabolize carbohydrate-rich foods will be low, which is exactly why increasing your level of insulin sensitivity is the most effective way to metabolize carbohydrate-rich foods and avoid high blood glucose and excess insulin.

**By increasing your insulin sensitivity, you will be able to eat carbohydrate-rich foods and experience excellent blood glucose control while simultaneously decreasing your risk for weight gain, obesity, high cholesterol, high blood pressure, and coronary artery disease.**

There are a few reasons that the prevailing wisdom in the world of diabetes has an overwhelmingly pessimistic view of foods containing carbohydrates. We ourselves were subjected to the following mistakes when we were first diagnosed with type 1 diabetes:

**Mistake 1:** Scientists, medical professionals, and people with diabetes erroneously use the word *sugar* when referring to both added sweeteners in processed foods as well as the natural energy contained in whole foods like fruits and starchy vegetables, reinforcing the concept that anything that creates more "sugar" in your body will negatively impact your health. The word *sugar* is misleading and fails to describe the fundamental difference between refined sweeteners and naturally occurring carbohydrate energy found in whole food.

**Mistake 2:** Many people believe that insulin is one of the most dangerous hormones in your body, and that insulin is to blame for fat synthesis, weight gain, high cholesterol, and high blood glucose. Because of this, low-carbohydrate dieters eat foods high in fat and protein because they stimulate your beta cells to secrete small amounts of insulin, or require only small amounts of exogenous (injected) insulin for those living with insulin-dependent diabetes. The truth is that insulin itself is not to blame for increased chronic disease risk. *Excess insulin* beyond a physiologically normal amount increases your risk for many chronic diseases and should be avoided at all costs.

**Mistake 3:** Scientists, medical professionals, and people with diabetes often lump all "carbs" into the same category, and do not adequately differentiate between packaged and processed foods like breads, cereals, and pastas and whole foods like fruits, starchy vegetables, legumes, and intact whole grains. But carbohydrates in food come in many forms, and differentiating between refined carbohydrates and whole carbohydrates is extremely important when understanding their true biological impact.

**Mistake 4:** Most scientific studies that directly compare the outcomes of low-carbohydrate diets to low-fat diets do not design their "low-fat" diet properly. We thoroughly researched studies commonly used by the low-carbohydrate community to debunk low-fat diets and found that every single one of these publications do not study a truly low-fat diet. They compare very low-carbohydrate diets against diets containing 25 to 35 percent fat (and containing significant amounts of animal foods), and erroneously conclude that eating carbohydrates worsens your long-term health. In contrast, scientific investigations performed in people eating a truly low-fat diet containing less than

15 percent of total calories result in increased insulin sensitivity, reduced oral medication and insulin needs, reduced fasting and post-meal blood glucose, reduced A1c, and significantly reduced risk for cardiovascular disease.

The truth is that there isn't a single study that shows that carbohydrate-rich whole foods eaten in a truly low-fat environment doesn't improve insulin sensitivity. In addition, studies performed in subjects fed a highly processed carbohydrate-rich diet *in a low-fat environment* also demonstrate significantly improved insulin sensitivity.

A closer look at the complex interplay between whole-food nutrition and diabetes reveals something very simple and extremely important that can profoundly affect your diabetes health for years to come:

**Your blood glucose is influenced by many variables, and is best understood when considering the amount and type of carbohydrate you eat, the amount and type of fat you eat, and, most important, the overall nutrient density of your diet.**

Because the amount and type of fat you eat plays a central role in your ability to control your blood glucose, failing to fully understand this connection can dramatically alter your risk for the development of other chronic diseases into the future and is an oversight that both healthcare professionals and people with diabetes repeatedly make. In most cases, medical professionals instruct people with type 1 diabetes, type 1.5 diabetes, type 2 diabetes, prediabetes, and gestational diabetes to eat a low-carbohydrate diet from the time they are first diagnosed, sometimes telling patients that diabetes is a *carbohydrate metabolism disorder*. It's easy to believe this to be the truth, especially when most of the diabetes world preaches the same message. Unfortunately, this methodology creates two serious problems:

1. Patients often receive a recommendation to eat a low-carbohydrate diet when they are first diagnosed, at a time when they're emotionally vulnerable and willing to follow any advice that could minimize their physical and emotional discomfort.

2. Following the carbohydrate-centric diabetes model sets into motion a dietary pattern that can last for many years, resulting in a diet that increases your risk for chronic diseases in the long term. Worst of all, many people think that they're doing the right thing by eating a low-carbohydrate diet, completely unaware that they're actually eating themselves toward more insulin resistance and increased chronic disease risk.

# Human Biology 101

Before going into how exactly insulin resistance works, let's first take a look at how a normal, healthy glucose metabolism functions—just in case you fell asleep during high school biology class.

When you eat food that contains carbohydrates, your body cuts long-chain carbohydrates into smaller pieces, and then eventually to chains that are 1, 2, or 3 *monosaccharide* pieces long, thanks to an enzyme called amylase that is secreted by your mouth and small intestine. These monosaccharide molecules end in *-ose* and include compounds like glucose, ribose, galactose, and fructose (just to name a few). Monosaccharides are commonly referred to as *sugar* in conventional textbooks, but we choose not to use the word *sugar* in this context, because the word *sugar* refers to a refined sweetener that you buy at the grocery store. For the remainder of this book, we will refer to natural sugars as *monosaccharides* and man-made sugars as *refined sugars,* because they have drastically different metabolic effects, and using them interchangeably causes unnecessary confusion. Don't worry; we'll revisit and expand on this concept in chapter 6.

When glucose enters your blood following a carbohydrate-rich meal, it first travels to your liver via a highway known as the portal vein. Your liver is given first crack at this fresh supply of glucose and can either take it up to burn immediately for energy, store it as *glycogen* (the stored form of glucose) for later use, or allow it to remain in your blood for other tissues to use. Your pancreas contains beta cells, a highly specialized group of cells found in clusters known as the islets of Langerhans that are the only cells in your body capable of manufacturing and secreting insulin. Beta cells release small amounts of *first-phase* insulin to help your liver take up glucose from the portal vein, then later release *second-phase* insulin once larger amounts of glucose get into general circulation. Insulin is an extremely powerful hormone that acts as a key to unlock millions of cellular doors located on the surface of cells all over your body, in tissues ranging from your muscle and liver to smaller tissues like your gallbladder and prostate gland.

Contrary to popular belief, insulin is not your enemy. Many medical professionals and people living with diabetes erroneously point their finger at insulin, claiming that insulin will make you fat, increase your cholesterol level, and increase your risk for diabetes. However, a closer look reveals two very important aspects of insulin biology that are often misinterpreted:

a. Insulin is absolutely necessary for life. If insulin were not present in your body at all, you would die in a short period of time—likely within weeks or months.

b. Insulin itself does not raise your risk for chronic disease. *Excess insulin* beyond your normal physiological level is what causes severe metabolic dysfunction and increases your risk for many chronic diseases over the course of time.

Your dog secretes insulin. Your neighbor's cat secretes insulin. Your nondiabetic coworker secretes insulin. Insulin is an absolutely essential biological hormone that is secreted by beta cells in all mammals, a critical hormone that is mandatory for life. Without insulin, your dog would die. Your neighbor's cat would die. Your coworker would, yes, die. Without insulin, the cells in your liver, muscles, and fat tissue would have a very difficult time recognizing that glucose is present in your blood, and would be able to uptake only a tiny fraction of what was present in circulation, resulting in chronically high blood glucose at all times.

**Think of insulin as an escort for glucose that tells cells in tissues all over your body, "Glucose is available in the blood—would you like to take some inside?"**

When insulin knocks on the door of cells inside tissues all over your

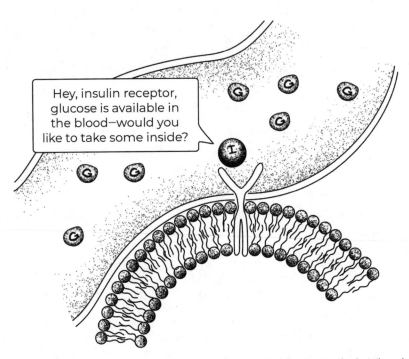

Insulin receptors are located on the surfaces of cells in tissues all over your body. When they recognize insulin in your blood efficiently, cells are given the opportunity to import large amounts of glucose.

body, they are given the opportunity to import glucose from your blood *if and only if they have the ability to recognize insulin's presence.* You run into trouble when cells in your liver, muscles, pancreas, and adipose tissue (fat tissue) fail to recognize insulin's signal, which then prevents them from importing large amounts of glucose from your blood. (Your muscles and liver are the largest insulin-dependent tissues in your body, accounting for the majority of glucose absorption. Your brain also uptakes large amounts of glucose but requires only a fraction of the insulin that your muscles and liver require.) Since insulin's job is to escort glucose into tissues, when cells can't recognize insulin well, they *reject* it. When cells reject insulin, glucose gets trapped in your blood for extended periods of time, causing high blood glucose. To compensate, your pancreas releases more insulin, in the hope of overpowering these cells to import more glucose.

**So what causes cells in your body to reject insulin in the first place?** When cells reject insulin, they are "resistant" to insulin and said to be in an "insulin resistant" state. The causes of insulin resistance are numerous and relate specifically to the amount of food you eat, the type of food you eat, your movement patterns, the nutrient density of your diet, and your stress levels (to name a few). Think of insulin resistance as a puzzle that contains different-sized pieces in which the larger pieces have more of an impact than the smaller pieces. Without question, the largest and most important puzzle pieces are those that relate to the amount of food you eat, the type of food you eat, and your macronutrient ratio (the ratio of carbohydrates to fat to protein). Don't worry, we'll cover all of this in detail in upcoming chapters.

Even though people will tell you that carbohydrates are dangerous, understand that *carbohydrates are not the enemy,* especially if they originate from whole plant foods. Carbohydrates were never the enemy, and they will never be the enemy. On the contrary, fatty acids *directly* inhibit the action of insulin, and the amount of fat you eat and type of fat you eat are the primary determinants of how insulin resistant you become over the course of time. That's right. The more fat you eat (especially saturated fat), the more insulin resistant you become.

If you are like most people living with diabetes, chances are you were never taught the fat-insulin connection, and it may surprise you to learn that dietary fat is one of the most important aspects of your diet that influences how effectively insulin operates in your body. Let's go into detail about this connection so that you have a clearer understanding of the biology of insulin resistance.

An overwhelming amount of scientific evidence shows that a high-fat diet is the single most effective method at *inducing* insulin resistance in both your liver and muscle. These studies clearly demonstrate that increasing your fat intake has an immediate negative impact on the ability of insulin to communicate with tissues, which can then develop into a chronic state of insulin resistance and diabetes if your fat intake remains high.

This isn't new information.

Scientists have known that dietary fat makes insulin less powerful for almost a hundred years. Starting in the early 1920s, researchers named Dr. William Sansum and Dr. J. Shirley Sweeney were some of the first to publish research about the fat-insulin connection. During the 1930s, Dr. I. M. Rabinowitch and Dr. Harold Percival Himsworth continued to conduct elegant experiments to demonstrate the detrimental effects of high-fat diets on insulin action. In the 1950s, Dr. Walter Kempner reversed type 2 diabetes in his patients using a diet low in dietary fat that was remarkably effective at also reversing long-standing retinopathy, kidney disease, and malignant hypertension. In the 1970s, Dr. James W. Anderson published experiments in which he reduced or eliminated the use of insulin in patients with type 2 diabetes by swtiching them to a low-fat, high-fiber diet. You'll have a chance to learn details about these studies (and more) in chapter 7, but for now suffice it to say that the fat-insulin connection is nothing new—it's just that it has been largely ignored for almost a hundred years.

One of the most important discoveries happened in 1963 when a scientist named Philip Randle described that carbohydrate and fat are mutually exclusive fuels, and that fatty acids and glucose compete for entry into cells. He demonstrated that fatty acids gain access to tissues and block insulin from working, leaving glucose trapped in your blood. Philip Randle told the scientific world that eating fatty acids sets the stage for insulin rejection in your muscle and liver. He called this effect the *fatty-acid syndrome,* which was later renamed the *Randle cycle.* More than fifty years later, this research is still considered one of the most profound observations in carbohydrate biology; however, the modern scientific world is quick to misinterpret this simple and very powerful insight. Let's start by defining the primary cause of insulin resistance as follows:

**Insulin resistance is caused by the accumulation of excess fat in tissues that are not designed to store large quantities of fat.**

In order to understand the fat-insulin connection in more detail, let's take a closer look at the effect of dietary fat inside your body.

# A Step-by-Step Overview of the Fat-Insulin Connection

### Step 1: Fat Enters Your Blood Before Glucose

When you eat foods containing fat-soluble nutrients (including triglycerides, phospholipids, and cholesterol), these fat-soluble nutrients travel down your esophagus until they reach your stomach. Your stomach releases hydrochloric acid (HCl) to kill potentially harmful bacteria, while the cells in your stomach lining secrete protein-digesting enzymes to begin unfolding protein chains. The smooth muscle in the walls of your stomach contracts vigorously in order to create a sludge known as *chyme,* which then exits your stomach bound for your small intestine, where the bulk of nutrients are absorbed.

In your small intestine, two important processes occur. First, cells in the lining of your small intestine absorb these fat-soluble nutrients and package them into particles called *chylomicrons,* which are then dumped into your lymphatic system, a collection of vessels that carry lymphatic fluid to the blood and clear waste compounds from tissues. When the lymphatic fluid ushers chylomicrons into your blood, they're circulated throughout your body so that your adipose tissue and muscle have the first chance to uptake triglycerides from your food.

When your small intestine detects fat-soluble nutrients in your food, it releases a collection of powerful hormones that communicate with your brain and stomach to control your appetite and slow your *gastric emptying rate,* or the rate at which food exits your stomach. In effect, your small intestine says, "Hey, stomach, slow down how quickly you process food. This fatty meal is going to take me some time to digest and absorb." A slowed gastric emptying rate results in an upstream traffic jam, slowing down the passage of chyme out of your stomach and into your small intestine. If you've ever noticed that a high-fat meal takes longer for your stomach to process than a lower fat meal, this is exactly why—because the presence of dietary fat slows the digestion of all food material, causing a temporary traffic jam in your stomach. This is one reason why diets high in fat are effective at curbing your appetite and making you feel full for long periods of time.

But back to your intestines. As a result of the simultaneous fat absorption into your lymphatic system and slowed gastric emptying rate, both carbohydrate and protein digestion are slowed. The net consequence is that fat-rich chylomicrons appear in your blood more rapidly than glucose (one of the building blocks of carbohydrates) and amino acids (the building blocks of protein).

## Step 2: Fat Enters Your Blood and Tissues

When fat-rich chylomicron particles have circulated throughout your body and offloaded triglycerides, your liver then uptakes the remaining particles, called *chylomicron remnants*. A simple way to understand this is to think of your liver as the post office of fat metabolism. In the same way that the post office receives mail at the loading dock from large mail trucks, sorts it, and then sends it out on smaller trucks to local residents and businesses, chylomicron remnants appear at the loading docks of your liver, where they're unpacked, sorted, and repackaged. The triglyceride molecules are then transferred into lipoprotein particles and sent out in your blood once again.

With the help of enzymes located on the surface of cells throughout your body, tissues absorb fatty acids and cholesterol from these lipoproteins. Unlike glucose, fatty acids can enter cells easily without requiring an escort like insulin. In effect, the lipoprotein particles in circulation say, "Hey, tissues, I'm here! I have a bunch of fatty acids for you to take up if you want." While insulin can certainly help fatty acids get out of lipoproteins and into tissues, insulin is not fully required because fatty acids can also enter tissues without insulin. Because of this, tissues have no choice but to absorb fatty acids when they appear in your blood in large amounts.

As soon as the fatty acids are absorbed by cells in your liver and muscle tissue, they are either burned for energy or stored for later use. Those that are burned for energy are immediately ripped apart and transported to the mitochondria to be turned into ATP (the cellular equivalent of energy), and those that are stored enter a pool of fatty acids inside the cell, known as a lipid droplet. Fatty acids will continue to enter cells as long as they are present in your blood, and unfortunately cells don't have sophisticated mechanisms to block large amounts from entering. In effect, the more fat you eat, the more fat you force cells in your liver and muscle to absorb.

**Step 1: Import Chylomicrons**

Liver

**Step 2: Repackage Lipids**

Chl

Chl

Chl

Chl

**Step 3: Secrete Lipoproteins**

Lipoprotein

Make room!

We're coming inside!

Blood Vessel

Adipose Tissue

Liver

Muscle

**Step 4: Tissues Uptake Lipids**

In the same way that the post office receives mail from large mail trucks, sorts it, and sends it back out on smaller trucks, your liver imports, repackages, and exports fatty acids at all times.

**Step 3: Fat Enters Your Adipose Tissue**

Unlike other tissues with a distinct location in your body such as your brain, heart, or lungs, your adipose tissue (also called fat) is located in many places. You can find small and large pockets of fat almost everywhere, including your abdomen, butt, thighs, lower back, chest, armpits, face, neck, and even ankles. Fatty acids enter your adipose tissue in the exact same way that they enter all other tissues—aided by enzymes known as *lipases* and *fatty acid transport proteins* (FATPs). Fatty acids are easily absorbed because your adipose tissue contains the perfect molecular machinery to uptake and store fatty acids for long periods of time; in fact that's exactly what your adipose tissue is designed to do.

While most people want to minimize the amount of adipose tissue on their body, it's important to point out that adipose tissue is actually a *protective* organ. Your adipose tissue is designed to grow and shrink in response to times of feast and times of famine, storing energy at times when there are excess calories available to protect you for when calories are sparse. In addition, your adipose tissue also protects tissues like your liver and muscle from accumulating excess fatty acids by giving them another location to end up.

The reason most people and health professionals consider adipose tissue dangerous is that, much like insulin, *excess* fat increases your risk for many chronic diseases—especially the deep abdominal fat that surrounds your internal organs—because the more fat you store in your abdomen, the higher your risk for obesity, cardiovascular disease, hypertension, diabetes, and insulin resistance.

**Step 4: Your Adipose Tissue Becomes Inflamed**

The biology of adipose tissue insulin resistance is fascinating and deserves a thorough explanation. To begin, fat cells are incredibly flexible and are designed to store large quantities of fat, but they cannot expand indefinitely. As a result, when fat cells are chronically overfed, they can become inflamed just like any other tissue, resulting in a low-grade chronic inflammation that triggers insulin resistance.

When you eat a high-fat diet, cells in your adipose tissue accumulate fatty acids. Over time, cells in your adipose tissue can burst open, spilling their

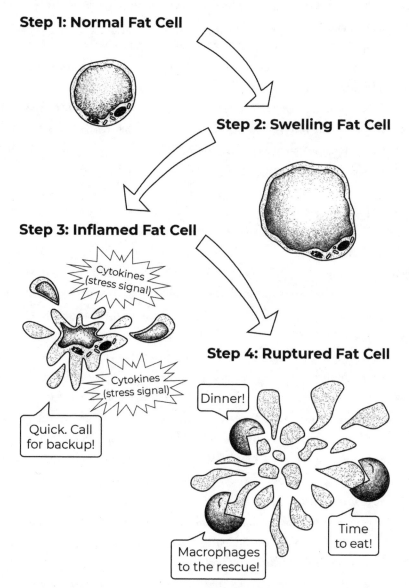

Macrophages are cells in your blood that engulf cellular debris from damaged and broken cells. Cells in your adipose tissue can swell and break when chronically overfed, triggering a low-grade inflammation that reduces the ability of insulin to function properly.

contents into the interstitial fluid that surrounds the tissue. This explosion re-leases cellular debris into your blood, and neighboring cells release stress signals called *cytokines* into your blood, which then recruits cells called *macrophages* to invade the tissue in search of unwanted cellular debris from ruptured cells. Think of macrophages as the biological version of Pac-Man, tasked with the job of cleaning up cellular debris by engulfing waste material. And there's no job too big for macrophages—if there's too much debris, they can signal for backup by secreting more cytokines. The problem is that these signals don't just recruit more hungry macrophages; they also trigger chronic inflammation, and in the process create a state of adipose tissue insulin resistance.

### Step 5: Fat Causes Insulin Rejection in Your Muscle and Liver

Even though your muscles and liver can generate ATP from glucose, fatty acids, and amino acids, your muscles and liver are designed to use glucose as their primary fuel. Both your muscle and liver cells have a similar construction—they can store small quantities of fat in lipid droplets and store glucose as glycogen. Your muscles and liver are specifically designed to remain "lean," with only small amounts of fatty acids in lipid droplets at all times.

But because these tissues absorb nutrients that appear in your blood, they remain unprotected against a large influx of fatty acids that occurs in the hours following a fat-rich meal. Since fatty acids appear before glucose during the digestion process, your muscles and liver are exposed to more fatty acids than glucose, setting the stage for insulin resistance when glucose becomes more readily available. When your muscles and liver uptake fatty acids from your blood, they also *upregulate* enzymes involved in all aspects of fatty acid metabolism and *downregulate* enzymes involved in all aspects of glucose metabolism—because fatty acids are now the predominant fuel.

When cells in your liver and muscles begin burning and storing fatty acids, just as Philip Randle described, they block glucose from entering be-cause the cellular machinery required to uptake, process, and store glucose has been deprioritized. In effect, cells in your liver and muscle alter their in-ternal enzymatic machinery based on the fuel that is most readily available.

How do these cells block glucose from entering? It's actually quite simple—they stop paying attention to insulin by downregulating insulin receptors located on the cell surface. Within hours of a single high-fat meal, insulin receptors become less numerous and less functional, perform less work, and have a very difficult time recognizing insulin in your blood. These dysfunctional insulin receptors keep glucose outside of cells, leaving glucose trapped in your blood for long periods of time. When you check your blood glucose two to six hours after eating a meal containing predominantly fat and protein with a small or medium amount of carbohydrate energy, you may see a high number and ask yourself, "Why is my blood glucose high? I didn't eat that much carbohydrate."

This is exactly when insulin rejection first takes place. Unlike your adipose tissue, which is specifically designed to store fat to protect other organs from fat overload, your muscle and liver tissues are designed to store small amounts of fat and large amounts of glycogen. But when your liver and muscles first absorb fat from your blood following a fat-rich meal, they respond by rejecting insulin to block glucose from entering, because they have already accepted fatty acids as their primary energy source. First come, first served.

## Excess Insulin Acts Like a Wrecking Ball

**A simple way to** understand insulin resistance is to imagine tissues constructing a brick wall to protect themselves against excess nutrients, and insulin as a wrecking ball specifically designed to knock it down. Under normal circumstances, insulin acts as a chaperone to help glucose enter tissues all over your body. Any time you eat a meal containing carbohydrates, insulin is *required* to get it inside of cells—namely, the other side of that brick wall.

In insulin-sensitive individuals, the brick wall is small, and therefore only small amounts of insulin are required to knock a hole in the wall and get glucose inside. In insulin-resistant individuals, the wall is high and thick, and in order to overpower the wall and get glucose inside cells, your pancreas is forced to secrete excess insulin. In effect, your pancreas says, "Hey, tissues, you need a larger wrecking ball? I'll just make more insulin!" As more and more insulin is secreted (or injected in the case of people with insulin-dependent diabetes), the strength of the wrecking ball increases until it's finally capable of breaking a hole in the wall. As soon as the insulin wrecking ball has created a hole, glucose can then flood into tissues, and the amount of glucose in your blood drops rapidly.

Ultimately, you have two options to allow glucose to enter tissues: (a) reduce the height and thickness of the brick wall by preventing excess fatty acid accumulation, or (b) rely on the excess insulin wrecking ball to knock the wall down. Technically speaking, both methods result in glucose entering tissues. However, the first method is the only one that minimizes your risk for long-term chronic disease, while the second method significantly increases your risk for cardiovascular mortality.

Take a look at the illustration on the next page for a visual representation of how excess insulin acts as a wrecking ball in response to the brick wall created by insulin resistance.

If we go back to the two options you have for encouraging glucose to enter cells in your muscle and liver, it probably goes without saying that we're fans of the first method: *Reduce the height and thickness of the brick wall by preventing excess fatty acid accumulation.* That's largely because eating a diet high in fat not only causes insulin resistance but increases your risk for many chronic diseases over the course of time.

One of the most common side effects of eating a high-fat diet is *fatty liver disease* (also known as non-alcoholic fatty liver disease, NAFLD). Fatty liver disease occurs when the amount of fat in your liver is more than 5 percent by weight, resulting in liver enlargement, which can then lead to *liver fibrosis,* a condition marked by the formation of scar tissue. Finally, *liver cirrhosis* occurs when connective tissue destroys dysfunctional liver cells. While it's certainly true that eating or drinking refined sugars like sucrose and high-fructose corn syrup (HFCS) can contribute to fatty liver disease, a growing body of research shows that a high-fat diet results in a progressive decline in liver function over time.

Your liver is a crucial part of the insulin resistance equation because cells in your liver are capable of exporting glucose into your blood to provide your brain with a constant supply of glucose at all times. And insulin is the signal that tells your liver exactly when to increase and when to decrease the amount of glucose it exports. When insulin is readily available following a meal, your

Insulin resistance functions like a brick wall, blocking the ability of insulin to communicate with cells, which traps glucose in your blood. Excess insulin acts like a wrecking ball, knocking a hole in the brick wall and allowing glucose to enter cells in tissues all over your body.

liver decreases the amount of glucose it exports. When insulin is less available after multiple hours of fasting, your liver increases the rate at which it exports glucose in order to drip feed your brain with a stable supply.

Here's the problem: When you develop insulin resistance in your liver due to the accumulation of excess dietary fat, your liver can't communicate with insulin very effectively, resulting in a chronically high rate of glucose export, high fasting blood glucose, and high post-meal blood glucose. In effect, an accumulation of excess fatty acids prevents your liver from accurately controlling how much glucose it releases into your blood.

### Step 6: Beta Cells Get Stressed

Beta cells in your pancreas have one function: to manufacture and secrete insulin into your blood. They make up less than 1 percent of your total pancreas by weight, representing a very small population of cells. Your body has no backup mechanism for producing insulin, so when your beta cell function is compromised, it presents a *disastrous* metabolic problem to tissues all over your body. In the same way that your liver and muscles are highly sensitive to the accumulation of fat, so are beta cells. The accumulation of excess fat in your beta cells leads to severe dysfunction known as *lipotoxicity*.

In comparison with cells in your liver and muscle, beta cells are particularly sensitive to fatty acids because they have a limited ability to protect themselves against damage. And when exposed to high fat concentrations for long periods of time, their antioxidant self-defense mechanisms are inadequate to protect them against dysfunction. In addition, an increasing demand for insulin forces your beta cells to manufacture insulin in overdrive, creating even more internal cellular stress, and eventually their ability to produce insulin gets maxed out. In some individuals, this process can take many years to develop, while in others this process can occur rapidly.

The result of chronic beta cell stress has a fittingly bleak name: beta cell suicide. There comes a point in the life of a stressed beta cell when it is more advantageous to commit suicide than to stay alive. At this point, beta cells undergo a process known as *apoptosis,* or programmed cell death. It is a point of no return that's the equivalent of saying, "That's it! We can't take it anymore!" When a large population of beta cells undergoes apoptosis, insulin production rapidly falls below normal physiological levels within a short period of time.

In the same way that peak insulin production varies between individuals, the extent of beta cell suicide is also a highly variable process. Some individuals retain 60 percent of their original beta cell mass, whereas others will drop to as low as 20 percent. Autopsies have revealed that in the majority of patients with type 2 diabetes, more than half of the beta cell population has died. In this state, only a small population of beta cells are then responsible for secreting enough insulin to satisfy the metabolic demands of your entire body. As you might guess, this job is extremely difficult unless you help your muscle and liver significantly reduce their insulin requirements.

After the age of 20, your body stops making new beta cells; therefore beta cell death is considered irreversible. The question then becomes: If you significantly reduce your level of whole-body insulin resistance, can the remaining beta cell population produce enough insulin to meet the demands of all tissues? Fortunately, the answer is almost always yes. Even when beta cell mass has been significantly compromised, the remaining beta cell population is often capable of producing sufficient insulin for all tissues, but *only if you take steps to reduce your body's insulin needs by increasing your insulin sensitivity.* This means that you will benefit from substantially reducing your body's need for excess insulin to protect beta cells from committing suicide. Luckily, the Mastering Diabetes Method teaches you how to prevent and reverse the accumulation of excess fat in nonfatty tissues and prevent beta cell suicide before it has the chance to begin.

## Insulin Resistance in Type 1 and Type 1.5 Diabetes

Many doctors, in addition to people living with type 1 and type 1.5 diabetes, believe that insulin resistance pertains only to people living with prediabetes, type 2 diabetes, and gestational diabetes. Furthermore, many people think that insulin resistance affects only overweight individuals, and that being slender or having a normal body mass index (BMI) is proof of being insulin sensitive. Unfortunately, these assumptions are incorrect. It is important to

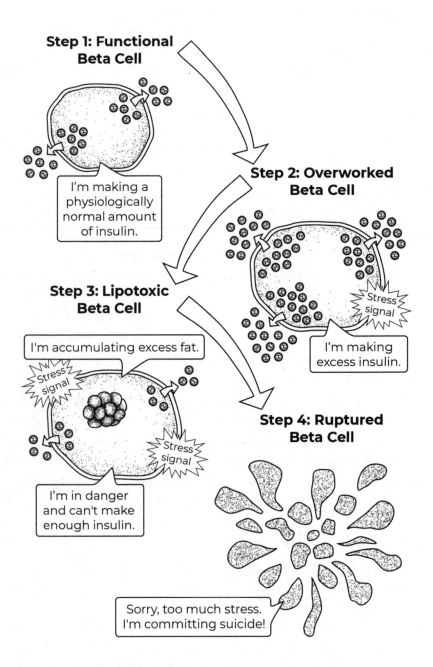

Functional beta cells can commit suicide when they are stressed and when they accumulate excess fatty acids over time. Since beta cell death is largely irreversible, taking the necessary steps to maximize beta cell function can make a dramatic difference in your overall health.

understand that insulin resistance cannot be seen from the outside—it is a condition that reflects the *internal* state of your liver, muscles, adipose tissue, pancreas, and blood vessels. It can affect you, no matter how much you weigh.

Unlike type 2 diabetes, type 1 and 1.5 diabetes occur when your own immune system targets beta cells for destruction, leaving them incapable of manufacturing enough insulin to maintain your blood glucose within the normal range (80–130 mg/dL). When your own immune system erroneously targets your own tissues for destruction, scientists call this an *autoimmune* condition. Given what scientists understand about autoimmunity, they believe that certain individuals have a genetic predisposition to type 1 and type 1.5 diabetes at birth, but develop autoimmunity only when exposed to one or more environmental "triggers," including a viral infection, a bacterial infection, or exposure to cow's milk protein at a very young age. We'll explain more about the link between dairy products and autoimmunity in chapter 5, but for now suffice it to say that living with an autoimmune version of diabetes does not exclude you from developing diet-induced insulin resistance.

Even though type 2 diabetes is *caused* by insulin resistance, and type 1 and 1.5 diabetes result from an autoimmune reaction, the diet-induced insulin resistance present in both conditions is biologically identical. In fact, a growing body of scientific evidence demonstrates that insulin resistance is a growing concern in autoimmune diabetes owing to less-than-ideal lifestyle choices, and eating a diet that consists of low-carbohydrate foods like meat, fish, dairy, eggs, and oils or a diet containing significant quantities of refined sugar and processed foods.

**When you're living with autoimmune diabetes and also develop insulin resistance from your diet, you develop *double diabetes,* a term used to describe people living with both autoimmune diabetes and the symptoms of type 2 diabetes.**

Double diabetes is a life-threatening combination of health conditions that makes controlling your blood glucose virtually impossible, as glucose routinely gets trapped in your blood, unable to enter your muscle and liver in large quantities. Double diabetes occurs when you already have type 1 or type 1.5 diabetes, and you then eat yourself into insulin resistance.

We have observed that many people living with type 1 and 1.5 diabetes experience double diabetes, frustrated by some combination of an elevated A1c, hard-to-control blood glucose, increasing insulin requirements, low energy, impaired digestion, high blood pressure, high cholesterol, a low tolerance for carbohydrates, and/or an inability to lose weight. If you're in this segment of the population, you're in luck because the Mastering Diabetes Method directly addresses double diabetes head-on, simplifies the process of living with autoimmune diabetes, and teaches you how to control your blood glucose with precision.

## Take-Home Messages

- Your doctors didn't learn nutrition in medical school (and it's not their fault!).
- The carbohydrate-centric diabetes model is an incomplete, flawed, and overly simplistic view of diabetes biology that keeps people with diabetes at a high risk for future complications.
- Insulin is not your enemy—*excess insulin* increases your risk for metabolic dysfunction in many tissues over time.
- Insulin resistance is caused by the accumulation of *excess* fat in tissues not designed to store large quantities of fat.
- High-fat diets cause whole-body insulin resistance that causes insulin rejection in your liver, muscles, and adipose tissue, in addition to promoting beta cell death.
- Insulin resistance can affect you even if you are slender, have a normal BMI, or are living with type 1 or type 1.5 diabetes.

To view the 150+ scientific references cited in this chapter, please visit us online at www.masteringdiabetes.org/bookinfo.

# Chapter 4

# All Fat Is Not Created Equal

## High Fat to High Plant: Lindsay

Lindsay Garcia was diagnosed with type 2 diabetes in 2014. Motivated by the desire to control her blood glucose and to improve her long-term health, she began eating a low-carbohydrate, high-protein diet as recommended by her naturopath, despite the fact that she had eliminated all animal products from her diet prior to her diagnosis. For the first few months, Lindsay saw excellent results. Her A1c dropped from 10.0% to below 6.0% and she was able to control her blood glucose with precision. But even though her numbers looked good, she felt terrible. She was consistently constipated and had to take laxatives every few days in order to go to the bathroom. After a few months following this low-carbohydrate, high-protein diet, she found it more challenging to control her cholesterol, and her blood glucose was constantly in the 300s and rarely dipped below 250 mg/dL. Her naturopath incorrectly diagnosed her with type 2 diabetes and prescribed metformin to reduce her blood glucose, but an appointment with an endocrinologist revealed that she was actually living with type 1 diabetes.

Feeling frustrated, she began looking for a plant-based coach to help her manage type 1 diabetes as an athlete. She enrolled in the Mastering

Diabetes Coaching Program in October of 2016 and immediately learned how to reduce her total fat intake, how to adjust her insulin timing strategy, how to manage her blood glucose before, during, and after exercise, as well as how to increase her intake of low-fat plant-based whole foods. After just a few weeks of transitioning to a low-fat plant-based whole-food diet, her carbohydrate-to-insulin ratio increased from 9:1 to between 25:1 and 35:1. She increased her carbohydrate intake from approximately 175 grams per day to 500 grams per day or more, and at the same time, decreased her total insulin use from 40 units per day to 30 units per day. Best of all, Lindsay's A1c is now 5.8%, and she also significantly improved her cardiovascular health. Following this approach, her total cholesterol dropped from 187 mg/dL to 126 mg/dL, and she no longer worries about her risk for cardiovascular disease. In November of 2018, Lindsay felt so good, she ran her first marathon fueled by nothing but plants. She considers herself transformed from the inside out, and loves the simplicity and effectiveness that the Mastering Diabetes Method has brought to her life.

---

While it is true that the *quantity* of fat in your diet influences your blood glucose values, so does the *quality* of the fat you eat. When it comes to managing your blood glucose and controlling insulin resistance, all fat is not created equal. There are significant and important differences in how trans fat, saturated fat, and unsaturated fat affect your metabolic health. Fat-rich animal foods (meat, fish, dairy, eggs, poultry, and processed meat products) and refined carbohydrates (sugar-sweetened beverages, pastries, cookies, crackers, and breads), as well as vegetable, nut, and seed oils, will have the most dramatic impact on the development of insulin resistance and will increase your risk for chronic disease. Plant-based fat-rich foods (nuts, seeds, olives, avocados, and coconuts) certainly have their place in the Mastering Diabetes Method in small proportions, but will also impact the development of insulin resistance when eaten in excess. Even though they are better alternatives than animal-based fat-rich foods, it is very important to pay attention to how many plant-based fat-rich foods you eat in order to control your blood glucose with precision. Understanding the source of fat in your diet is vitally important in taking the next step in adopting a low-fat plant-based whole-food diet.

---

### A Word About the Importance of Dietary Fat

It's important to point out that even though the fat-insulin connection is an underappreciated biological phenomenon, we want to be very clear that fatty acids and fat-soluble compounds play a necessary role in tissues all throughout your body. The Mastering Diabetes Method encourages you to *reduce* your overall fat intake, not to *eliminate* your fat intake, while increasing the quality of your fatty acid supply for exceptional insulin sensitivity and reduced chronic disease risk.

---

Despite the fact that eating excess total fat can set the stage for insulin resistance and high blood glucose, it's important to differentiate between different types of fat, because not all types of fat behave the same way in your body and each has different effects on insulin resistance and your ability to control your blood glucose.

## 1. Trans Fatty Acids

Trans fatty acids are a type of fat that occurs naturally in very small quantities in beef, pork, lamb, butter, and milk (between 1 and 10 percent of total fat content). However, the overwhelming majority of trans fats in most people's diets originate from a process known as *hydrogenation,* a chemical manufacturing process that food manufacturers use to convert unsaturated fatty acids into saturated fatty acids. Hydrogenation was invented to turn liquids into solids for the purpose of creating spreadable products that have long shelf lives. Exhibit A: margarine.

Trans fats are hidden everywhere in processed foods and are also found in products containing *partially hydrogenated vegetable oils,* including cakes, pies, cookies, biscuits, breakfast sandwiches, margarine, crackers, microwave popcorn, cream-filled candies, doughnuts, ready-to-use dough, and both dairy and nondairy coffee creamers. Trans fats are likewise found in both unprocessed and processed meats, with processed meats containing significantly more trans fats than the unprocessed meat from which they originated.

For many years, products containing partially hydrogenated vegetable oils have been deceptively marketed as being "healthier" because they contain less cholesterol (or zero cholesterol). The truth is that the trans fatty acids created by partial hydrogenation actually cause more metabolic damage than cholesterol, but this important fact remains hidden from consumers searching for healthier ways to eat.

Trans fatty acids are associated with an increasing list of cardiovascular conditions, including congestive heart disease, stroke, atherosclerosis, high cholesterol, and high blood pressure. Studies show that industrial trans fats can significantly increase your risk for congestive heart disease, and that even small amounts of trans fats can directly elevate your LDL cholesterol, reduce your HDL cholesterol, cause vascular inflammation, and accelerate the development of atherosclerotic plaques, both in your heart and in peripheral blood vessels. Trans fats have also been implicated in cognitive decline, including conditions like Alzheimer's disease, dementia, and depression. Studies have shown that those who eat more industrial trans fats have a greater risk for Alzheimer's disease than those who eat the fewest, either due to direct damage to neurons in your brain or indirectly by increasing your cholesterol levels, which are known to be associated with Alzheimer's disease.

When it comes to the connection between trans fats and insulin resistance, ample evidence has shown that trans fats directly impair the ability of beta cells to respond to glucose in both animals and cell culture. The Nurses' Health Study, in which researchers from the Harvard T. H. Chan School of Public Health performed an analysis on data from more than 200,000 individuals taken over the course of nineteen years, showed that a higher intake of trans fatty acids was associated with a higher risk of type 2 diabetes over the course of fourteen years.

## 2. Saturated Fatty Acids

Saturated fatty acids are naturally occurring fatty acids that are found in all whole foods, but mainly in meat, poultry, fish, shellfish, dairy products (butter, cheese, milk, yogurt, sour cream, ice cream, and whipped cream), and eggs, but are also present in higher amounts in plant foods including vegetable oils, coconut oil, palm oil, palm kernel oil, cocoa butter, avocados, coconuts, nuts, and seeds.

There is currently a massive debate about whether saturated fat improves or worsens your diabetes health. Proponents of low-carbohydrate diets, the Paleo diet, and the ketogenic diet argue that diets high in saturated fat promote optimal metabolic health and actually *improve* your diabetes health, whereas proponents of a whole-food plant-based diet contend that diets high in saturated fat *increase* insulin resistance, promote atherosclerosis, and increase your risk for coronary artery disease, high cholesterol, and cancer. Reading science from both sides of the argument can be quite convincing, even though the conclusions conflict with one another. So who's correct? Are diets high in saturated fat optimal or dangerous? Do they increase longevity or increase your risk for premature death?

A large body of scientific information has clearly documented that saturated fats are powerful triggers for insulin resistance, and that diets high in saturated fat may result in a fantastic blood glucose level and a low A1c value, but they do so at the expense of significantly increased insulin resistance, which in turn increases your overall risk for chronic disease and all-cause mortality (premature death) in the long term. This single fact has helped thousands of people make the switch to a low-fat diet, and is one of the most misunderstood aspects of diabetes biology altogether.

**Diets high in saturated fat are effective *short-term* treatments to lose weight and normalize blood glucose, but they significantly increase your level of insulin resistance, which in turn increases your risk for many chronic diseases and premature death in the *long term*.**

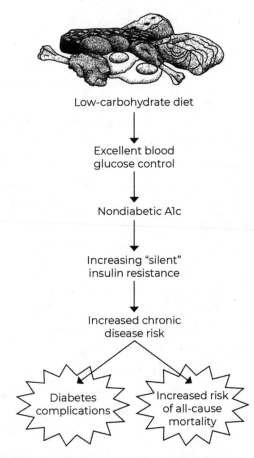

Low-carbohydrate diet

↓

Excellent blood
glucose control

↓

Nondiabetic A1c

↓

Increasing "silent"
insulin resistance

↓

Increased chronic
disease risk

Diabetes
complications

Increased risk
of all-cause
mortality

A low-carbohydrate diet is very effective at improving your blood glucose control in the short term, but it can lead to "silent" insulin resistance, which in turn increases your risk for long-term diabetes complications and premature death.

In fact, the scientific world is so knowledgeable about the detrimental effects of saturated fat that scientists actually induce obesity and insulin resistance in animals and humans using diets high in saturated fat. Cyrus first recognized this in his PhD program, and was shocked that the standard protocol for creating insulin resistance in laboratory animals involved the use of a diet high in saturated fat and low in carbohydrate. This was the first time Cyrus recognized that the way people in the real world are told to eat to prevent and reverse diabetes is unfortunately the same protocol that scientists use to *create* insulin resistance in controlled scientific experiments.

Saturated fatty acids directly interfere with insulin signaling within hours of entering muscle and liver cells, inhibiting the ability of your muscle and liver to uptake glucose from your blood. While small amounts of saturated fat (1–5 grams per day) do not pose a significant threat to your glucose metabolism, the consumption of large amounts of saturated fat (more than about 10 grams per day) triggers a series of adverse biochemical reactions in your muscle, liver, pancreas, and adipose tissue, which rapidly create an insulin-resistant state that can last for a minimum of one to two days and continue for weeks, months, or years, depending on the amount of saturated fat in your diet and how frequently you eat foods containing it.

Inside muscle and liver cells, the presence of excess saturated fatty acids activates a series of intracellular signals that:

- Reduce the number of insulin receptors that appear on the cell surface
- Impair insulin receptors by modifying their structure on the inside of the cell membrane
- Reduce the ability of glucose transport vesicles (GLUT vesicles) to migrate to the surface of cells to import glucose from your blood
- Increase free radical production in mitochondria

And remember from chapter 3—when your adipose tissue accumulates excess fatty acids over time, macrophages invade and secrete inflammatory *cytokines.* These inflammatory signals create chronic low-grade inflammation and directly inhibit the action of insulin. So the cumulative result of excess saturated fatty acids in your muscle and liver is a reduced ability of both tissues to utilize glucose as a fuel, which traps glucose and insulin in your blood for extended periods of time. If you've ever wondered why people with pre-diabetes often experience high blood glucose and high insulin levels at the same time, this is exactly why—both insulin and glucose get trapped in your blood simultaneously. In addition to the direct negative impact on your muscle, liver, and adipose tissue, excess saturated fatty acids also directly impair the ability of pancreatic beta cells to manufacture and secrete insulin. As we

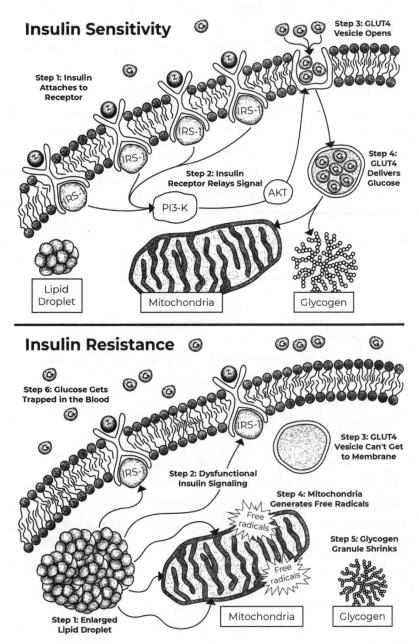

A schematic diagram of how the storage of excess fatty acids in muscle and liver cells disrupts insulin signaling and reduces the ability of glucose to enter, resulting in high blood glucose.

covered in chapter 3, lipotoxicity is extremely dangerous for beta cells because of their limited antioxidant self-defense mechanisms, which makes them easy targets for programmed cell death.

Diets high in saturated fat are also especially dangerous for your liver, as they are extremely effective at promoting fatty liver disease, which can eventually lead to liver cirrhosis and induce an advanced state of liver insulin resistance and liver inflammation. When excess saturated fat accumulates in liver cells over the course of time, it increases the rate at which the cells offload glucose and triglycerides into your blood, leading to increased glucose production, increased triglycerides, and increased LDL cholesterol.

To demonstrate this conclusively, large-scale research and controlled clinical trials have demonstrated that increasing your intake of saturated fat will increase your LDL cholesterol (the "bad" cholesterol—see the box below). The connection is so strong that researchers have developed a mathematical model (called the Hegsted equation) that specifically predicts how the saturated fat in your diet impacts the cholesterol level in your blood. Although the specifics of the equation are beyond the scope of this book, the most important thing to understand is that *saturated fat in your diet increases your LDL cholesterol (more than dietary cholesterol itself)*!

## Cholesterol 101

**There are two main** types of cholesterol in your blood. **Low-density lipoprotein (LDL)** cholesterol is considered "bad" cholesterol because scientists have discovered that the more LDL cholesterol you have in your blood, the higher your risk for an acute cardiac event. This is because LDL particles *deliver* cholesterol to tissues, and LDL particles can often get trapped in the lining of blood vessels, increasing your risk for atherosclerosis. **High-density lipoprotein (HDL)** cholesterol, on the other hand, is considered your "good" cholesterol because it is involved in *reverse cholesterol transport,* pulling cholesterol out of tissues and returning it to your liver. For years, the medical world has focused on reducing cardiovasuclar disease risk by finding ways to increase HDL cholesterol, but research now shows that reducing your LDL cholesterol is significantly more effective at preventing and reversing cardiovascular disease.

Both saturated fat and cholesterol in your diet are known to increase your LDL cholesterol level. In people with low LDL cholesterol, eating a single meal containing dietary cholesterol can dramatically increase blood cholesterol within hours. Pharmaceutical companies and animal food lobbyists often publish misleading studies that deny this connection by reporting that foods high in cholesterol do not raise blood cholesterol levels. How do they get away with this? By enrolling subjects with high cholesterol at baseline. In such people, meals containing high-cholesterol foods don't have a dramatic or immediate impact on LDL cholesterol.

Despite compelling scientific evidence, many medical professionals and people remain confused about whether LDL cholesterol increases your risk for heart disease or not. Have no doubt about it: Data from more than *one million* participants enrolled in more than a hundred studies have demonstrated a strong positive relationship between your total LDL cholesterol level and your risk for coronary artery disease. Much like the Hegsted equation, which predicts how increasing amounts of dietary saturated fat increase your total and LDL cholesterol, the relationship between LDL cholesterol and coronary artery disease is so strong that it is well worth your time to understand inside and out. Without question—the more LDL you have in your blood, the greater your risk for coronary artery disease.

While many people understand that lowering your LDL cholesterol is an important strategy to reduce your risk for an *acute coronary event* (heart attack or sudden cardiac death), many advocates of low-carbohydrate diets argue that the total number of LDL particles is less important than the size of LDL particles, and that just having a high LDL cholesterol does not mean that you are at an elevated risk for a heart attack. They refer to large, buoyant LDL particles as *protective* against heart disease, and only caution against increasing small, dense LDL particles.

Even though this may seem reasonable at first glance, a deep dive into the evidence-based research shows that analyzing your LDL particle size does not actually add much value to your basic lipid panel. Here are a few things that are extremely important to understand:

1. All LDL particles increase your risk for heart disease, regardless of whether they are small or large.
2. Large, buoyant LDL particles increase your risk for heart disease by approximately 31 percent.
3. Small, dense LDL particles increase your risk for heart disease by approximately 44 percent.
4. The most effective way to reduce your LDL cholesterol is by reducing your saturated fat intake, reducing or eliminating your cholesterol intake, and increasing your intake of carbohydrate-rich whole foods.

Any dietary habit that increases the number of LDL particles in your blood increases your risk for an acute coronary event, regardless of whether they are large or small LDL particles. And as it turns out, eating saturated fat abundantly raises your LDL cholesterol more than any other nutrient in your diet, including dietary cholesterol itself!

So if you're interested in reducing your total and LDL cholesterol to lower your risk for atherosclerosis and coronary artery disease, focus on reducing your intake of saturated fat to ensure the most dramatic and lasting effect. Making these lifestyle changes will not only reduce your heart disease risk in the long term but can begin reducing your LDL cholesterol within weeks.

## 3. Unsaturated Fatty Acids

Unsaturated fatty acids are the least harmful of the three fat types and offer significant protection against the development of insulin resistance when eaten in small quantities. In fact, a comprehensive review conducted on this topic suggests that substituting higher quality unsaturated fatty acids for lower quality saturated fatty acids and trans fatty acids dramatically improves your insulin sensitivity within weeks, in addition to reduced LDL cholesterol and reduced body fat.

Within the unsaturated fat family are two types of fatty acids: monounsaturated fatty acids (MUFAs) and polyunsaturated fatty acids (PUFAs). MUFAs are considered nonessential fatty acids because your body can synthesize them endogenously (translation: your body has the ability to make them in-house). PUFAs, on the other hand, are considered essential because your body cannot manufacture them. Even though they're both from the same family of fatty acids, PUFAs have a greater association with reduced diabetes risk than do MUFAs.

Evidence for this came from a 2011 paper published in the *American Journal of Clinical Nutrition*, which analyzed data from the Nurses' Health Study. Researchers discovered that higher PUFA intake correlated with less type 2 diabetes risk, but that higher MUFA intake did not. Similarly, an article in *Diabetes Care* from the Iowa Women's Health Study found that substituting PUFAs for saturated fatty acids significantly decreased type 2 diabetes risk. Researchers have also found that substituting foods rich in PUFAs for foods rich in saturated fatty acids improves your insulin sensitivity within as little as four to five weeks, without changing any other aspect of your diet. Studies also consistently show that replacing foods rich in saturated fats with those high in unsaturated fats is a simple and powerful way to lower your LDL cholesterol, raise your HDL cholesterol, and protect against sudden cardiac death.

An elegantly conducted meta-analysis involving more than 395 metabolic ward experiments found that replacing only 10 percent of your calories from saturated fat with equal amounts of polyunsaturated and monounsaturated fat can reduce your total cholesterol by approximately 25 mg/dL. This same collection of experiments showed that replacing 10 percent of your calories from saturated fat with carbohydrate-rich whole foods can reduce your total cholesterol by about 20 mg/dL and your LDL cholesterol by about 14 mg/dL. The beauty here is that small changes in your intake of saturated fat lead to large changes in your total and LDL cholesterol. The good news is that replacing saturated fat with carbohydrate-rich whole foods happens naturally when you follow the Mastering Diabetes Method, and is not something that you have to think about when constructing your meals the way we recommend.

While it may be tempting to start replacing foods high in saturated fat with foods high in unsaturated fat, please understand that *all* whole foods contain unsaturated fat, without exception. There is no single whole food that does not contain fat, even unusual suspects like bananas, carrots, lettuce, potatoes, and beans. If you base your diet around low-fat plant-based whole foods, then you will intake small amounts of fat from each whole food you eat, resulting in a larger total fat intake than you may suspect. Many people are surprised that foods like squash, quinoa, papaya, tomatoes, and celery contain any fat at all, but the truth is that they contain not only fat but primarily unsaturated fat, and they all contribute to helping you meet your daily essential fatty acid requirements.

Nuts and seeds (walnuts, almonds, cashews, hempseeds, chia seeds, flaxseeds) contain significant sources of unsaturated fat. They have a high nutrient density and are rich in protective phytochemical compounds, including lignans, sterols, antioxidants, fiber, polyphenols, minerals, and bioflavonoids. Even though you may be tempted to begin eating large amounts of nuts and seeds instead of meat and dairy products, we strongly encourage you to eat no more than 15 percent of your total calories in fat in order to maximize your insulin sensitivity. That means that we recommend eating small quantities of nuts, seeds, and other high-fat plants like avocados, coconuts, and olives in order to keep your total fat intake below this threshold. We will address this in much more detail later in the book, and will also show you which foods can act as an insurance policy to make sure you meet your essential fatty acid requirements every day.

# Take-Home Messages

The most important things to understand when it comes to dietary fat are:

- The most effective way to increase your insulin sensitivity through diet is to reduce your total fat intake to a maximum of 15 percent of total calories.
- The second most effective way to increase your insulin sensitivity is to replace foods that are rich in saturated fat and trans fat (including meat, poultry, fish, dairy, eggs, oils, and processed foods) with carbohydrate-rich whole foods that are low in saturated fat and trans fat.
- High-fat plants like nuts, seeds, avocados, coconuts, and olives are nutrient-dense foods rich in PUFAs, but will contribute to increasing insulin resistance if your total fat intake exceeds approximately 15 percent. Feel free to eat these foods, but be aware that a little bit goes a long way!
- All whole foods contain fat, even if they have a sweet flavor. To calculate your total fat consumption from whole foods, add up the total fat from each food you've eaten throughout the day using diet-logging software that we describe in chapter 8.

To view the 40+ scientific references cited in this chapter, please visit us online at www.masteringdiabetes.org/bookinfo.

# Chapter 5

# Contributing Culprits: Animal Foods

## From Meathead to Plant-Based: Marc

Marc Ramirez is not your typical vegan. He was raised in Texas "meat country" and spent the majority of his early life playing football, where a high-protein meat-based diet is not only the status quo, it's practically a requirement.

Throughout his childhood, Marc's mother struggled with type 2 diabetes. He watched as her health progressively declined, requiring larger doses of insulin and eventually a kidney transplant. Of his eight brothers and sisters, only one sister avoided developing type 2 diabetes, and in 2002, Marc himself was diagnosed the same year his brother died of pancreatic cancer and his mother died after struggling with diabetes complications for over 33 years. Marc expected to experience the same struggles as his mother and siblings—a lifetime of "managing" diabetes and its resulting complications, including cardiovascular disease, organ transplants, and limb amputations. But diabetes was not his only concern. He also struggled with erectile dysfunction, psoriasis, heartburn, insomnia, and obesity.

In December 2011, Marc and his wife were given a DVD of the documentary *Forks Over Knives* by his in-laws. From watching the movie, he learned about a physician named Neal Barnard, MD, who had many years of experience helping patients reverse prediabetes and type 2 diabetes using a low-fat plant-based whole-food diet. Marc immediately purchased Dr. Barnard's book, *Dr. Neal Barnard's Program for Reversing Diabetes,* read it cover to cover, and set out to try to reverse type 2 diabetes. He started eating the way Dr. Barnard described and has never looked back.

After two months, Marc eliminated insulin altogether as well as four oral medications. By the third month, Marc had lost a total of 50 pounds and no longer experienced heartburn, psoriasis, insomnia, or erectile dysfunction. What's interesting is that Marc realized that his "manly" meat-heavy diet was actually the cause of the sexual dysfunction he had been experiencing for years. Seven years later, Marc has maintained his weight loss of more than 50 pounds, is medication-free, and does not count calories or limit his portion sizes. At the age of 51, he is in the best shape of his life, both metabolically and physically, and has been so inspired by his health changes that he generously shares his experience with others. Marc has joined the Mastering Diabetes team as a coach, and he and his wife are both Food for Life Instructors, regularly educating people about the benefits of low-fat plant-based whole-food nutrition.

---

In the world of diabetes, there is significant debate about the effect of meat and dairy products on your risk for developing insulin resistance and diabetes. The prevailing wisdom is that eating carbohydrate-rich foods causes rapid insulin secretion, increases insulin resistance, and causes weight gain. As a result, many people turn to high-fat, high-protein foods such as meat and dairy with the explicit intent of reducing their carbohydrate intake.

While this may work in the short term to reduce the amount of insulin your pancreas secretes, it also causes a number of "hidden" cellular effects that target tissues all over your body, which end up causing significant long-term damage and increase your risk for premature death. In fact, there is a large body of compelling research that demonstrates how eating meat and dairy not only increases your risk for high blood glucose, insulin resistance, weight gain, increased fasting glucose, and increased fasting insulin concentrations, but also causes inflammation and promotes heart disease and hypertension over the course of time.

## What Large-Scale Studies Have to Say About It

Over the past thirty years, the research world has taken a great interest in understanding what dietary and lifestyle factors contribute to insulin resistance. We, of course, would never force you to read all of these studies—and make sense of them—so we've taken the liberty of doing it for you. We've highlighted the following studies not only because they were undertaken by reputable scientific groups but also because they are large scale and conducted over long periods of time, making them some of the most credible studies that the nutrition world has to offer. Thus you can begin to understand the long-term effects of specific foods on chronic disease risk and deviate from the "tunnel vision" approach of only paying attention to your blood glucose meter.

We understand that the studies below suggest a *correlation* between specific foods and your risk for chronic disease rather than a *causation*. The types of studies outlined below are large-scale research studies that required following large numbers of people over long periods of time. Studies designed this way are not designed to show cause and effect; they can only demonstrate associations and correlations. Despite this, these studies highlight the fact that there is an extremely strong association between increasing animal food intake and chronic disease risk, and that these associations are very consistent across many large-scale studies. In other words, when you see a correlation *this* strong, it's worth paying attention to.

- **EPIC study:** The EPIC (European Prospective Investigation into Cancer and Nutrition) study is one of the largest investigations ever performed to investigate the connection between nutrition and chronic disease, involving hundreds of researchers, more than

500,000 participants, and twelve years of data. What researchers discovered was very straightforward: Meat (especially processed meats like bacon, cold cuts, sausage, hot dogs, and hamburgers) increases your risk for type 2 diabetes, while eating a diet rich in fruits and vegetables reduces your diabetes risk. The EPIC study also revealed that replacing 5 percent of saturated fat with fructose (from fruits or refined sources) reduces your diabetes risk by 30 percent, and that replacing 5 percent of protein with fructose reduces your diabetes risk by 28 percent. Even though mainstream recommendations suggest that eating glucose and fructose (from fruits) will increase your risk for type 2 diabetes, after studying more than half a million people, EPIC researchers concluded that these monosaccharides actually *decrease* your risk for type 2 diabetes, especially when they are eaten as substitutes for saturated fat and protein-rich foods.

- **Adventist Health Studies:** Members of the Seventh-day Adventist Church follow a wide range of diets, including omnivores, pesco-vegetarians, semi-vegetarians, lacto-ovo-vegetarians, and vegans. An analysis of more than 8,000 people in this community over the course of seventeen years found extremely strong relationships between meat consumption and diabetes. In comparison with people who ate zero meat, people who ate meat as infrequently as once per week were 29 percent more likely to develop diabetes and those who ate salted or processed meats were 38 percent more likely to develop diabetes. Most important, those who ate a vegetarian diet in the long term were 74 percent less likely to develop diabetes, even when compared with those who ate meat only once per week.

- **Health Professionals Follow-Up Study:** In 2002, researchers analyzed data from more than 42,000 male subjects over twelve years and found that men who ate more total and saturated fat developed significantly more cases of type 2 diabetes. They found that men who ate processed meats (bacon, hot dogs, hamburgers, sausage, salami, and bologna) at least 5 times per week were

46 percent more likely to develop type 2 diabetes than those who ate meat once a month.

- **Nurses' Health Study:** To this day, this study is one of the largest and most comprehensive on meat and diabetes risk ever performed. In 2011, researchers from the Harvard T. H. Chan School of Public Health performed an analysis on data from more than 200,000 men and women taken over the course of nineteen years. Their results were tremendous. They found that both unprocessed and processed red meat consumption increased the risk of developing type 2 diabetes. Eating just one serving per day of unprocessed red meat increased diabetes risk by 12 percent and eating one serving per day of processed red meat increased diabetes risk by 32 percent.
- **Women's Health Study:** The Women's Health Study followed more than 37,000 women over 45 years old for 8.8 years and found that those who ate the most red meat were 28 percent more likely to develop diabetes, and those who ate the most total processed meat were at a 43 percent increased risk for diabetes.

Even though these studies do a great job of explaining the connection between red and processed meat and diabetes risk, chicken is often left out of the conversation. Recent data from Spanish researchers, observed in more than 18,000 people over the course of fourteen years, shows that eating three or more servings of either processed *or* unprocessed meat (including chicken) was associated with a significantly higher risk for the development of type 2 diabetes, and that switching from processed meat to unprocessed meat did not reduce diabetes risk.

The puzzle piece that connects each of these studies is simple: There is a consistent and strong positive association between all meat consumption and type 2 diabetes risk, regardless of the type or degree of processing. Most important, *every one of these studies found a positive association between meat consumption and diabetes risk*, removing significant doubt about the detrimental effect of eating any type of meat, whether red or white, processed or unprocessed. A meta-analysis published in 2013 provides a comprehensive summary of large-scale studies on the risk of developing type 2 diabetes from various types of meat, and the results are summarized in the table below.

| Type of Meat | Amount per Day (g) | Change | Relative Risk of Type 2 Diabetes |
|---|---|---|---|
| Poultry (chicken, duck, goose, turkey) | 100 grams | Increased Risk | 4-8% |
| All Red Meat (beef, pork, veal, horse, lamb, sausage, salami, bacon, and ham) | 100 grams | Increased Risk | 13-17% |
| Unprocessed Red Meat (beef, pork, veal, horse, and lamb) | 100 grams | Increased Risk | 15-19% |
| Processed Meat (sausage, salami, bacon, and ham) | 50 grams | Increased Risk | 13-57% |
| Total Meat (chicken, duck, goose, turkey, beef, pork, veal, horse, lamb, sausage, salami, bacon, and ham) | 100 grams | Increased Risk | 12-21% |

# Are Eggs Safe to Eat?

Over the past forty years, there has been significant debate about the safety of including eggs in your diet. In the 1970s, the public was told to reduce dietary cholesterol in order to reduce the risk of developing heart disease, and given that eggs are a highly concentrated source of dietary cholesterol, people were cautioned against consuming more than one egg per day. Later, the association between dietary cholesterol and heart disease was scrutinized, and research indicated that eggs were harmful only if you ate more than one per day. Now eggs are making a comeback as a "nutritious" food. So who is right?

In order to fully understand egg nutrition, you should ask yourself a simple question: *How do eggs affect my risk for long-term disease, including heart disease, diabetes, and cancer?* By understanding the metabolic effect of eating eggs, we gain insight into how eggs promote or reduce your risk for chronic disease. The Physicians' Health Study found that people with diabetes significantly elevate their risk for all-cause mortality after eating about five eggs per week, and two other studies involving more than 80,000 people found that eating more than six eggs per week significantly increases the risk of cardiovascular disease in people with diabetes.

In addition, recent studies have linked egg consumption with an increase in arterial plaque. Researchers found that three eggs per week significantly increased arterial plaque formation in carotid arteries, which in turn elevated the risk for hypertension, stroke, and heart attack. Studies have also shown that eating more than two and a half eggs per week increases the risk for the development of prostate cancer by more than 81 percent. A meta-analysis published in the *European Journal of Nutrition* containing more than forty-four studies performed in over 400,000 subjects found that the risk for gastrointestinal cancers increased linearly with increasing egg consumption. The authors found that the strongest correlation was between egg consumption and colon cancer, and that eating more than five eggs per week increased colon cancer risk by 42 percent. Eggs promote the development of cancer because they are high in both cholesterol and choline, both of which may promote tumor formation and tumor progression. Cholesterol is elevated in tumor cells in all tissues, and increasing blood cholesterol has been shown to promote tumor growth and metastases. Choline is also elevated in tumor cells and is metabolized in the large intestine into pro-inflammatory compounds that may promote cancer development.

Finally, findings from the 2008 Physicians' Health Study found that consumption of more than one egg per day resulted in a 23 percent increase in the risk of all-cause mortality, or death from any cause. Data from the Nurses' Health Study indicates that eating more than seven eggs per week doubled the risk of all-cause mortality in male subjects, and that eating more than seven eggs per week increased the risk for heart disease in males living with diabetes. So when it comes to eggs, we recommend reducing or eliminating them altogether, and instead eating nutrient-dense anti-inflammatory plant-based foods.

## What's Actually in the Animal Foods You Eat?

Given the above evidence, it's easy to point a finger at animal foods and think, "It's the saturated fat that makes them so dangerous," or "The animal protein is what causes insulin resistance." In truth, unprocessed meat products, processed meat products, cooked meat, and dairy products contain many metabolites that have documented negative effects on your metabolic health, including trans fat, saturated fat, leucine, heme iron, sodium, nitrites, and advanced glycation end products (AGEs). Understanding the effect of each of these nutrients on your risk for all forms of diabetes is well worth discussion, as it will give you a clearer idea of why we recommend steering clear of these foods as much as possible.

### Leucine

Meat and dairy products contain high amounts of leucine, an amino acid that activates a high-energy biochemical pathway known as mTOR in your beta cells, muscle, liver, adipose tissue, and brain. Frequently eating meat and dairy products can overstimulate the mTOR pathway in these tissues, and when this happens, the tissues enter a prolonged high-energy state in which many biochemical pathways go awry. This includes (a) fatty acid accumulation in muscle and liver, (b) chronic liver glucose export, (c) increased insulin secretion, (d) increased beta cell reproduction, and (e) eventual beta cell suicide. Leucine promotes more insulin production than any other amino acid, and some scientists believe that increased leucine intake from both meat and dairy products stimulates beta cells to chronically overproduce insulin. To be fair, some plants also contain leucine, but per 100 grams of weight, the leucine content between commonly eaten animal and plant foods is dramatically different, suggesting that even modest amounts of animal products can put you at risk for excess leucine intake. Four ounces of beef contains 3,200 milligrams of leucine and a quarter cup of Gouda cheese contains 1,600; whereas 1 cup of corn contains 410, 1 cup of rice contains 430, and 1 cup of potatoes contains 250.

## Heme Iron

Iron is an essential mineral that plays key roles in critical biochemical pathways, including mitochondrial energy metabolism, oxygen transport, and the production and release of neurotransmitters, as well as the synthesis of DNA, collagen, and steroid hormones. Even though iron facilitates thousands of critical reactions in your body, ample research has uncovered the detrimental effects of *excess* iron in many tissues. It has been well established that iron is a potent pro-oxidant that not only is associated with insulin resistance but can actually *cause* insulin resistance by antagonizing multiple tissues. In beta cells, iron can induce oxidative stress that results in apoptosis (programmed cell death) and eventually insulin deficiency. In adipose and muscle tissue, excess iron dramatically reduces glucose uptake, trapping glucose in your blood and causing high blood glucose. In your liver, excess iron interferes with insulin signaling, leading to excess glucose production. The metabolic effects of iron in many tissues is very clear—iron itself is not dangerous; it's the intake and storage of *excess* iron that leads to biochemical complications that significantly increase your risk for type 2 diabetes.

Iron in food is found in two forms: heme iron and non-heme iron. Heme iron is found predominantly in animal foods including meat, poultry, and fish, whereas non-heme iron is found in plant foods including fruits, starchy vegetables, legumes, intact whole grains, non-starchy vegetables, leafy greens, nuts, and seeds. Interestingly, people who eat non-heme iron *do not* increase their risk for the development of beta cell death and insulin resistance, suggesting that both the *amount* and the *type* of iron are important indicators of your risk for elevated blood glucose. What's incredible is that even small amounts of heme iron have been shown to have a dramatic effect on type 2 diabetes risk. Studies involving more than 185,000 people showed that as little as 5 milligrams per day of dietary heme iron from animal foods can elevate type 2 diabetes risk by as much as *224 percent*, suggesting that even small amounts of animal products can significantly increase your risk for elevated blood glucose and whole-body inflammation.

## Nitrates and Nitrites

Nitrates are naturally occurring compounds found in certain vegetables. Nitrates and nitrites are compounds that are added to meat products because they act as antimicrobials and enhance the color and flavor of cured meats. In food as well as in your digestive system, nitrate is converted into nitrite by bacteria, and then further converted into a family of molecules known as N-nitroso compounds or nitrosamines. Nitrosamine compounds are known to be beta cell toxins that can directly trigger oxidative stress and beta cell death. Research has shown that consumption of foods with a high nitrite and nitrosamine content has been associated with the development of type 1 diabetes.

New research published in the *British Medical Journal* in 2018 investigated the effect of meat, heme iron, and added nitrates and nitrites in more than half a million people aged 50 to 71. Their findings indicated that the intake of nitrate and nitrite from processed meat increased the risk for all-cause mortality by 15 percent, and was associated with an increased risk for death from cancer, heart disease, respiratory diseases, stroke, diabetes, infections, kidney disease, and liver disease. The strongest associations were death from diabetes, respiratory diseases, and kidney disease.

It's important to keep one thing clear: Nitrate-rich vegetables like beets, spinach, arugula, and Swiss chard contain large amounts of nitrate compounds that stimulate the production of nitric oxide in your blood, reduce your blood pressure, and improve oxygen delivery to muscles. These nitrate compounds found in vegetables come prepackaged with a host of micronutrients, including vitamins, minerals, antioxidants, and phytochemicals thought to block the conversion of nitrate into nitrosamine compounds. A randomized control trial from 2003 revealed that heme iron found only in meat may actually accelerate the conversion of nitrate into nitrosamine compounds, but that non-heme iron found in plants did not. Given the strength of evidence implicating nitrosamine compounds with insulin resistance, coronary artery disease, and cancer, it's no surprise that reducing your intake of meat can dramatically improve your diabetes health and reduce your risk for premature death.

## Sodium

Sodium is another sneaky compound that is added to meat products to act as a preservative and flavor enhancer. If you've ever analyzed the ingredients in packaged foods, you may have seen sodium disguised as *sodium acetate, sodium ascorbate, sodium benzoate, sodium lactate, sodium nitrate, sodium nitrite, sodium phosphate, sodium propionate,* or *sodium sulfite.* These compounds are everywhere, and you can easily find them in salad dressings, canned foods, cheese, baked goods, jams, and jellies, as well as in cured and canned meats.

There is little debate that excess dietary sodium increases blood pressure, damages the inside of blood vessels (known as your endothelium), and promotes the hardening of blood vessels all around your body. A single pinch of salt can impair the flexibility of blood vessels by as much as 50 percent within one to two hours of eating a meal, and a quarter of a teaspoon of salt can block blood vessel dilation by as much as 75 percent. Because of this, it's important to minimize your intake of added sodium from salt and packaged foods, to protect yourself against cardiovascular complications down the road.

Processed meat contains on average four times the amount of sodium as unprocessed meat, and researchers have calculated that eating just one 50-gram serving of processed meat per day could increase your risk for cardiovascular disease by as much as 27 percent. In 2010, a large-scale study from researchers in Finland and the National Institutes of Health (NIH) examined the relationship between many compounds found in meat and the development of type 2 diabetes. Researchers from Finland analyzed the data of more than 24,000 people over the course of twelve years to determine which compounds were the most predictive of type 2 diabetes, and found that sodium was the strongest predictor of type 2 diabetes risk.

## Advanced Glycation End Products (AGEs)

Advanced glycation end products (AGEs) are a diverse collection of compounds that are created in your body and are also found in the food you eat. In your food, AGEs are formed when you cook at high temperatures and when you cook in low-moisture environments. Frying, broiling, grilling, and roasting increase AGE production in food, while boiling, poaching, stewing, and steaming limit AGE production substantially. In 2010, researchers at the Mount Sinai School of Medicine tested the AGE content of almost 550 foods at various temperatures to determine which foods posed the highest risk for many chronic diseases. They found that the foods with the highest AGE content were beef, cheese, poultry, pork, fish, and eggs, whereas the foods with the lowest AGE content were those that were highest in carbohydrate content, including grains, legumes, breads, vegetables, and fruits.

AGEs can also be formed in your body when sugar molecules combine with lipids or amino acids. AGEs form in a similar manner as glycated hemoglobin (the molecule that gets measured when you test your A1c level). Both AGEs and glycated hemoglobin form when a monosaccharide molecule attaches to a protein, forming a compound that can alter the function of critical biochemical pathways in many tissues. One of the reasons why it's important to control your blood glucose carefully is because the higher your glucose level, the more AGEs form and the higher your A1c value becomes.

People living with diabetes have higher levels of AGEs than nondiabetic individuals because of higher circulating glucose and oxidative stress. Studies have shown that this can be 20 to 30 percent higher in those with both type 1 diabetes and type 2 diabetes, and 40 to 100 percent higher in those who have both diabetes and coronary artery disease. In addition to causing or exacerbating type 2 diabetes, high AGE levels also promote atherosclerosis, neuropathy, inflammation, endothelial damage, and kidney disease. Therefore, limiting your exposure to dietary AGEs and controlling your blood glucose with precision are two extremely important things that you can do to help prevent diabetes complications.

# How Meat and Dairy Affect Your Risk for Autoimmune Diabetes

While the information we've covered so far primarily addresses the connection between eating meat and the risk for developing prediabetes and type 2 diabetes, it does not answer a simple question: *Do particular foods increase your risk for autoimmune (type 1 and type 1.5) diabetes?*

Given that type 1 diabetes has doubled in prevalence over the past twenty-five years, scientists are constantly on the lookout for environmental and genetic triggers that might help explain why the rate of type 1 diabetes diagnosis is higher today than it has been at any point in human history and why the prevalence of type 1 diabetes is increasing by about 3 percent per year.

Even though many people think of autoimmune conditions as being caused by poor genetics, a collection of fascinating research now shows that drinking milk and eating meat can both increase your risk for type 1 diabetes and type 1.5 diabetes—in addition to Crohn's disease—via a specific pathogen known as mycobacterium avium paratuberculosis (MAP). MAP is a mycobacterium, or a bacteria that grows like a fungus, and has been shown to influence susceptibility to autoimmune type 1 diabetes. In fact, the connection between MAP and type 1 diabetes is so strong that a recent review of current scientific literature showed that *100 percent* of human studies analyzed detected the presence of MAP bacteria in those living with type 1 diabetes.

So how does MAP enter our food supply? Well, it's a little . . . unsavory. MAP infects the gastrointestinal tract of industrialized cows (cows being raised for food or milk), causing an often fatal condition known as Johne's disease. While the MAP bacteria lives in the intestines of cows, it is also present in the fecal matter of infected cows, which means that the MAP bacteria can easily be passed between animals exposed to one another's fecal material—a common occurrence when hundreds or thousands of cows are living together in close quarters, as is common in large industrialized farms.

Under ideal conditions, MAP present in the intestines and fecal matter of livestock would pose no threat to human health, assuming that (a) their intestines were removed after slaughter and (b) their fecal matter remained separated from the slaughterhouse.

However, when animals are slaughtered, fecal residue from the soil ends up clinging to the boots, clothes, and gloves of slaughterhouse workers, which then cross-contaminates the carcasses of the animals, contaminating both the milk and the meat products en route to the grocery store. No matter how stringent the conditions are at industrial slaughterhouses, MAP migrates into dairy and meat products; avoiding this fecal contamination when animals are slaughtered is virtually impossible at large scale.

This means that MAP is present in milk and dairy products that you purchase at the grocery store, including raw milk, bulk milk, pasteurized milk, infant food formula, cheese, ice cream, and flavored milk drinks. A study published in 2007 revealed that more than 68 percent of all US dairy operations housed cows infected with MAP, and that more than 95 percent of farms containing more than 500 cows housed animals infected with MAP. Even though milk must be pasteurized (treated at high heat to kill off disease-causing bacteria) prior to being sold at the grocery store, a small fraction of live MAP bacteria can actually survive pasteurization. Approximately 3 out of every 100 milk products purchased in the United States contain living MAP bacteria, meaning that milk and milk products are a vehicle that transports infectious bacteria directly from cows to humans, increasing your risk for developing various autoimmune diseases, including type 1 diabetes.

MAP is also present in the meat you buy at the grocery store or butcher, including beef, pork, chicken, and organ tissues. Studies have shown that between 15 and 20 percent of commonly eaten meat products test positive for MAP DNA, and that ground beef presents the greatest risk for transporting MAP into the human food chain. A recent investigation in 298 children in Sardinia, Italy, found that those who ate more meat before the age of 2 years old developed significantly more cases of type 1 diabetes and that "high meat consumption tends to be an important early life cofactor for type 1 diabetes development." This same research team also showed that both milk consumption and meat intake are significantly correlated with the incidence of type 1 diabetes in children younger than 15 years old in forty countries around the world.

But how exactly does autoimmunity happen in the first place? The process is known as *molecular mimicry*, a sneaky tactic used by various bacteria and viruses in which pathogenic proteins attempt to evade detection by the human immune system by "disguising" themselves as mammalian proteins. In both young children and adults, microscopic holes in the lining of your gut wall allow pathogenic proteins to pass directly from your digestive system into your blood before they have been sufficiently cut by digestive enzymes. Once these pathogenic proteins are present in your blood, your immune system recognizes them as foreign proteins and mounts an immune response that targets them for destruction. But because these pathogenic proteins contain specific regions that mimic proteins found in your body, your immune system can mistakenly target proteins on human cells in tissues all over your body for destruction, setting the stage for an autoimmune reaction.

**Think of autoimmunity as a form of biological "friendly fire" in which your immune system is hijacked by a pathogenic protein that tricks your immune system into destroying critical human cells containing proteins with a similar structure.**

When infected with MAP, your immune system manufactures antibodies that mistakenly attack the ZnT8 protein on the surface of beta cells, targeting them for destruction. In order to target these proteins for destruction, your immune system activates the same macrophages that infiltrate your adipose tissue, causing a low-grade inflammation and insulin resistance. These macrophages engulf and destroy entire beta cells, leading to a near or complete loss of insulin production.

# How Protein from Animal Sources Affects Your Risk for Premature Death

A growing body of scientific evidence shows that diets low in carbohydrate energy actually increase your risk for all-cause mortality. While this may seem hard to believe at first, a collection of large-scale studies consistently show that plant and animal protein behave very differently in your body, affecting your risk for premature death in opposing ways. This fascinating research clearly illustrates that foods high in animal protein pose significantly more metabolic risk than foods high in plant protein, increasing your risk for chronic disease and early death.

One of the most impressive studies to demonstrate the detrimental effects of animal protein consumption was performed at the University of Southern California and published in *Cell Metabolism*. Researchers divided more than 6,000 adults into one of three groups—(a) low-protein (less than 10 percent of calories from protein); (b) moderate-protein (10 to 19 percent of calories from protein); or (c) high-protein (20 percent or more calories from protein)—and then studied their risk for death from cancer and diabetes over the course of eighteen years.

In participants aged 50 to 65 years old, people eating the most protein were 74 percent more likely to die from any cause and were more than four times as likely to die from cancer, as compared with those in the low-protein group. When the researchers separated those who ate animal-based protein from those who ate plant-based protein, they found that "high levels of animal proteins promote mortality and that plant-based proteins have a protective effect."

In people who did not have diabetes at the beginning of the study, those in the low-protein group had the lowest incidence of diabetes mortality; those in the moderate-protein group had a 23-fold increase in their risk for death from diabetes; and those in the high-protein group had a 73-fold increase in their risk for death from diabetes. These numbers indicate that there is a strong connection between the amount of animal protein you eat and your risk for death from diabetes, and that both moderate- and high-protein intake can substantially increase your risk of death.

## How Fish Increases Your Risk for Diabetes

In comparison with meat and dairy products, understanding the connection between fish intake and diabetes risk is more challenging, due to a high degree of variability among fish types, geographical differences in fish quality, different preparation methods, and varying levels of environmental contaminants.

Research involving more than 4,000 Dutch participants showed that eating more than 28 grams of fish per day significantly increased diabetes risk by 32 percent, with lean fish being more problematic than fatty fish, which admittedly seems counterintuitive. In contrast, a few meta-analyses published in 2012 and 2013 found no significant association between fish intake and type 2 diabetes risk—researchers found neither a positive nor negative correlation. All authors commented on a large degree of variability between studies, making it challenging to uncover consistent results. Another meta-analysis, published in 2018, that investigated how fish consumption influences type 2 diabetes risk in more than 250,000 people found that fish consumption was weakly correlated with type 2 diabetes risk, much less than has been observed with white meat, red meat, unprocessed meat, and processed meat.

So while a top-down view of the research may suggest that eating fish is less problematic than eating meat, the environmental pollutants present in many waterways around the world present another danger altogether. Toxic substances commonly found in fish include heavy metals, dioxin, PCBs (polychlorinated biphenyls), PBDEs (polybrominated diphenyl ethers), and pesticides. The most common heavy metal found in fish is mercury, which enters lakes and oceans mainly through industrial runoff from coal-fired power plants, and which with bacteria in the water is then converted into *methylmercury*. Elevated mercury levels are associated with a host of metabolic and neurologic conditions, including hypertension, cardiovascular disease, coronary artery dysfunction, and atherosclerosis, and studies in mice show that elevated blood mercury levels can directly interfere with beta cell function, contributing to beta cell death.

Dioxins and PCBs are two other environmental contaminants that are often found in high levels in marine and freshwater fish, and are by-products of burning waste, paper bleaching, pesticide production, and plastics manufacturing that persist in the environment for long periods of time. Dioxins are carcinogenic compounds that cause reproductive and developmental problems, damage your immune system, and interfere with hormonal signaling. PBDEs are a class of flame retardants whose presence is steadily increasing in marine mammals and fish. They are associated with thyroid hormone disruption, neurodevelopmental deficits, and cancer. Finally, pesticide residues normally considered to be present only in fruits and vegetables are steadily increasing in fish products, salmon being the most contaminated of all. Persistent ingestion of pesticide residue in humans leads to nervous system disorders, disrupted hormones and endocrine system functioning, and cancer.

Even though plant foods can also be contaminated with organic pollutants, the reason why fish consistently tests higher for mercury, dioxins, PCBs, PBDEs, and many organic pesticides is because of a process known as bioaccumulation. These *persistent organic pollutants* (POPs) enter waterways aided by rain, and many of them settle to the bottom of lakes, rivers, and ocean floors along with other sediment. Small fish ingest these compounds while bottom feeding. Larger fish eat those bottom-feeders, ingesting not only the flesh but also the contaminants within the flesh. Larger fish then eat those fish, and the process continues all the way up the food chain. The problem is that these POPs accumulate in the muscle and fat of fish at every level in the food chain and become more concentrated in fish at the top of the food chain as the pollutants bioaccumulate from one level to the next.

For this very reason, farmed fish often contains more POPs than wild-caught fish. A study published in 2005 in the journal *Science* analyzed over two metric tons of farmed and wild salmon from around the world and found that concentrations of DDT (a banned pesticide), PCBs, and dioxins in farmed salmon were significantly higher than their wild-caught counterparts.

Eating fish can certainly provide you with the beneficial omega-3 essential fatty acids EPA and DHA. However, given the problems mentioned above, we will show you another way to optimize your omega-3s using freshly ground chia seeds and/or flaxseeds. Our recommendation is to minimize or completely eliminate your fish intake altogether to limit your intake of environmental pollutants and maximize your total body health while preserving your insulin sensitivity. Given the status of today's environment and the strength of the scientific evidence, the metabolic risks of eating fish seem to exceed the benefits, especially when you can obtain the essential nutrients from low-fat plant-based whole foods instead.

## Take-Home Messages

- All meat products (including chicken) increase your level of insulin resistance and therefore raise your risk for prediabetes and type 2 diabetes, while complicating your blood glucose control in type 1 and type 1.5 diabetes.
- Eggs increase the risk of cardiovascular disease and all-cause mortality in people with diabetes.
- Leucine, heme iron, nitrates and nitrites, sodium, and AGEs present in meat contribute to the development of insulin resistance and increase your risk for chronic disease.
- MAP in meat and dairy products is strongly suspected to play a causative role in the development of autoimmunity in type 1 diabetes.
- Persistent organic pollutants like mercury, dioxins, PCBs, PBDEs, and organic pesticides in fish significantly raise your risk for diabetes and other chronic diseases.

To view the 130+ scientific references cited in this chapter, please visit us online at www.masteringdiabetes.org/bookinfo.

# Chapter 6

# Your Carbohydrate Master Class

## Low-Carb Rehab: Jessica

Since the time she was diagnosed with type 1 diabetes at the age of 3, Jessica had worked hard to follow a strict low-carbohydrate diet in order to control her blood glucose to the best of her ability, as commonly recommended for people living with type 1 diabetes. However, she found that no matter how few carbohydrate-rich foods she ate, her blood glucose was quite unpredictable, to say the least. No matter how diligently she ate a low-carbohydrate diet, whenever she checked her blood glucose—either before or after a meal—she often saw values in the high 200s or low 300s. As a result, she began injecting more insulin to bring her blood glucose down.

In order for Jessica to cope with increasing insulin requirements, her doctor recommended starting 1,000 mg of metformin on a daily basis in addition to basal and bolus insulin. Jessica found her doctor's advice quite strange, given that metformin is prescribed for people with prediabetes and type 2 diabetes. Despite this, she followed her doctor's advice, desperate for any solution that would help improve her diabetes health. In a short period of time, Jessica began losing energy rapidly and found that staying awake became increasingly difficult during the day. Exercise was almost entirely out of the question, because she simply couldn't muster up enough energy. She knew something was terribly wrong, but she didn't know what to do to improve her health, her blood glucose control, and her energy levels. For a woman in her early twenties, this situation was quite overwhelming.

While perusing the internet, Jessica stumbled across our website and was extremely intrigued by the prospect of improving her insulin sensitivity. This was the first time she'd observed anyone recommending eating fruit for people with type 1 diabetes. She became very curious as to why our recommendations went against the mainstream. She found our evidence-based approach to nutrition intriguing and decided to enroll in our coaching program. In the first three weeks, Jessica significantly increased her intake of fruits and vegetables while reducing her intake of animal products. She gradually went from eating about 20 grams of carbohydrates a day to 325 grams per day. Initially, she was nervous that eating carbohydrate-rich foods would dramatically increase her insulin use, but despite that, she began the program with an open mind, hopeful to experience positive change. In the first thirty days, she found that her blood glucose had become significantly more predictable, and in an effort to avoid hypoglycemia, she stopped using metformin altogether.

But the most surprising effect was how quickly her basal and bolus insulin requirements fell. **After all, she was eating fifteen times more carbohydrate energy than she had in the previous twenty years, yet her insulin use was decreasing quickly!** On a low-carbohydrate diet, she averaged 20 units of basal insulin and 17.5 units of bolus insulin per day, for a total of about 37.5 units of total insulin per day. When she was eating only 20 grams of dietary carbohydrate per day, her 24-hour baseline insulin sensitivity had been approximately 0.5 grams/unit. By the end of her first three months in the Mastering Diabetes Coaching Program, her basal insulin requirements had fallen to 14 units per day and her bolus insulin requirements had fallen to about 15 units per day, for a total of approximately 29 units of total insulin per day. At 325 grams of carbohydrate per day, her 24-hour insulin sensitivity was now more than 11 grams/unit, 21 times higher than when she began. And at the six-month mark, she had lost 15 pounds; her basal insulin requirements had fallen to 11 units per day and her bolus insulin requirements had fallen to approximately 14 units per day, for a total of 25 units of total insulin per day. Today she feels better than she has ever felt and has more energy than she could have ever expected—thanks to the power of the Mastering Diabetes Method.

---

Since the Atkins diet first gained popularity in the early 2000s, carbohydrates have been blamed for a host of metabolic disorders including diabetes, obesity, heart disease, cancer, and insulin resistance. The resulting anti-carbohydrate literature would lead you to believe that these issues could be solved only by eliminating carbohydrates from your diet. It's easy to believe these claims because they are always backed up by seemingly credible scientific research and communicated confidently. Because of this, low-carbohydrate diets have taken the world by storm, resulting in millions of people who actively avoid eating carbohydrate energy, whether from refined sources like bread, cereal, pasta, cookies, and crackers or from whole sources like fruits, starchy vegetables, legumes, and whole grains.

As a society, we have come to fear carbohydrates. The words *low-carb* and *no-carb* are printed prominently on food packaging everywhere you turn, further feeding the anti-carbohydrate frenzy and strengthening the stance against this alleged dietary criminal. Visit your nearby bookstore and you'll find entire sections containing books on the dangers of carbohydrates, with authors making wild claims that "there is no biological need for carbohydrates in your diet" and arguing that our Paleolithic ancestors lived for thousands of years on low-carbohydrate or no-carbohydrate diets.

Is any of this true? Are carbohydrates the cause of our generation's ailing health? Does eating carbohydrate-rich food cause weight gain, obesity, and diabetes? Are carbohydrates responsible for the epidemic of statin medication?

**If you spend time researching the scientific evidence with a fine-tooth comb, you'll find that blaming carbohydrates as the cause of insulin resistance and diabetes is short-sighted and lacks scientific rigor.**

But before we exonerate all carbohydrate-rich foods as "healthy," let's dive into the details of carbohydrate biology so that you can see that much like fatty acids, all carbohydrates are not created equal, and that subtle differences in the way carbohydrates exist in food can make a dramatic difference in your overall health. If you've ever wanted to learn more about what carbohydrates are and how they function in your body, this is your chance.

## Breaking Down Carbohydrates

As we discussed in chapter 2, carbohydrates are nothing more than chains of *monosaccharide* molecules. Most people don't use the word *monosaccharide* because it's cumbersome, and instead use the word *sugar*. Technically speaking, this is correct, but the word *sugar* has a completely different connotation in our modern world. *Sugar* is used to refer to a refined sweetener you buy at the grocery store that increases your risk for many chronic diseases. In an effort to clear up any confusion, we refer to natural sugars as *monosaccharides* and man-made sugars as *refined sugars*. Table sugar, otherwise known as sucrose, is a classic example of a refined sugar. Table sugar is the end product of a manufacturing process that began with a whole food like sugarcane or sugar beets and is a crystalline substance that contains only glucose and fructose. The manufacturing process stripped the original whole food of protective micronutrients, including vitamins, minerals, fiber, water, antioxidants, and phytochemicals, rendering the final product nutritionally useless.

Most likely, we aren't the first to tell you that sucrose, other refined sugars, and most artificial sweeteners can dramatically increase your disease risk. This has been the subject of many books, scientific articles, conferences, YouTube videos, and podcasts, and the message is very clear: *Refined sugars* accelerate weight gain, obesity, heart disease, atherosclerosis, high cholesterol, diabetes, and cancer.

Carbohydrates found in whole food exist in a three-dimensional matrix of many other nutrients and are extremely complex packets of information that your digestive system has the ability to interpret, unpackage, and distribute to other tissues in your body. All whole foods have a similar three-dimensional construction, but differ in the types and amounts of carbohydrate, fat, protein, vitamins, minerals, fiber, water, antioxidants, and phytochemicals inside. Fiber acts like rebar in concrete structures—it reinforces the structure of a whole food, and the rest of the nutrients are interspersed throughout the three-dimensional space. Macronutrients are what account for the calories in each food, and micronutrients offer disease protection and add nutrient density.

When you eat foods containing carbohydrates, these chains are broken down into their individual monosaccharide units by digestive enzymes known as *amylases*. Beginning in your mouth and continuing all the way to the small intestine, these enzymes act like scissors, cutting carbohydrate chains into smaller monosaccharide chains at every step of the process. Once inside your small intestine, single monosaccharide molecules are absorbed through the walls of your intestine and passed to capillary blood vessels, to be distributed all throughout your body. Think of your blood as a sophisticated highway system that nutrients use to travel to every tissue in your body.

A simple way to understand carbohydrates is to think of monosaccharides as letters and carbohydrates as words. In the English alphabet there are twenty-six letters that can be arranged to form millions of words. Words are formed by a specific sequence of letters, resulting in a vocabulary that we use to communicate thoughts and ideas with one another. In the carbohydrate world, there are more than twenty commonly occurring monosaccharides that can be combined in many ways to create a virtually endless array of carbohydrate chains of varying length. Short-chain carbohydrates are formed by combining between two and ten monosaccharide sugars, whereas long-chain carbohydrates are formed by combining hundreds to thousands.

Glucose and fructose are the most abundant monosaccharides found in plants. Glucose is found in both short-chain carbohydrates like *sucrose* (found in table sugar) and *lactose* (found in dairy products like milk and soft cheeses). When it comes to long-chain starchy carbohydrates like *amylose* and *amylopectin* (commonly found in potatoes, squash, beans, lentils, and intact whole grains), as well as *cellulose* (fiber), glucose is not only abundant, it is the only monosaccharide building block.

The difference between the structure of starchy carbohydrates and that of fiber is the way in which the glucose molecules are linked together. Starchy carbohydrate molecules can be cut by your digestive enzymes; fiber cannot because humans don't make the required enzyme *cellulase*. But that's okay, because trillions of bacteria in your microbiome can fully metabolize fiber and use it for energy to help them replicate and colonize the inside lining of your large intestine.

## What Are Refined Carbohydrates?

At some point, you have most likely been advised to reduce or completely eliminate refined products in your diet to lose weight, improve your mood, strengthen your immune system, or sleep better. It's very important to understand what the term *refined* means so that you can objectively decide whether to eat or pass on a given food. Lucky for you, when it comes to carbohydrates, the term *refined* is quite straightforward. Let's dive into detail to understand a bit more about the manufacturing process of carbohydrates.

### Refined Sweeteners

Refined sweeteners like sucrose, high-fructose corn syrup (HFCS), and dextrose result from a manufacturing process in which a whole fruit, vegetable, or grain is subjected to a combination of steps involving cutting, milling, cracking, grinding, washing, extracting, boiling, steaming, condensing, and drying. The final product is a solid crystal, powder, flour, or syrup that is then either sold as is or added to products such as cereals, pastries, sodas, sauces, condiments, crackers, pastas, breads, and dressings to make them appealing to customers.

Food manufacturers spend millions of dollars developing inexpensive methods to refine whole carbohydrates into sweeteners, flours, texturizers, and flavors. Sweeteners are added to an otherwise bland food; texturizers are used to create specific consistencies for chips, crackers, sauces, and glazes; flours are sold as flour or added to baked goods; and flavors are added in measured proportions and often disguised with the word *natural*. The end result of adding refined carbohydrates to packaged food products is a pleasurable eating experience, which in turn creates a subconscious addiction that lures you back to the store to buy more.

Often food manufacturers sneak refined sweeteners into processed foods and disguise their names, while trying to convince consumers they are "healthy," "low-carb," or "zero-calorie" alternatives. While it may seem overwhelming that a majority of the foods in the grocery store contain refined ingredients, understanding how to differentiate between whole carbohydrates and refined carbohydrates will provide you with insight that will set you apart from the average uninformed shopper.

Refined sweeteners can be made in a laboratory from artificial ingredients or made from natural sources. Examples of laboratory-made refined sweeteners include aspartame, Equal, Splenda, and Sweet'N Low. Examples of natural foods that have been turned into refined sweeteners include stevia (from the leaves of a stevia plant) and agave (from the aguamiel plant). Stevia is often refined into a powder or liquid sweetener, and agave is often refined into agave nectar. Refined sweeteners made from artificial ingredients and from natural foods are added to many packaged items in the grocery store, and some of them are specifically marketed as "diabetic-friendly" options because they are "sugar free" or because they contain few or no calories. Regardless of whether a refined sweetener is made from artificial ingredients or from natural sources, we encourage you to minimize or eliminate them altogether.

We recommend staying clear of refined sweeteners because they can make your blood glucose extremely difficult to control. In addition, refined sweeteners can overstimulate your taste buds, which in turn programs neurological signals in your brain to expect unnaturally sweet flavors when you eat. In effect, refined sweeteners numb your taste buds to the flavors present in natural whole foods, making whole foods seem less appetizing. In addition, refined sweeteners are nutritionally *void*, and do not contain valuable and protective micronutrients that we will talk about in the remainder of this chapter.

## Refined Grains

Intact whole grains are often refined into flours and added to pastas, baked goods, snack foods, pastries, cereals, and breads. Refined grains are what most people think of when they hear the word *carb,* even though they represent only a small subset of carbohydrate-rich foods.

The difference between intact whole grains and refined grains is simple. Intact whole grains keep their outside bran and germ intact, whereas refined grains are stripped of both, leaving you with just the inside endosperm. Food manufacturers remove the bran and germ in intact whole grains in order to prolong their shelf life. Refined grains are just the starchy inside, containing significantly less fiber and fewer antioxidants, vitamins, minerals, and protective phytochemicals than their intact whole-grain counterparts. These components not only aid in optimal nutrient absorption and transport but are *essential* for it.

The problem is that food-labeling laws do not regulate the use of the words *whole grain.* Food manufacturers can label a food as "whole grain" even though the food contains as little as 15 percent whole grain and as much as 85 percent refined grains. Marketing phrases like "whole grain," "multigrain," "stone-ground," "100% wheat," "cracked wheat," "seven grain," or "bran" are terms used to lure you into a purchase.

Refined grains and products made from flour are metabolized and absorbed very quickly, resulting in a large rush of glucose into your blood in a short period of time. If you've ever experienced a high blood glucose within a few hours of eating a product containing refined grains, that's likely because the flour used to make the food absorbed into your blood extremely quickly, overpowering the ability of your liver and pancreas to control your blood glucose. Simply switching to a true intact whole grain product not made from flour can dramatically improve your blood glucose control in the hours following your meal.

The net result of a single meal containing refined carbohydrates is a cascade of adverse effects to your liver, blood vessels, heart, adipose tissue, and muscle. The consumption of refined carbohydrates is very effective at causing liver insulin resistance, fatty liver, increased LDL cholesterol, increased triglycerides, increased adipose tissue fat, and increased muscle fat. The combination of these factors creates insulin resistance mainly in your liver but also in your muscle, and significantly increases your risk for heart disease.

Refined carbohydrate-rich foods are also processed differently by your digestive system than whole carbohydrate-rich foods, which in turn affects the health of many tissues. The reason for this is simple: Whole foods are broken down less efficiently by your digestive system than are products made with flour. But don't worry, that's actually a good thing because you benefit from eating foods with a high nutrient density and your gut bacteria benefit from the fiber-rich core. When you eat your food in a processed state, your bacteria don't get as many nutrients, they don't multiply as rapidly, and they don't bulk your stool nearly as much as when you eat the same foods in their unprocessed whole state. Given that the majority of your stool is composed of pure bacteria, the more food you eat in its whole state, the happier your bacteria become, the more immune-boosting short-chain fatty acids they produce, the more they multiply and colonize your gut, and the more regularly they are replaced by new bacteria.

## What Are Whole Carbohydrates?

In sharp contrast to foods containing refined carbohydrates, whole carbohydrate-rich foods are made up of long-chain molecules and are found mainly in plant foods like fruits, vegetables, beans, lentils, and peas and in whole grains like brown rice, buckwheat, millet, and barley. The carbohydrate chains in whole foods come prepackaged with micronutrients including vitamins, minerals, fiber, water, antioxidants, and phytochemicals, and these vital behind-the-scenes players play an incredibly important role in directing how nutrients are utilized in tissues all over your body.

Carbohydrate-rich whole foods are some of the most nutrient-dense on the planet, providing you with lasting energy, as well as high-quality micronutrients that refined carbohydrate foods do not. Micronutrients present in whole foods are potent and highly bioactive compounds that reduce inflammation, boost immune function, help digested food material move through your digestive tract, help blood to clot at the site of an injury, and improve the function of your brain, sexual organs, eyes, and heart—and that's only scratching the surface. Think of micronutrients as "information" that cells require to perform thousands of chemical reactions at every moment of every day, allowing them to work around the clock to optimize tissue function and slow the rate of aging.

**In the same way that blueprints contain the information necessary to build a house, micronutrients provide the *information* that tissues use to digest, absorb, transport, uptake, and oxidize nutrients from the food you eat. And carbohydrate-rich foods are the most micronutrient-dense foods on the planet.**

There are many classes of micronutrients, and each has a specific function. They include vitamins, minerals, fiber, water, antioxidants, and phytochemicals. Let's zoom into each micronutrient class to understand more about why they're so beneficial for optimal cellular function.

### Vitamins

Vitamins are essential compounds that assist in thousands of biochemical reactions in tissues all throughout your body. There are thirteen known vitamins, and they are classified into two groups: fat-soluble vitamins and water-soluble vitamins. Fat-soluble vitamins A, E, and K are widely available in fruits, starchy vegetables, legumes, intact whole grains, non-starchy vegetables, and leafy greens. Vitamin D is generated by exposing your skin to the sun, and we cover this in more detail in chapter 8.

Water-soluble vitamins are present in fruits, starchy vegetables, legumes, intact whole grains, non-starchy vegetables, and leafy greens. These include the B vitamins as well as vitamin C, which have a diverse collection of functions in many tissues in your body. Because vitamins B and C are water-soluble, they are easily secreted in your urine and therefore need to be replaced more often from your diet.

All vitamins have a diverse collection of functions that are vital to optimal cellular function. Vitamins are required for thousands of metabolic reactions, including (but not limited to) DNA synthesis and repair, protein synthesis and repair, RNA synthesis and repair, glycogen synthesis, fatty acid synthesis, hormone synthesis, and neurotransmitter synthesis. By eating the foods that we recommend in the Mastering Diabetes Method, you maximize your chances of meeting (and exceeding) your fat- and water-soluble vitamin requirements (vitamin $B_{12}$ is the exception to this rule, and we'll cover that in chapter 8).

## Minerals

Minerals are essential nutrients that originate from the earth and cannot be made by living organisms. In humans, the major minerals we require include calcium, potassium, sodium, phosphorous, and magnesium, and the trace minerals iron, sulfur, molybdenum, chlorine, copper, zinc, manganese, cobalt, iodine, and selenium. All of these minerals play vital functions in your body. In the same way that vitamins assist in a wide variety of biological processes, minerals also have a diverse collection of functions including (but not limited to) maintaining electrolyte balance in your blood; synthesizing digestive enzymes; maintaining a regular heartbeat; producing ATP; transporting oxygen throughout your body; building bones and teeth; and promoting fetal development, hair growth, thyroid hormone synthesis, DNA synthesis and repair, and antioxidant enzyme activity. Every tissue in your body requires minerals to support its biological orchestra, and plants contain more minerals than any other food group.

## Fiber

Fiber is one of the most interesting nutrients in food, and our understanding of how fiber behaves in your digestive tract is an ever-evolving process that is intricately connected to the health of your microbiome. Scientists used to believe that fiber merely helped sweep undigested food material and excess cholesterol into the toilet, promoting normal digestive function and helping to protect you against heart disease, hypertension, and certain types of cancer. However, we now know that fiber is actually food—not for you, but for the microbiome housed in your large intestine.

Your body is home to approximately 38 trillion bacteria, and the majority of those bacteria live in your large intestine and on your skin, but other bacterial populations exist in your mouth, your small intestine, and your stomach. The most recent estimates suggest that your body is composed of about 45 percent human cells and 55 percent bacterial cells, and these bacteria exist in a friendly symbiotic relationship with human cells. Maintaining excellent gut health is critical for maintaining total body metabolic health, and a dysregulated gut microflora has been linked with many chronic diseases, including autism, depression, Hashimoto's thyroiditis, inflammatory bowel disease, and type 1 diabetes.

Carbohydrate-rich whole foods contain ample fiber, which provides digestible material for your microbiome. When bacteria in your large intestine metabolize fiber for energy, they make compounds known as short-chain fatty acids that have broad anti-inflammatory effects, help boost immune function, and minimize your risk for chronic disease. Some research shows that short-chain fatty acids can even prevent macrophages from entering your adipose tissue and creating an insulin-resistant state, as we discussed in chapter 3.

Fiber also helps slow the rate of glucose absorption into your blood, which is great news for you because it protects you against large blood glucose elevations when you are eating foods rich in carbohydrate energy. In addition, fiber helps bulk your stool, which is tremendously helpful in moving undigested food material through your large intestine to keep you going to the bathroom regularly. That being said, fiber supplements do not behave the same way as fiber-rich foods. Studies have shown that the addition of fiber powder (like Metamucil or psyllium husk) to a poor diet does not protect against colon cancer, but that diets high in fiber-rich foods do.

## Water

Many people would call us crazy for labeling water as a micronutrient. The reason we do so is because much like vitamins and minerals, water assists in thousands of chemical reactions in your blood and in your tissues, and is an underappreciated component of whole foods that rarely gets mentioned. Every second of every day, thousands of chemical reactions are taking place in your body simultaneously, and water is an essential participant that enables them to be carried out efficiently.

Water helps in many aspects of nutrient digestion and absorption. In your stomach, water helps facilitate the digestion and unfolding of intact food material. In your small intestine, water helps facilitate the continued digestion and absorption of food material, and plays a significant role in the absorption of glucose, fatty acids, and amino acids into your blood. In your large intestine, water plays a vital role in bulking your stool, feeding your microbiome, and helping to regulate the electrolyte balance in your blood. Water is an essential nutrient required for optimal nutrient digestion, absorption, transport, and oxidation.

Refined and processed foods are significantly lower in their water content than whole foods. For example, cornflakes contain 4 percent of water by mass and a typical whole-wheat bagel is 34 percent water by mass. On the other hand, whole foods generally contain between 60 and 95 percent water by mass. This means that when you eat plants, you actually *eat* water, which helps keep you hydrated, improves both mental and physical performance, and may reduce the amount of water you need to drink in order to stay fully hydrated. Take a look at the table below to see the water content of a collection of fruits, starchy vegetables, legumes, intact whole grains, non-starchy vegetables, and leafy greens.

| Food Name | Water Content (%) |
| --- | --- |
| Raw zucchini | 95 |
| Raw green leaf lettuce | 95 |
| Raw white mushrooms | 92 |
| Raw arugula | 92 |
| Raw spinach | 92 |
| Raw watermelons | 91 |
| Boiled collard greens | 90 |
| Raw peaches | 89 |
| Baked butternut squash | 88 |
| Boiled beets | 87 |
| Raw mangoes | 83 |
| Raw grapes | 81 |
| Raw figs | 79 |

| Food Name | Water Content (%) |
|---|---|
| Cooked green peas | 78 |
| Cooked buckwheat groats | 76 |
| Raw bananas | 75 |
| Baked potato | 74 |
| Cooked brown rice | 73 |
| Boiled corn | 73 |
| Boiled yam | 70 |
| Boiled lentils | 70 |
| Boiled chickpeas | 60 |

**Antioxidants**

Antioxidants are compounds found in brightly colored plant foods (and in animal foods to a much smaller extent). They neutralize *free radicals* in your blood and tissues and protect you against inflammation. Free radicals are unstable molecules that are generated by a wide range of experiences, both harmful and beneficial, including breathing, eating, exercising, stress, alcohol consumption, ultraviolet radiation, and exposure to environmental chemicals. Free radicals are created when a molecule loses an electron, resulting in a highly unstable compound that bombards neighboring molecules in search of stability. In the hunt for stability, free radicals bombard DNA, proteins, and lipids, and are capable of causing extensive cellular damage.

Even though free radicals are generated every second of every day just by living, tissues also possess the ability to repair free radical damage by using antioxidants found in whole food. Antioxidants are electron donors that hand out electrons to "quench" dangerous free radicals that are in search of electrons. Antioxidants are invaluable nutrients that assist in the repair of damaged mitochondria, cell membranes, and DNA, and dramatically extend the lives of cells in all tissues. Antioxidant compounds are excellent at reducing oxidative stress in inflamed cells.

Plants contain the highest concentration of antioxidants of any type of food, and this is one of many reasons why health experts agree that eating more fruits and vegetables reduces inflammation and protects against chronic disease. Just how antioxidant rich are plant-based whole foods?

**Plant foods contain on average 64 times more antioxidant content than animal foods.**

In general, the antioxidant content of plant foods trumps that of animal foods. You can actually see the distinction because antioxidants are pigments that are easily recognizable as bright colors in fruits and vegetables. At some point in your life you may have been told to *eat the rainbow,* which is actually excellent advice, because it ensures that you get a wide variety of highly potent and biologically active antioxidants every time you eat.

### Phytochemicals

The final class of micronutrients are called phytochemicals, which are an extremely diverse collection of compounds found only in plants that have an extensive portfolio of biological activities. Plants manufacture phytochemicals to grow and to protect themselves against competitors, pathogens, and predators. Phytochemicals are absolute biological powerhouses that inhibit tumor growth, prevent platelet aggregation and blood clots, relax blood vessels, improve insulin sensitivity, stimulate insulin production, improve neurological activity, fight against harmful bacteria, reduce cholesterol, and improve immune function. There are many classes of phytochemical compounds, and some of these subgroups include carotenoids, which are usually found in yellow, orange, and red fruits and vegetables; alkaloids, which are found in nightshade vegetables; organosulfur compounds, which are found in onions and garlic; and phenolic compounds, which are found in berries, tea leaves, and cacao.

Diets rich in phytochemicals are associated with reduced risk of cardiovascular disease, cancer, stroke, and diabetes, and an increase in bone mineral density and brain function in elderly patients. In fact, ample research shows that diets rich in phytochemicals reduce the risk of prenature death. The good news is that rather than searching for specific foods with high phytochemical content, eating a wide variety of carbohydrate-rich whole foods will provide you with a diverse collection of phytochemicals that can improve the health of many organ systems simultaneously. In contrast to a diet containing predominantly animal foods with low phytochemical content, a low-fat plant-based whole-food diet is the most phytochemical-rich option at your disposal.

When you eat carbohydrate-rich whole foods, you naturally ingest vitamins, minerals, fiber, water, antioxidants, and a wide variety of phytochemicals without trying. Now that you have an understanding of how these foods provide a broad range of health benefits to all tissues, let's understand how the carbohydrate energy from these nutrient-dense foods is metabolized in your body in a step-by-step manner.

## Step 1: Your Liver Absorbs Glucose Slowly

Foods containing intact whole carbohydrate chains require considerably more time to break down into single monosaccharide units than do foods containing refined carbohydrates, and this limits the rate and amount of glucose that your liver is exposed to during and after a meal. The presence of fiber molecules—which remain fully or partially intact in the absence of a refining process—slows down the digestive process altogether, resulting in a delayed rise in blood glucose following your meal. Ample large-scale research studies show that simply increasing your intake of intact fiber from whole foods can dramatically reduce the frequency and magnitude of high blood glucose following a meal and reduces your risk for insulin resistance, type 2 diabetes, and cardiovascular disease. Controlling the rate at which your liver is exposed to glucose following a meal by choosing slower-digesting carbohydrate-rich whole foods can dramatically improve the health of your liver, blood vessels, muscle, and adipose tissue while decreasing your level of insulin resistance.

In contrast, foods containing refined carbohydrates and refined sweeteners may lead to large increases in glucose in your blood immediately following a meal. When your liver is exposed to large concentrations of glucose in a short period of time, your brain responds by increasing your total energy expenditure to "waste" excess calories.

Plagued by a rapid and large influx of glucose, your liver does its best to absorb as much glucose as possible to protect other tissues from experiencing the same thing, and your muscles and liver slow the rate at which they burn fatty acids. In effect, multiple organs communicate with one another and say, "Help! Let's all do our part to get rid of this excess glucose as efficiently as possible. Liver—you absorb as much as you can. Brain—increase energy output. Muscles and liver—temporarily reduce your dependence on fatty acids and use this glucose as fuel."

In an effort to dispose of this excess glucose, your liver seeks alternative biochemical pathways, too. One of those pathways results in the conversion of glucose to fat, known as *de novo lipogenesis (DNL)*. De novo lipogenesis is a very well studied (and unnecessarily controversial) phenomenon in animals and humans and occurs to a small extent either when you increase your intake of refined carbohydrate foods or when you massively overeat calories. In reality, DNL occurs to a very small extent in humans and is a biologically expensive process that is considered a "pathway of last resort" when no other options exist. A thought-provoking paper published in the *American Journal of Clinical Nutrition*, written by one of the world's experts on DNL, explains that the process of converting carbohydrate to fat in humans is an extremely inefficient process and generally occurs for about 1 to 2 percent of all the carbohydrate energy you eat.

**Many low-carbohydrate nutrition experts** claim that your liver converts large amounts of carbohydrate energy into fat every time you eat carbohydrate-rich foods and therefore suggest that you avoid eating carbohydrate-rich foods to prevent this unwanted carbohydrate-to-fat conversion. Even though this may sound plausible, the truth is that DNL is an active pathway in pigs, rats, mice, cows, dogs, cats, and birds and a largely inactive pathway in humans. Extremely rigorous scientific experiments using state-of-the-art methods (stable isotope tracers) consistently demonstrate that *DNL does not occur in humans nearly as much as scientists once believed.* Using extremely sophisticated mass spectrometers and the most rigorous analytical techniques, Dr. Marc Hellerstein (one of the world's foremost authorities on DNL) and colleagues at the University of California at Berkeley have conclusively demonstrated the following:

- **High-Fat Diet:** In people who eat a high-fat, low-carbohydrate diet containing between 100 and 200 grams of fat per day, less than 1 gram of newly synthesized fatty acids is made from DNL per day.

- **Low-Fat Diet:** In people who eat a high-carbohydrate diet containing between 65 and 75 percent carbohydrate and 10 to 20 percent fat per day, DNL accounted for less than 10 grams of newly synthesized fatty acids per day.
- **Massive Overfeeding:** Experiments have shown that DNL occurs in substantial quantities only in people who massively overeat carbohydrate energy. Experiments show that people who eat approximately 2,000 grams of carbohydrate energy per day (4,500 calories of excess energy) for 7 to 10 days at a time manufacture about 150 grams of newly synthesized fatty acids from DNL per day.

But what about in the setting of insulin resistance—does eating carbohydrate-rich foods increase DNL? While it is true that excess insulin can certainly stimulate DNL, a study performed in insulin-resistant obese men demonstrated that the amount of newly synthesized fatty acids is so small that it does not account for even a minor part of excess body fat present in obesity. In other words, even in the insulin-resistant state when DNL rates are increased, the amount of newly synthesized fatty acids created from DNL in response to eating carbohydrate-rich foods is so small that it is biologically irrelevant.

What these experiments demonstrate is critically important—when you eat carbohydrate-rich foods, your liver does *not* convert carbohydrate into fatty acids in substantial quantities unless you massively overeat carbohydrate energy to the tune of 2,000 grams per day (or 4,500 excess calories per day) for a minimum of 7 to 10 days at a time!

**The next time you hear someone tell you to avoid carbohydrates in food because "carbs turn into fat," recognize that this statement is a gross overexaggeration of the truth, is biologically inaccurate, and demonstrates a fundamental lack of understanding of human biochemistry and human bioenergetics.**

## Step 2: Your Liver Burns Glucose

When you eat whole carbohydrate-rich foods, glucose enters your liver at a physiologically acceptable rate, slowed mainly by the presence of intact fiber molecules. As soon as glucose enters your liver, cells in your liver choose to either burn glucose for energy or store it for later use as glycogen. Glucose that is burned for energy immediately is sent through a series of complex reactions that eventually creates ATP, the cellular equivalent of energy.

A simple way to understand ATP is to think of it as the biological equivalent of money. Money is used to purchase items, pay for services, conduct trade, and power economies. In the same way, ATP is used in biological systems to power chemical reactions, allow pathways to function, manufacture hormones, stimulate muscle contraction, generate electrical impulses in nerves, and much, much more.

Think of your liver as metabolic command central—a supercomputer that oversees thousands of chemical reactions every second of your life. Given that your liver is involved in a wider range of metabolic activities than any other tissue in your body, cells in your liver have a high demand for ATP, which means they also have a high demand for vitamins, minerals, antioxidants, and phytochemicals. Whole carbohydrate-rich foods are an excellent source of glucose for ATP as well as a diverse collection of micronutrients to facilitate an organized and perpetual biochemical orchestra.

## Step 3: Your Liver Stores Glucose as Glycogen

The glucose that is stored for later use is stored as glycogen, a densely packed treelike structure containing thousands of glucose molecules. Think of liver glycogen as a glucose fuel tank that can be accessed whenever liver cells need it. Only your liver and muscle can store large quantities of glycogen, and the amount of glycogen stored in both tissues directly relates to the amount of carbohydrate in your diet. People who eat diets containing more carbohydrate energy increase the size of their liver and muscle glycogen stores over time, whereas people who eat diets low in carbohydrate energy have limited glycogen stores in both their liver and muscle.

The main reason your liver stores glycogen is to maintain a backup supply of glucose for your brain, because your brain is incapable of storing glucose for energy and requires a steady supply of glucose in order to function as designed. Your brain is unique in that it has an extremely strong preference for glucose as fuel, as evidenced by a high reliance on enzymatic machinery that is perfectly designed to extract ATP from glucose at all times. When you restrict the amount of carbohydrate energy in your diet, not only do you shrink the amount of glycogen in your liver and muscle but your brain is forced to adapt to a new fuel called *ketone bodies,* which your liver manufactures as an *emergency backup fuel* to maintain mental function. We'll cover ketone bodies in more detail in chapter 7 when we talk about the short- and long-term effects of ketogenic diets. For now it's important to understand that maintaining a large glycogen reserve in your liver is an excellent way to "drip feed" your brain with a stable supply of glucose twenty-four hours a day for optimal function.

In addition to feeding your brain, liver glycogen can be used to power itself during times of limited glucose availability—namely, when you're sleeping, when you're exercising, or when you're fasting. Think of liver glycogen as a protective glucose storage tank designed to provide glucose to tissues in need to cover a wide range of daily activities.

## Step 4: Your Muscles Store Glucose as Glycogen

When you eat a carbohydrate-rich diet, your liver absorbs some of the glucose that enters your blood, but also allows other tissues like your brain and muscle to uptake their own supply. In a given day, your brain will burn up to 60 percent of all the glucose in circulation because it is the largest consumer of glucose in your body and does not possess the ability to burn amino acids from protein or fatty acids from lipids.

Your muscles are the second largest consumer of glucose and will absorb 20 to 30 percent of the glucose in your blood with the help of insulin. Just like your liver, your muscle can either burn glucose immediately for ATP or store glucose as glycogen for later use. Some fraction of all the glucose your muscle absorbs will be burned for energy immediately and the remainder will be stored as glycogen for later use, during rest and while performing exercise, as you will learn about in chapter 14.

# Take-Home Messages

- All carbohydrate-rich foods do *not* cause insulin resistance—differentiating between the type of carbohydrate is essential in understanding a food's metabolic effect.
- Refined grains, refined sweeteners, and artificial sweeteners can overload your liver with excess glucose in a short period of time, causing a cascade of adverse metabolic reactions in many tissues.
- Carbohydrate-rich whole foods including fruits, starchy vegetables, legumes, and intact whole grains come prepackaged with a collection of micronutrients that protect against insulin resistance, rapid blood glucose elevations, and the secretion of excess insulin.
- Carbohydrates in plant-based whole foods are contained in a three-dimensional matrix with fat and protein, as well as vitamins, minerals, fiber, water, antioxidants, and phytochemicals that slow the rate of glucose absorption into your blood.
- Micronutrients are essential compounds that act as *information* that tissues use to digest, absorb, transport, uptake, and oxidize nutrients from the food you eat.
- Phytochemicals are found only in plants and are some of the most powerful disease-fighting compounds in all of nature.
- Contrary to popular belief, your liver does not convert carbohydrates into fatty acids via DNL in large quantities unless you massively overeat carbohydrates to the tune of 4,500 calories per day for 7 to 10 days at a time.
- Your brain, liver, and muscle have a strong preference for glucose as a fuel, and are capable of utilizing glucose very effectively when you eat whole carbohydrate-rich foods.

To view the 70+ scientific references cited in this chapter, please visit us online at www.masteringdiabetes.org/bookinfo.

# Chapter 7

## The Ketogenic Diet vs. a Low-Fat Plant-Based Whole-Food Diet: A Comparison of Short-Term and Long-Term Results

### Kicking Keto: Patricia

Patricia does not have a typical diabetes diagnosis story, but it is one that is becoming more and more common. She lived diabetes-free for most of her life, but at age 62 suddenly found herself diagnosed with type 1.5 diabetes, an adult-onset, slow-progressing version of type 1 diabetes that affects people over the age of 30. As Patricia adjusted to her new reality, she tried hard to manage her blood glucose. Realizing that the food she ate was an integral part of controlling her blood glucose, she tried one dietary approach after another, searching for one that "worked." Eventually, she adopted a ketogenic diet that restricted her intake of carbohydrate-rich food drastically while increasing her intake of low-carbohydrate, high-protein foods, including chicken, eggs, fish, and dairy products. She followed the ketogenic diet religiously, with 100 percent compliance for six months. But Patricia found that as time went on, she became increasingly exhausted and wasn't able to lose a single pound. She ate about 30 to 40 grams of carbohydrate energy and injected 30 units of basal insulin and 5 units of bolus insulin per day, for a 24-hour carbohydrate-to-insulin ratio of about 1:1.

One day, while reading posts in a low-carb group on Facebook, she watched a video that ridiculed Cyrus's video explaining the power of the Mastering Diabetes Method for people living with diabetes. Even though it went against what she thought she knew to be true, she was intrigued by the idea of eating the foods that she loved—less meat and more fruits and vegetables. Excited by the possibility of becoming more plant-based, she decided she had nothing to lose by trying Cyrus's program. She approached the program with an open mind, looking to achieve the four following goals:

- Lose approximately 30 to 40 pounds
- Gain better control of her blood glucose
- Reduce her insulin needs
- Gain energy

Patricia turned her diet on its head, switching from eating foods low in carbohydrate and high in protein and fat to foods high in carbohydrate and low in protein and fat. She stopped eating all animal foods, including meat, dairy, and eggs. She started eating the nutrient-dense plant foods that she craved—fruits, vegetables, intact whole grains, beans, lentils, potatoes (yes, potatoes!), and squash. In the first four months of her new diet, her A1c dropped from 7.1% to 6.4%, and by eight months her A1c was 5.8%. She ate as much as 300 grams of carbohydrate per day; decreased her daily basal insulin use from 30 units to 12 units; and injected approximately 8 to 10 units of bolus insulin per day, for a 24-hour carbohydrate-to-insulin ratio of 14:1.

Two years after her transition, Patricia maintains an A1c of 6.3%, has lost a total of 50 pounds, and her LDL cholesterol has dropped by more than 40 percent. She is eternally grateful for watching Cyrus's video and listening with an open and hopeful mind to the testimonials of others who completed the program. Following the Mastering Diabetes Method has helped her gain full control of type 1.5 diabetes, control her blood glucose with precision, and live her life with the vigor that she lacked when eating a ketogenic diet. Even though she did not experience the dramatic short-term improvements that many experience when they adopt a ketogenic diet, Patricia took the steps that she describes as "miraculous," dramatically improving both her short-term results and long-term health, backed by almost 100 years of evidence-based science that you'll read about below.

---

If you are living with diabetes, you may have been told to eat a low-carbohydrate diet to control your blood glucose or you may have been told to eat a *very* low-carbohydrate diet, otherwise known as a *ketogenic diet*. Regardless of which form of low-carbohydrate nutrition you may have come across, in this chapter we'll discuss the pros and cons of low-carbohydrate and ketogenic diets so that you have the information you need to choose what's right for you.

In the world of ketogenic diets, people are told to eat a very low-carbohydrate diet in order to achieve a metabolic state known as *ketosis*, in which your muscles and liver derive the bulk of their energy from fatty acids and amino acids instead of from glucose found in carbohydrates. To do so, people are told to eat 70 to 90 percent of calories of fat from meat, eggs, sausages, heavy cream, cheeses, fish, nuts, butter, oils, seeds, non-starchy vegetables, avocados, coconuts, and small amounts of berries, while avoiding almost all fruits, starchy vegetables, breads, pastas, legumes, milk, and yogurt.

Many people around the world who eat a ketogenic diet are able to lose weight, achieve a flat-line blood glucose profile, greatly reduce or eliminate their need for oral medication and insulin, and reduce their total cholesterol. So why aren't we recommending this diet ourselves? Because despite these advantages, there are four very important points to take into consideration:

- Evidence-based research conducted in large numbers of people over long periods of time consistently demonstrates that eating more animal products *increases* your risk for premature death, no matter what short-term benefits may unfold in the process. Similar large-scale research demonstrates that eating more whole plant foods *reduces* your risk for premature death.

- The short-term benefits associated with a ketogenic diet can also easily be achieved using a low-fat plant-based whole-food diet, as seen in research dating back to the 1920s.
- Low-fat plant-based whole-food nutrition is the only approach shown to *reverse* heart disease (the leading cause of death of people living with all forms of diabetes), whereas diets high in saturated fat and cholesterol have been shown to *promote* heart disease.
- There are many examples of long-lived societies around the world who eat plant-based diets, and *zero* examples of long-lived societies who eat a low-carbohydrate or ketogenic diet with a high intake of animal products.

While the ketogenic diet may seem like a logical approach to reducing blood glucose fluctuations, it is based on the outdated and incorrect carbohydrate-centric model of diabetes that we covered in chapter 3, which points a finger at carbohydrates as the *cause* of insulin resistance and type 2 diabetes, even though overwhelming evidence shows that low-carbohydrate, high-fat diets are actually the cause of insulin resistance and type 2 diabetes. To make sure you're completely clear on why that is, let's travel back in time.

The ketogenic diet was originally developed in the 1920s as a treatment to reduce the frequency of seizures in children suffering from intractable epilepsy. At the time, researchers thought that they could induce ketosis as well as a condition known as metabolic acidosis, both of which were known to have anticonvulsant effects.

What researchers also noticed was that a ketogenic diet often stimulated rapid weight loss, flat-line blood glucose, reduced cholesterol, and reduced blood pressure. As a result, researchers and medical professionals began experimenting with a ketogenic diet in people living with metabolic conditions like prediabetes, type 2 diabetes, obesity, fatty liver disease, Alzheimer's disease, chronic kidney disease, and cancer in an effort to reverse chronic disease.

But that's not the whole story. In 2004, researchers in Korea reported on the side effects of 129 epileptic children who were administered a ketogenic diet in a hospital setting. Within six months, more than half of the patients stopped the ketogenic diet (even those who experienced anticonvulsant benefits) owing to symptoms such as dehydration, nausea, vomiting, diarrhea, and constipation. About a third of the patients experienced high triglyceride values, and a third were put on cholesterol-reducing medication to counteract increasing cholesterol levels. The researchers reported a complete list of early- and late-onset side effects that also included acid reflux, hair loss, kidney stones, muscle cramps or weakness, hypoglycemia, low platelet count, impaired cognition, an inability to concentrate, impaired mood, renal tubular acidosis, disordered mineral metabolism, stunted growth, increased risk for bone fractures, osteopenia and osteoporosis, increased bruising, sepsis, pneumonia, acute pancreatitis, hyperlipidemia, high cholesterol, insulin resistance, elevated cortisol, increased risk for cardiovascular disease, increased risk for atherosclerosis, cardiomyopathy, heart arrhythmia, myocardial infarction, menstrual irregularities, amenorrhea (loss of period), and an increased risk for all-cause mortality.

Even though this study demonstrated strong evidence that a ketogenic diet may decrease seizure incidence, it was one of the first to demonstrate a strikingly low adherence rate and comprehensive list of undesirable side effects. Despite these findings more than fifteen years ago, many doctors today are quick to recommend a ketogenic diet to patients with type 2 diabetes based predominantly on short-term studies. In 2005, scientists from Temple University followed 10 obese patients living with type 2 diabetes for two weeks and observed that in this condensed time period, patients reduced their A1c by 0.5 percent and increased their insulin sensitivity by 75 percent. That same year, another team of researchers from Duke University found that sixteen weeks of a ketogenic diet in 28 different overweight patients led to dramatic reductions in A1c, diabetes medication needs, body weight, and triglyceride levels.

In 2006, researchers at the University of Kuwait studied the effect of a ketogenic diet on 66 obese subjects and observed significant weight loss, reduced total cholesterol, reduced LDL cholesterol, reduced triglycerides, and reduced blood glucose. The same research group admitted 64 obese individuals with and without high blood glucose into a study lasting thirteen months to determine the effect of a ketogenic diet on body weight, blood glucose, and cholesterol levels. In this time frame, the participants on average lost 50 to 66 pounds and significantly dropped their total cholesterol, LDL cholesterol, triglycerides, and blood glucose, while increasing their HDL.

And most recently, a team of researchers reported on the effects of an online ketogenic nutrition and lifestyle coaching program in 238 participants with type 2 diabetes over ten weeks. The researchers found that a ketogenic diet dropped the participants' A1c by 1.0 percent while reducing or eliminating common oral diabetes medications, along with significant reductions in fasting glucose, body weight, BMI, and triglycerides. Many of the participants continued to use metformin. The same researchers extended their findings to 349 people living with type 2 diabetes over the course of a year and found that a ketogenic diet dramatically reduced insulin and oral medication needs, as well as body weight, and led to a 1.3 percent reduction in A1c.

Ketogenic and low-carbohydrate diets have also been studied in people living with type 1 diabetes, demonstrating many positive benefits. A 2003 study from Duke University retroactively analyzed the results of 30 patients who ate a ketogenic diet consisting of 30 grams of carbohydrate energy per day; 10 of the 30 patients had type 1 diabetes. After an average of nineteen months, patients with type 1 diabetes experienced an A1c reduction of 1.3 percent (from 6.8 % to 5.5 %). Researchers observed modest improvements in the patients' lipid panel—their total cholesterol reduced by 11 mg/dL, their triglycerides reduced by 9 mg/dL, and their HDL cholesterol increased by 16 mg/dL. Their total insulin use dropped from 47 units per day to 30 units per day, resulting in a 24-hour carbohydrate-to-insulin ratio of 1:1 (30 grams of daily carbohydrate to 30 units of daily insulin).

A study published in 2005 found that a ketogenic diet significantly reduced the number of hypoglycemic episodes, insulin requirements, and A1c values in 22 individuals living with type 1 diabetes over a twelve-month period. And in 2012, researchers in Sweden found that eating less than 75 grams of carbohydrate per day for four years helped people with type 1 diabetes drop their A1c from an average of 7.8% to 6.0%. Over the course of those four years, all participants lost an average of 2 pounds, but only 48 percent of them adhered to the low-carbohydrate diet.

## What About LDL Cholesterol on a Ketogenic Diet?

**One notable exception to** the list of short-term improvements mentioned above is that a ketogenic diet almost always *raises* LDL cholesterol levels. And remember, LDL particles are the lipid particle known to have the highest correlation with cardiovascular disease, which means that irrespective of other health benefits, a ketogenic diet is likely to raise your cardiovascular mortality risk. Many ketogenic professionals aren't concerned by the total LDL concentration and focus instead on the types of LDL particles, but as we covered in chapter 4, *all LDL particle sizes increase your risk for atherosclerosis and coronary artery disease, regardless of particle size.*

But what about people who do drop their LDL cholesterol on a ketogenic diet? Are they just lucky? Do they have excellent genes helping them out? No, in fact the reason is actually quite simple. When you lose weight, many aspects of your cardiovascular health improve naturally, including lower total cholesterol, lower LDL cholesterol, lower triglycerides, higher HDL cholesterol, and reduced blood pressure. More often than not, people who reduce their LDL cholesterol on a ketogenic diet aren't just lucky; weight loss itself reduces their LDL cholesterol level despite a high intake of saturated fat and/or cholesterol. But here's the problem—as soon as your weight loss stops, many aspects of your cardiovascular health are likely to stall or move in the opposite direction, often leading to an increase in LDL cholesterol and atherosclerosis risk once again. This discrepancy between short-term and long-term effects on LDL cholesterol is one of many reasons why the ketogenic diet is a highly controversial topic in the world of nutrition today.

# Ketogenic Diets in the Long Term: A Less Positive Outlook

Based on the short-term evidence, a ketogenic diet is a very effective tool at promoting short-term improvements in body weight, blood glucose, A1c, and triglyceride levels. In the long term, however, eating a ketogenic diet is unlikely to provide the same results, and it's more likely to pose risks, as is the general class of low-carbohydrate diets. In large-scale studies performed over long periods of time, the evidence-based literature consistently shows that low-carbohydrate diets *worsen* long-term health, *increase* the risk for many chronic diseases, *increase* the risk for infectious diseases, and *increase* mortality.

The truth is that there are no long-term studies on the effect of a truly ketogenic diet in large numbers of people (greater than approximately 20,000) over long periods of time (five to twenty years). This is concerning, to say the least, and some researchers believe that this is because the ketogenic diet is very challenging to adhere to beyond the first year. Despite this, the scientific literature has ample data about the long-term effects of reducing carbohydrate intake and increasing intake of fat- and protein-rich foods from animal sources, which provides evidence for what is likely to happen to those eating a ketogenic diet over the course of time.

Researchers at the Harvard T. H. Chan School of Public Health analyzed the data of more than 129,000 people over more than twenty years and found that a low-carbohydrate diet based on animal foods was associated with higher all-cause mortality and higher cancer mortality, and that simply substituting plant foods for animal foods (while still eating a low-carbohydrate diet) dropped total and cardiovascular mortality.

In 2014, researchers from Loma Linda University summarized the results of three separate Adventist health studies conducted between 1960 and 2014, including the California Adventist Mortality Study (23,000 people), the Adventist Health Study-1 (34,000 people), and the Adventist Health Study-2 (96,000 people). They segregated participants between non-vegetarian, vegetarian, lacto-ovo-vegetarian, and vegan to determine how increasing amounts of meat and dairy products affected their risk for death from cancer, heart disease, and diabetes. Their findings from these three studies were very consistent—those who ate more meat and dairy increased their risk for all-cause mortality and disease-specific causes. They found that those who ate meat and dairy products experienced a 10 to 20 percent higher risk for all-cause mortality, a 28 to 68 percent increase in the risk of death from ischemic heart disease, cardiovascular disease, and cerebrovascular disease (which can lead to stroke), and a 48 percent increase in the risk of death from breast cancer as compared with vegetarians who eliminated meat but included dairy products in their diet. In comparison with their meat-eating counterparts, lacto-ovo-vegetarians were 38 to 61 percent less likely to develop diabetes, and vegans were 47 to 78 percent less likely to develop diabetes. They concluded that vegetarian and vegan diets offer significant protection against death from cancer, heart disease, and diabetes, and that those who chose to eat more meat and dairy products in the long term significantly increased their risk for death.

The EPIC study showed a very strong association between meat consumption and all-cause mortality that sheds some light on exactly why a ketogenic diet is a questionable strategy in the long term. After analyzing more than 448,000 men and women who were free of cancer, stroke, or a previous heart attack over an average time of twelve years, EPIC researchers found that a high consumption of processed meat was associated with an 18 percent increase in all-cause mortality.

Research published in the *Journal of Internal Medicine* analyzed the cardiovascular mortality of more than 40,000 Swedish women over the course of more than fifteen years. They found that women who ate the highest amount of protein were 60 percent more likely to die of cardiovascular disease than those who ate the lowest amount of protein. They estimated that simply increasing protein intake by 10 grams per day and dropping carbohydrate intake by 40 grams per day increases cardiovascular disease risk by 10 percent. And to be accurate, the total amount of protein that people in the study ate is highly representative of the amount of protein that free-living ketogenic dieters eat on a typical day. Ketogenic dieters eat between 1.0 and 1.5 grams of protein per kilogram of their "ideal" body weight, which translates to approximately 60 to 88 grams of protein per day for a 130-pound woman. In this study, those eating the lowest amount of protein (who had the lowest risk for cardiovascular death) ate approximately 40 grams of protein per day, while those who ate the highest amount of protein (who had the highest risk for cardiovascular death) ate approximately 90 grams of protein per day.

These findings are very similar to a study from 2007 that analyzed more than 22,000 adults from Greece who were followed for an average of ten years. Similar to the 40,000 Swedish women mentioned above, diets containing 20 percent protein (corresponding to about 76 grams per day) were associated with a significantly higher risk for premature death in comparison with diets containing about 10 percent protein. They calculated that replacing 50 grams of carbohydrate with 15 grams of animal protein per day (replacing 2 medium apples with 2 ounces of chicken breast) was associated with a 22 percent increased risk of premature death from any cause. As you can see, the amount of animal protein required to increase your risk for premature death is not large, and that the sustained intake of significant quantities of animal protein over the course of many years can dramatically reduce your metabolic health and increase your risk for premature death.

A carefully controlled meta-analysis of seventeen observational studies of more than 270,000 people concluded that low-carbohydrate diets increase mortality risk. The authors indicated that a "systematic review and meta-analyses of worldwide reports suggested that low-carbohydrate diets were associated with a significantly higher risk of all-cause mortality in the long run." The authors further stated that "these findings support the hypothesis that the short-term benefits of low-carbohydrate diets for weight loss are potentially irrelevant." The researchers reasoned that low-carbohydrate diets result in less fruit intake and less fiber intake, and often coincide with an increased intake of protein from animal sources, cholesterol, and saturated fat. Some combination of these factors is likely what contributes to an increase in cardiovascular disease and all-cause mortality observed in low-carbohydrate eaters.

In 2016, researchers from Massachusetts General Hospital and Harvard Medical School added a critical piece of information to the puzzle by analyzing how diets heavy in either animal protein or plant protein affect mortality risk. To do so, they analyzed the data of more than 130,000 participants from the Nurses' Health Study and Health Professionals Follow-Up Study over the course of a minimum of twenty-six years. Similar to the other studies mentioned above, they found that animal protein intake was associated with a significantly increased risk of cardiovascular mortality and that plant protein intake was associated with a significantly reduced risk of cardiovascular mortality and all-cause mortality.

The authors of this study did something very interesting—they analyzed how replacing 3 percent of the energy from animal protein with plant protein affected the participants' risk for death from cardiovascular disease, cancer, or any cause. What they found was fascinating. Replacing *every* type of animal protein with plant protein was associated with a reduced risk of death from cardiovascular disease and cancer, regardless of whether the animal protein came from processed red meat, unprocessed red meat, poultry, fish, eggs, or dairy. It didn't matter which type of animal protein was in question—replacing 3 percent of those calories with plant protein was associated with a reduced risk of premature death.

In addition, they found that for those who were already living with diabetes, eating more animal protein raised the risk of all-cause mortality, whereas eating more plant protein reduced the risk of all-cause mortality. This is exactly the crux of the argument—most mainstream diabetes recommendations encourage eating more animal protein as a means of losing weight and "stabilizing blood glucose," but large-scale research shows exactly the opposite.

**Eating more animal protein is associated with an increased risk of early death, especially for people living with diabetes.**

Finally, another large-scale study published in 2018 evaluated the risk of all-cause mortality of more than 15,000 adults over the course of twenty-five years. They found that animal foods high in protein and fat such as lamb, beef, pork, and chicken were associated with a higher risk for premature death, and that plant foods high in protein and in fat such as vegetables, nuts, peanut butter, and whole-grain breads were associated with a lower risk for premature death, suggesting that the type of food you eat may be as important as the percentage of carbohydrate, fat, and protein in your overall diet.

No matter how hard you look for long-term evidence to support a diet including more animal protein, more saturated fat, and fewer carbohydrates, the results tell the same story—carbohydrate restriction in the long term is associated with increased risk for chronic disease and all-cause mortality. No matter how you slice it, the supposed long-term health benefits of eating a low-carbohydrate diet simply don't add up.

## Animal- vs. Plant-Based Ketogenic Diets

This discussion brings up an obvious question: If eating an animal-protein-heavy ketogenic diet is associated with an increased risk of premature death, what effects does a purely plant-based ketogenic diet have on diabetes outcomes in both the short and long term? In other words, is eating a plant-based ketogenic diet safe?

Once again, short-term research on plant-based low-carbohydrate diets does exist, but long-term studies don't. A study performed by researchers in Toronto of 47 men and women with high cholesterol for four weeks showed that a plant-based low-carbohydrate diet (also called the Eco-Atkins diet) produced greater reductions in total cholesterol and LDL cholesterol than did a high-carbohydrate lacto-ovo-vegetarian diet containing low-fat dairy products. The same research group then studied what happened over the course of six months in the same two groups and found that Eco-Atkins dieters lost more weight and reduced their total cholesterol, LDL cholesterol, and triglycerides more than the lacto-ovo-vegetarian group.

Given that the long-term data above shows that eating more plant protein in substitution for animal protein is associated with increased longevity, it stands to reason that modifying the typical animal-based ketogenic diet with a plant-based version could benefit you both in the short and long term. Since plant foods have a dramatically higher nutrient density than animal foods, a plant-based ketogenic diet is likely to dramatically increase your intake of anti-inflammatory vitamins, minerals, fiber, water, antioxidants, and phytochemicals than an animal-based ketogenic diet. However, as we have covered extensively in chapter 3, eating a diet with a significant amount of total fat (even if it is completely plant-based fat) can dramatically increase your level of insulin resistance, make you intolerant of carbohydrate-rich foods, and make it more challenging to exercise than eating a low-fat plant-based whole-food diet containing ample energy from carbohydrate-rich whole foods.

Just like an animal-based ketogenic diet, a plant-based ketogenic diet often results in a dramatic reduction in total insulin use, which is beneficial for many people living with insulin-dependent diabetes. People living with insulin-dependent autoimmune diabetes greatly benefit from a sharp reduction in insulin use and more predictable blood glucose values, as it greatly improves their quality of life and reduces the anxiety of controlling blood glucose at all times. People living with insulin-dependent prediabetes or type 2 diabetes also greatly benefit from reducing their biological need for insulin and oral medications.

**It's critically important to understand that the total amount of insulin injected per day is not the most important metric of your diabetes health.**

Many medical professionals and people with diabetes focus their efforts on reducing total insulin use instead of paying attention to a more valuable metric that directly influences your risk for chronic disease—your 24-hour carbohydrate-to-insulin ratio.

Your carbohydrate-to-insulin ratio is an excellent indicator of your overall insulin sensitivity and is easily measurable for those living with insulin-dependent diabetes. The higher your carbohydrate-to-insulin ratio, the higher your insulin sensitivity and the lower your risk for chronic disease. Conversely, the lower your carbohydrate-to-insulin ratio is, the lower your insulin sensitivity and the higher your risk for chronic disease. Even though a plant-based ketogenic diet is extremely effective at reducing your total insulin use, it does so at the expense of reduced carbohydrate intake, resulting in a low carbohydrate-to-insulin ratio, a high degree of insulin resistance, and a greatly diminished carbohydrate tolerance. And remember what we covered in chapter 1—any lifestyle choice that increases your level of insulin resistance can also increase your risk for many chronic diabetes complications, so taking measures to keep your nutrient density and insulin sensitivity high will greatly benefit you today and in the long term. We both suffered from a 24-hour carbohydrate-to-insulin ratio between 1:1 and 4:1 when following a low-carbohydrate diet, and those numbers quickly increased to between 22:1 and 28:1 within months of switching to the Mastering Diabetes Method. In chapter 8, you'll learn how to calculate and track your carbohydrate-to-insulin ratio over time to use as a marker of your daily insulin sensitivity.

We understand that the short-term benefits of a ketogenic diet can make a tremendous positive difference in your metabolic health. However, turning a blind eye to the long-term risks that may evolve over time may be a very costly decision. We recommend asking yourself a simple question:

**Are the short-term benefits of a ketogenic diet worth the increased long-term chronic disease risks, or is there another way to achieve excellent short-term health *and* reduce your long-term chronic disease risk at the same time?**

If a ketogenic diet was the *only* way to improve your metabolic health in the short term, then the benefits would certainly outweigh the prospect of no improvements at all. However, practically all "diets" work in the short term, because diets prompt you to pay attention to the quality of the food that you're eating, how much you're eating, when you're eating, and how you feel between meals. The difference between dietary approaches becomes much more apparent over the course of time, and those that create long-term sustainable habits and provide lasting metabolic fitness will always beat out those that are unsustainable as well as those that negatively impact your long-term metabolic health.

And this is exactly why we strongly caution you against adopting a ketogenic diet without understanding that the short-term metabolic improvements can easily trick you into believing that it is a smart long-term option, when the evidence-based research demonstrates that people who reduce their intake of carbohydrate-rich foods and substitute more fat- and more protein-rich foods from animal sources are at a greater risk for chronic disease and premature death.

## Now for the Good News

Unlike ketogenic diets that haven't been studied in depth for long periods of time, almost a hundred years of evidence-based research has demonstrated that a low-fat plant-based whole-food diet is an excellent option for simultaneously maximizing your overall metabolic health, reversing insulin resistance, and dropping your chronic disease risk.

Studies that clearly debunk the carbohydrate-centric model of diabetes date back as far as the 1920s. Prior to the discovery of insulin in 1922, doctors used a low-carbohydrate diet to keep people with diabetes alive. In 1926, William D. Sansum, MD, was one of the first doctors to observe that increasing carbohydrate-rich foods did not increase his patient's need for insulin, as was commonly believed at the time. Instead, his patients resumed their normal state of physical and mental activity, their cardiovascular health improved, and their food cravings subsided.

A year later, in 1927, J. Shirley Sweeney, MD, published a brilliant study that demonstrated how the function of insulin is compromised in a high-fat environment. Dr. Sweeney fed young, healthy male medical students one of four diets for two days, followed by a carbohydrate challenge to measure how their diet affected their carbohydrate tolerance and insulin sensitivity. Study participants were randomized into a high-protein group, a high-fat group, a high-carbohydrate group, or a water fasting group. Participants in the high-protein group ate only lean meat and egg whites; those in the high-fat group ate olive oil, butter, mayonnaise, and cream; those in the high-carbohydrate group ate white sugar, candy, pastries, white bread, baked potatoes, syrups, bananas, rice, and oatmeal; those in the fasting group drank only water for two days.

On the morning of the third day, Dr. Sweeney measured the participants' fasting blood glucose, then again at 30, 60, and 120 minutes after administering a glucose challenge. What Dr. Sweeney discovered was remarkable—those who ate the high-fat diet and those who fasted both experienced the worst carbohydrate tolerance. All subjects in the high-fat group experienced abnormally high blood glucose values, and all blood glucose values remained greater than 140 mg/dL after 120 minutes. Subjects in the high-protein group also experienced elevated blood glucose values as well, albeit less pronounced than those in the high-fat and fasting groups. Subjects who ate the high-carbohydrate diet experienced modest rises in their blood glucose, and all high-carbohydrate eaters experienced blood glucose values between

80–140 mg/dL after 120 minutes. Even though the sample size was small, these results were part of a collection of early, detailed investigations that demonstrated the power of a low-fat, high-carbohydrate diet on increasing carbohydrate tolerance and insulin sensitivity, contrary to what many researchers hypothesized to be true.

In 1930, Israel Rabinowitch, MD, and his colleagues at the Montreal General Hospital discovered that plant-based diets low in fat improve insulin sensitivity. Dr. Rabinowitch observed that patients who were switched from a low-carbohydrate diet to a high-carbohydrate diet containing large quantities of vegetables, fruits, grains, and beans reduced their need for insulin rapidly, both with and without calorie restriction. His team performed several studies and a five-year randomized control trial in patients with diabetes, and found that a high-carbohydrate diet significantly reduced insulin needs very quickly, and patients looked and felt well, had more energy, adhered to the diet more easily compared to a strict low-carbohydrate approach, and had improved cardiovascular health. In a paper published in 1935, Dr. Rabinowitch concluded, "Suffice it to say that it now appears to be fairly well established that carbohydrates improve whereas fats impair carbohydrate tolerance; and that carbohydrates increase whereas fats decrease the sensitivity of the individual, animal and man, to insulin."

Next, a renowned clinician and researcher named Sir Harold Himsworth, MD, conducted a series of experiments in England to further demonstrate the effect of a low-fat diet on insulin sensitivity. He conducted oral glucose tolerance tests on healthy young men fed either a high-fat diet or a high-carbohydrate diet, and observed dramatic differences in their response to drinking a glucose challenge containing 50 grams of glucose. Those eating a high-fat diet experienced blood glucose values as high as 200 mg/dL within the first hour, and their final blood glucose at the three-hour mark was still elevated, at 140 mg/dL. Those who ate a high-carbohydrate diet experienced a peak blood glucose value of 120 mg/dL, and their final blood glucose at the three-hour mark was slightly over 100 mg/dL. Dr. Himsworth referred to insulin sensitivity as *insulin efficiency,* and concluded, "It is evident that on the high-fat diet insulin takes longer to act, and then acts more slowly, on the blood sugar than when the subject is given a high-carbohydrate diet."

Dr. Himsworth also performed a study where subjects ate one of seven different diets, ranging from 13 percent of calories from fat to 80 percent of calories from fat. Using this experimental setup, he observed that subjects became more insulin sensitive as the fat content of their diet dropped, and that those in the group eating 13 percent of their calories from fat experienced the highest level of insulin sensitivity.

In 1955, Inder Singh conducted a study on 80 patients with type 2 diabetes who injected insulin to control their blood glucose. He placed subjects on a diet consisting of 20 to 30 grams of fat, 120 to 150 grams of protein, and the remainder from carbohydrate energy. Most patients ate 1,600 to 2,200 calories per day, and a few underweight patients ate 4,000 to 4,500 calories per day. All patients were instructed to eat enough to prevent weight loss. After only three to six weeks, Singh observed that 63 percent of his patients became nondiabetic and no longer required insulin. After eighteen weeks, 80 percent of his patients were nondiabetic and no longer required insulin. Six patients who initially required 80 to 120 units of insulin per day gained full control of their blood glucose using 20 to 40 units of insulin per day following six weeks of the low-fat, high-carbohydrate diet. He concluded this study by stating: "There is no indication that healthy people taking a diet high in carbohydrates are especially liable to diabetes; in fact, numerous observations show improvement of carbohydrate tolerance following its greater intake."

At approximately the same time, Walter Kempner, MD, at Duke University demonstrated that high-fat diets not only caused insulin resistance and type 2 diabetes, but that patients could begin reversing long-standing diabetic retinopathy in a matter of days by eating a highly processed diet that included fruit and fruit juice. Dr. Kempner is famous for inventing the rice-fruit diet, in which he allowed his patients to eat only white rice, fruit, fruit juice, and added sugar—*four foods that mainstream diabetes nutrition experts condemn entirely.*

The rice-fruit diet was Dr. Kempner's attempt at creating a no-salt, no-cholesterol diet containing almost pure carbohydrate energy. His original intention was to reverse malignant hypertension, a condition thought to be incurable at the time, but in the process of teaching his patients how to dramatically reduce their blood pressure by eating the rice-fruit diet, he also reversed type 2 diabetes, heart disease, kidney disease, and diabetic neuropathy.

Take a moment and think about this carefully. Conventional diabetes wisdom states that foods high in carbohydrate energy will exacerbate diabetes and increase your insulin and oral medication requirements, especially if the source of carbohydrate energy includes refined foods like white rice and white sugar. Therefore, Dr. Kempner's rice-fruit diet should have resulted in metabolic disaster for his patients living with type 2 diabetes because it consisted of mainly fast-acting carbohydrate energy. The rice-fruit diet should have increased insulin requirements, caused unwanted weight gain, and promoted cardiovascular disease. But it didn't. In fact, it did the exact opposite. Why? Because the rice-fruit diet was so low in total fat that his patient's insulin sensitivity increased rapidly, resulting in a significantly higher ability to utilize glucose for fuel in their muscles and liver.

Despite the research conducted by Sansum, Sweeney, Rabinowitch, Himsworth, Singh, Kempner, and others, many scientists criticized their investigations, claiming that improvements in insulin sensitivity occurred not because subjects ate a low-fat diet but because they lost weight, and that performing a study without weight loss would negate increases in insulin sensitivity and improvements in carbohydrate tolerance. To uncouple weight loss from a low-fat diet, James W. Anderson, MD, and Kyleen Ward, RD, conducted a study in 1979 in which they enrolled twenty subjects who had been living with type 2 diabetes for up to twenty years. They fed participants a low-fat plant-based whole-food diet and demanded that their patients eat enough to prevent weight loss. Some subjects complained of physical discomfort from eating so much food, but the protocol ensured that all subjects remained weight stable. By doing this, they could then study how insulin requirements changed on a low-fat diet, independent of weight loss.

The results of this study were nothing short of remarkable. Insulin requirements plummeted by an average of 58 percent in the group that ate a low-fat diet, whereas insulin requirements did not change in those eating a conventional diabetes diet. Despite eating a substantially larger amount of carbohydrate energy, ten out of twenty subjects were able to discontinue taking insulin altogether, and those who continued insulin therapy were able to reduce their dosages between 7 and 98 percent. The most surprising result was that subjects who discontinued insulin completely were able to do so after only *sixteen days* on a low-fat diet, even after having lived with type 2 diabetes for at least a year. As a convenient side effect of a reduced intake of dietary fat, cholesterol levels dropped an average of 29 percent. Most important, all patients in this study reduced or discontinued insulin therapy and reduced their cholesterol levels without any changes in body weight, clearly disproving their critics and demonstrating that less dietary fat not only results in less biological insulin need, but also that a reduction in insulin requirements begins to occur within days.

In 1994, James Barnard, PhD, published the results of participants who attended the Pritikin Longevity Center 26-day residential program. His research team sifted through 4,587 medical charts and found 652 patients living with diabetes. During the program, participants walked on a regular basis and ate a diet containing approximately 10 percent of calories from fat, 15 percent of calories from protein, and the remaining calories from carbohydrate energy. In just over three weeks, 39 percent of the participants using insulin to manage their blood glucose were able to discontinue insulin altogether, and 71 percent of those using oral medications discontinued their use.

More recent evidence from Neal Barnard, MD, demonstrates how a low-fat plant-based whole-food diet containing approximately 10 percent fat outperformed a conventional diet based on the 2003 American Diabetes Association guidelines. Researchers followed participants for 22 weeks and observed larger reductions in A1c, body weight, and LDL cholesterol. When they followed these individuals for a total of 74 weeks, those in the plant-based group reduced their A1c more than those in the conventional diet group despite equivalent weight loss.

An excellent review article published in the *Journal of Geriatric Cardiology* in 2017 documented the evidence showing how plant-based diets have been shown to prevent and reverse type 2 diabetes in both randomized control trials and large-scale studies. They explain how whole grains, legumes, fruits, vegetables, and nuts each have been shown to be protective against type 2 diabetes, and demonstrate overwhelming evidence that a whole-food plant-based diet containing these elements together can both protect against the development of type 2 diabetes and reverse insulin resistance in those already living with type 2 diabetes. In addition, they demonstrate how a whole-food plant-based diet can reduce the incidence of diabetes complications including coronary artery disease, high cholesterol, high blood pressure, chronic inflammation, chronic kidney disease, and peripheral neuropathy, and review potential mechanisms by which diets rich in whole plant foods and low or absent in animal foods reduce diabetes risk and insulin resistance.

As far as large-scale research is concerned, we run into a similar problem as we did when analyzing ketogenic diet studies: There are no available long-term studies that demonstrate the effect of a *truly* low-fat plant-based whole-food diet in large numbers of people over long periods of time. With that said, we can look to large-scale evidence that analyzes the long-term effects of people who increase their intake of fruits, vegetables, legumes, and intact whole grains in substitution for fat- and protein-rich foods from animal sources, because it provides excellent context for what is likely to happen to those eating a truly low-fat plant-based whole-food diet over the course of time.

A recent study published in *PLOS Medicine* tracked the health of 512,891 Chinese men and women between the ages of 30 and 79, for an average of seven years, to understand the effect of their diet on their overall health. For those who did not have diabetes at the beginning of the study, those who had a higher fruit consumption were 12 percent less likely to develop diabetes compared with those who ate zero pieces of fruit per day. The researchers found a dose-response relationship, which means that the more frequently these non-diabetic individuals ate fruit, the lower the risk for developing diabetes.

Among those living with diabetes at the beginning of the study, those who ate fruit three times per week reduced their risk of all-cause mortality by 17 percent compared with those who ate zero pieces of fruit per day. In addition, researchers uncovered that those who ate fresh fruit three days per week were 13 to 28 percent less likely to experience macrovascular complications (heart disease and stroke) and microvascular damage (kidney disease, retinopathy, and neuropathy) than those who ate zero fruit.

Evidence from the EPIC study in more than 500,000 people over the course of twelve years demonstrates that eating glucose and fructose found in food does not increase your risk for diabetes; instead it *decreases* your risk for diabetes—as long as your intake of saturated fat and/or protein decreases. They concluded that replacing 5 percent of a diet containing saturated fatty acids with fructose (from either fruit or refined sources) is associated with a 30 percent decreased risk of diabetes, and that replacing 5 percent of protein with fructose is associated with a 28 percent reduction in diabetes risk.

## Heart Disease and a Low-Fat Plant-Based Whole-Food Diet

In addition to being a potent treatment option for all types of diabetes, a low-fat plant-based whole-food diet can also dramatically reduce your risk for the complications of diabetes including (but not limited to) coronary artery disease, fatty liver disease, chronic kidney disease, stroke, hypertension, high cholesterol, cancer, and Alzheimer's disease, and also help you attain a normal body weight, increase your activity levels, increase your energy levels, and dramatically improve your digestive health. This is particulary noteworthy because living with diabetes dramatically increases your risk for heart disease, regardless of the type of diabetes you may be living with. In fact, heart disease is the leading cause of death for people living with diabetes. Therefore it's essential to eat a diet that not only helps you control your blood glucose but also protects your heart and blood vessels both today and into the future. That's because a low-fat plant-based whole-food diet is the only diet documented to both arrest and *reverse* heart disease. By contrast, low-carbohydrate diets high in animal products may help you control your blood glucose but actually increase your risk for heart disease.

To help you understand how this works, we'll break it down further. Heart disease is caused by a buildup of atherosclerotic plaque in blood vessels all over your body. When you eat either a diet high in fat or a diet high in fat and cholesterol, blood vessels all throughout your body begin to accumulate plaque that covers the single-cell internal blood vessel lining known as your *endothelium*. A diet high in saturated fat is the worst offender because saturated fat not only accelerates the development of insulin resistance but increases your total cholesterol, LDL cholesterol, and speeds up the rate at which atherosclerotic plaque accumulates inside blood vessels in all tissues.

As arterial plaque accumulates over time, many problems begin to occur, all of which contribute to an increased risk for a heart attack. First, endothelial cells become dysfunctional and inflamed, limiting the ability of glucose and insulin to access tissues. LDL particles then invade the blood vessel wall and eventually become oxidized, resulting in the formation of *foam cells,* which attract pro-inflammatory macrophages. As this process continues, the cross-sectional diameter of blood vessels becomes smaller and the pressure inside the blood vessel increases. The net result is a high-pressure hardened blood vessel that can eventually become fully occluded, resulting in a complete loss of blood flow.

The great news is that rigorous scientific research has consistently demonstrated that eating a diet low in saturated fat and cholesterol is the most effective way to prevent and reverse heart disease and protect against atherosclerosis, high blood pressure, high cholesterol, and stroke. The scientific evidence is in fact so strong that a low-fat plant-based whole-food diet is the only diet known to reverse heart disease.

In 1956, researchers from UC Berkeley performed a five-year study on 470 patients, 351 of whom had previously experienced a heart attack and 119 patients previously diagnosed with angina (chest pain). Over this five-year period, the researchers observed that patients who ate a low-fat, low-cholesterol diet experienced the lowest risk for atherosclerosis, and that those who were not compliant experienced a recurrence and a death rate that was four times greater. Those in the low-fat, low-cholesterol group were advised to limit their dietary fat intake to less than 50 grams per day and their cholesterol intake to less than 200 milligrams per day. Even under these moderate dietary restrictions, patients in the low-fat, low-cholesterol group reduced their recurrence of a heart attack by 71 percent.

Soon after, in 1959, an article published in *The Lancet* analyzed blood cholesterol, dietary habits, and the incidence of heart disease in Africans and Asians living in Uganda, where the staple foods included green plantains, sweet potatoes, cassava, yams, corn, millet, pumpkins, tomatoes, and leafy greens. The diet of the African subjects contained between 10 and 15 percent of their total calories from fat, whereas the Asian subjects ate between 30 and 45 percent of their calories from fat. Vegetarian Africans over the age of 40 eating a traditional Ugandan diet maintained lower cholesterol values than Asians eating a non-vegetarian diet, which cannot be explained by differences in physical activity alone. The authors conclude that "in the African population of Uganda coronary heart disease is almost non-existent," and have strong evidence that a low-fat plant-based whole-food diet is the main reason why.

In 1998, Dean Ornish, MD, and colleagues published the results of the Lifestyle Heart Trial, a randomized, controlled clinical trial designed to determine if outpatients with documented coronary artery disease could halt or reverse atherosclerosis. The experimental group followed a lifestyle program that included a low-fat vegetarian diet (8.5 percent of calories from fat), moderate aerobic exercise, stress management, no smoking, and group emotional support. Control group patients were asked to continue with their current lifestyle and received standard care from their physician, but were given the opportunity to modify their lifestyle if they chose.

After five years, the experimental group experienced a 3.1 percent average reduction in arterial blockage, whereas the control group experienced an 11.8 percent increase in arterial blockage and a 2.5 times increased risk for a cardiac event. It may seem that a 3.1 percent reduction is quite small, but it's important to note that small increases in blood vessel diameter result in significant reductions in cardiac events. Those taught to eat a low-fat diet high in carbohydrate-rich foods such as fruits, starchy vegetables, legumes, and whole grains experienced a regression in coronary artery disease and experienced fewer cardiac events.

In 1985, Caldwell B. Esselstyn Jr. began treating 22 patients with a plant-based diet containing a maximum of 10 percent of calories from fat. His dietary protocol eliminated oil, dairy products (except for skim milk and no-fat yogurt), fish, fowl, and meat, and all vegetable, nut, and seed oils, and included large amounts of whole grains, legumes, lentils, vegetables, and fruit. In the following 5.5 years, 11 patients who adhered to his dietary protocol had clinically arrested heart disease, determined by a 40 percent reduced cholesterol level (from an average of 246 mg/dL to below 150 mg/dL) in combination with zero cardiac events. After 10 years, the 6 patients who remained compliant experienced a total of zero cardiac events. Five patients who dropped out of the study went on to experience a total of ten more cardiac events!

In 2014, Dr. Esselstyn published results of 198 consecutive patients who followed this same dietary protocol. After 3.5 years of follow-up, 177 of the 198 patients remained adherent to the diet. Of those 177 patients, 99.4 percent of adherent patients had avoided major cardiac events, and only 1 patient experienced stroke. Researchers reported an average of 18.7 pounds of weight loss, a 93 percent improvement in angina, and avoidance of 27 coronary artery bypass surgeries. More important, of the 21 patients who did not comply, 13 participants experienced adverse cardiac events, resulting in a 62 percent recurrence rate.

In 2011, Dr. Satish K. Gupta published the results of a lifestyle intervention program similar to the Lifestyle Heart Trial but conducted in India. Dr. Gupta enrolled 123 patients with moderate to severe coronary artery disease into a lifestyle change program including a low-fat diet, moderate aerobic exercise, and stress management through meditation. Patients with the highest level of adherence experienced an 18 percent reduction in arterial blockages, and 91 percent of patients showed a trend toward complete regression of coronary artery disease. Most important, those who were the most compliant dropped their risk for a cardiac event more than fourfold.

In addition to these powerful studies performed in small sample sizes, researchers have studied the cardiovascular health of long-lived people who have eaten a high-carbohydrate diet their entire life. In 2017, Dr. Hillard Kaplan and colleagues performed research on the indigenous South American Tsimane population in Bolivia. They conducted coronary artery calcium tests on 705 Tsimane people over the age of 40 who ate a low-fat, high-carbohydrate diet containing approximately 72 percent of calories from carbohydrate, 14 percent of calories from fat, and 14 percent of calories from protein from mainly rice, plantains, cassava, and corn. An overwhelming 97 percent of those studied showed no signs of atherosclerosis, with an extremely low total cholesterol and LDL cholesterol. While this study does not prove that their diet is responsible for low rates of cardiovascular disease, given that the Tsimane "have the lowest reported levels of coronary artery disease of any population recorded to date," it's certainly worth paying attention to their lifelong dietary habits.

The truth is that there are many populations around the world who eat plant-rich diets that have extremely low rates of heart disease, including the Bantu peoples of Central and Southern Africa, natives of New Guinea, certain Ecuadorian villages, and Native Americans in Mexico, as well as the five Blue Zones as originally documented by Dan Buettner, including Ikaria (Greece), Okinawa (Japan), Sardinia (Italy), Loma Linda (California), and the Nicoya Peninsula (Costa Rica).

So instead of thinking about how to follow a specialized "diet" to specifically address insulin resistance, think about this lifestyle as a nutrient-dense dietary solution not only to prevent and reverse diabetes but also to prevent and reverse chronic diseases that affect your heart, blood vessels, liver, kidney, brain, pancreas, and other vital organs. Eating a diet rich in unprocessed plants is designed to flood every cell of your body with bioavailable micronutrients required for optimal tissue function.

That said, we know how frustrating it can be to make large-scale changes to your lifestyle. We know how overwhelming it can be to get a new set of recommendations that may or may not echo what your doctor has prescribed. But we have taught thousands of people how to successfully transition to this time-tested program, and many individuals have seen firsthand how this process dramatically improved their overall health. The key is focusing on making sustainable changes and letting patience be your best friend. That's why we have made sure that our method is also easy to follow.

As you'll begin reading about in the next chapter, our approach to wellness is designed to help you introduce a series of simple changes that are meant to unfold over the course of months, not days. This is to help you change your habits in a sustainable manner and equip you for long-term success. This is not a contest, and the rewards of transitioning to a plant-based diet will come as you make slow, steady, and sustainable improvements to your overall lifestyle. We encourage you to take your time and avoid the temptation to sprint through these changes, no matter how rapidly you may want to progress. We are very confident that if you follow the program as we have outlined, your health will improve dramatically!

# Take-Home Messages

- In the short term, evidence-based studies show that a ketogenic diet is very effective at promoting rapid weight loss, reduced fasting blood glucose, reduced A1c, reduced medication needs, and reduced triglycerides in patients with type 1 diabetes and type 2 diabetes, but often raises LDL cholesterol significantly.

- In the short term, a low-fat plant-based whole-food diet is an excellent option for simultaneously maximizing your overall metabolic health, reversing insulin resistance, and cutting your chronic disease risk, independent of weight loss.

- Large-scale studies show that consuming animal products worsens long-term health, increases the risk for many chronic diseases, increases the risk for infectious diseases, and reduces life expectancy.

- Large-scale studies show that people who increase their intake of fruits, vegetables, legumes, and whole grains improve their diabetes health and dramatically reduce their risk for chronic disease in the long term.

- Researchers and doctors have known since 1926 that a low-fat diet is an extremely powerful way to increase insulin sensitivity, yet this information remains largely hidden from the public.

- A low-fat plant-based whole-food diet is the only diet known to prevent and *reverse* heart disease, the leading cause of death for those living with diabetes.

- There are many examples of long-lived societies around the world who eat plant-based diets, and *zero* examples of long-lived societies who eat a low-carbohydrate or ketogenic diet with a high intake of animal products.

To view the 85+ scientific references cited in this chapter, please visit us online at www.masteringdiabetes.org/bookinfo.

# Chapter 8

# Getting Started with the Mastering Diabetes Method

## 90 Days to Great: Tina

In October 2017, Tina was diagnosed with type 2 diabetes. Though she had been experiencing high stress, chronic fatigue, and weight gain in recent years, this diagnosis took Tina completely by surprise. She had been conscious of nutrition for years and thought that she was eating healthfully to prevent diabetes and other chronic diseases. Unfortunately, she fell into the trap of believing that low-fat dairy products and "lean meats" were health foods. Fortunately, Tina had heard Robby speak on a podcast and became aware that eating a plant-based diet was a great option to reduce her A1c dramatically and give her the best chance at reversing type 2 diabetes. She knew fruits and vegetables were safe and healthful, but she wasn't sure how to navigate this way of eating. This led to anxiety after her diagnosis. After having watched her aunt's health deteriorate as a result of uncontrolled diabetes, Tina was determined to do everything in her power to maximize her health and avoid the same fate. She reached out to Mastering Diabetes, committed to trying the Mastering Diabetes Method, and never looked back.

Almost immediately, her skin began clearing up, her energy levels increased, she began sleeping better, she began losing weight, and her fasting blood glucose decreased significantly. These benefits trumped the temptation of fried foods and refined carbohydrates. After exactly 108 days, Tina had lost 53 pounds and her A1c had dropped from 10.6% to 5.4%. Having gained some control over her health, Tina no longer feels like a victim. She also discovered that the human body does not heal selectively and believes that everything—body, mind, and spirit—has improved dramatically. One year after diagnosis Tina's A1c is now 5.0%

---

As we've learned firsthand—and as we've witnessed thousands of times with our clients—the food you eat is the single most important variable when it comes to reversing insulin resistance. If you are nervous about changing your diet or concerned that eating more carbohydrate-rich food will increase your blood glucose values, don't worry. We don't recommend making sudden, drastic changes. This method is designed to help you ease into this lifestyle step by step, monitoring how your blood glucose responds along the way.

As the quantity of stored fat in your muscle and liver decreases, your muscle and liver will regain their ability to respond to insulin, allowing glucose to enter tissues easily. As both your liver and muscle become better at recognizing and responding to insulin, your blood glucose is likely to decrease significantly. In chapter 9, we will address how to manage your use of oral medications and insulin for maximum success, including how to recalculate and reduce your basal insulin needs, how to adjust your carbohydrate-to-insulin ratio, and how to reduce your use of oral medications safely. While we recommend partnering with your doctor, we also want to give you the tools necessary to make informed decisions on a day-to-day basis. Feeling your best is well within your control, and as long as you're making smart decisions and listening to your body, we'll do our best to help you take full control of your diabetes health, from head to toe.

# The First 30 Days

Because your body is unique, you are likely to respond to this transition in your own way, which may be different even from the way someone else of the same sex, height, and weight would respond. What we've found is that during the first 30 days of this program, most people fall into one of the following three categories: slow responder, medium responder, or fast responder. These categories do not indicate whether you're winning or losing; they are an indicator of how your body responds to the Mastering Diabetes Method. If you find that your blood glucose is a bit erratic at the beginning of this transition, don't worry because fluctuations in your blood glucose are perfectly natural in the first few weeks of adopting a plant-based diet. Your blood glucose values are certainly important; however, the *trend* in your blood glucose values is most important at the beginning.

## Category 1: Slow Responder

If you are a slow responder, you may experience variability in your fasting and post-meal blood glucose values as you begin to eat carbohydrate-rich foods. This occurs in approximately 10 to 15 percent of all people:

- Your fasting blood glucose may increase (by 25–50 mg/dL).
- Your post-meal blood glucose may increase (between 140 and 200 mg/dL).
- Your blood glucose may take about three hours to return to baseline after finishing your meal.

## Category 2: Medium Responder

If you are a medium responder—which about 10 to 15 percent of all people are—you may either experience no change or small increases in your fasting blood glucose and post-meal blood glucose values. For the first 14 to 21 days, your fasting and post-meal blood glucose values may be slightly variable and hard to predict:

- Your fasting blood glucose may not change significantly.
- Your post-meal blood glucose may not change or will be slightly elevated (140–170 mg/dL).
- Your blood glucose may take about two to three hours to return to baseline after finishing your meal.

### Category 3: Fast Responder

Some 70 to 80 percent of all people are fast responders, even after years of eating a high-fat, nutrient-poor diet. If you are in this category, you may experience a sudden reduction in your blood glucose values in the first few days. Fast responders will greatly benefit from reducing their dosage of both oral and injectable diabetes medications in order to protect against frequent hypoglycemia:

- Your fasting blood glucose may drop quickly, and even fall below the hypoglycemic threshold of 70 mg/dL.
- Your post-meal blood glucose may be between 80 and 120 mg/dL, or it may fall below 70 mg/dL.
- You may experience multiple hypoglycemic episodes per day, prompting the immediate necessity to reduce your oral and/or injectable medication doses.

## How Long Will It Take for Your Blood Glucose to Drop?

The length of time that it takes to reduce your fasting and post-meal blood glucose likewise differs among individuals. There is a long list of genetic and lifestyle considerations that influence the speed of your response, most notably:

- How active you are on a daily basis
- The length of time you have been living with diabetes
- Your body's insulin production (indicated by your C-peptide value)

- What types of foods you've been eating over the past few years
- Your body fat percentage at the beginning of your transition
- Your body fat distribution (abdomen vs. upper body vs. lower body)
- Whether you are also living with other metabolic health conditions (high blood pressure, coronary artery disease, chronic kidney disease, fatty liver disease, etc.)

Given that exercise is one of the most powerful insulin-sensitizing tools you have at your disposal, the more active you are—and the more active you have been in the years preceding this transition—the more quickly you are likely to respond, and the stronger your chances of being able to reduce oral medications and insulin.

**The truth is that it doesn't really matter how quickly you respond. The most important thing is that you remain *consistent* in your approach to the Mastering Diabetes Method.**

Even the slowest responders who experience elevated blood glucose immediately following their transition will ultimately benefit from sticking with the new plan. As you follow the method over the course of the first 30 days, your fasting and post-meal blood glucose values are likely to decrease. We've seen plenty of clients frustrated when they don't see immediate progress. But in every situation, we do our best to encourage them to trust the process and allow the biological symphony to play out as it's supposed to. Those that heed this advice are greatly rewarded by their patience and are incredibly grateful that they stayed on course.

## How to Properly Interpret Your A1c

Your hemoglobin A1c is used as a marker of your average blood glucose values and is routinely used to track your blood glucose control over time. Your hemoglobin A1c measures the percentage of hemoglobin molecules in red blood cells that have glucose attached to them, and as the amount of glucose in your blood increases, so does the amount of *glycosylated hemoglobin*. Hemoglobin's job is to transport oxygen in your blood, and because red blood cells have an average lifespan of about 100 to 120 days, doctors recommend that you measure your A1c value approximately every three to four months to understand how your lifestyle is affecting your blood glucose control. Doctors use the hemoglobin A1c to diagnose prediabetes and type 2 diabetes according to the following criteria:

- **Nondiabetic:** 5.6% or below
- **Prediabetes:** 5.7–6.4%
- **Type 2 diabetes:** 6.5% and above

While it's certainly important to track your A1c value, one of the most important things you will learn in this book is that *your A1c is an incomplete indicator of your diabetes health.* While maintaining a low A1c is certainly important, dropping your A1c does not necessarily indicate that your long-term health is improving.

The truth is, there are many ways to drop your A1c effectively, including calorie restriction, frequent exercise, a low-carbohydrate diet, a low-fat diet, weight loss, the injection of insulin, and the use of oral medications (to name a few). Each of these methods can certainly reduce your blood glucose values and A1c, but as you now know, some of these methods increase your long-term disease risk while others reduce it.

Common dogma in the low-carbohydrate world is that every time your blood glucose increases above 120 mg/dL, your risk for neuropathy, retinopathy, and kidney damage increases. In addition, low-carbohydrate dieters commonly argue that any A1c value greater than 5.3% is associated with diabetes complications, even though the threshold for prediabetes is 5.7%. As a result, many adopt a ketogenic diet and are very successful at maintaining their blood glucose between 80 and 100 mg/dL at all times and dropping their A1c to less than 5.3%. This is one of the reasons low-carbohydrate diets are so popular— because they are very effective at improving many diabetes-related biomarkers.

But here's the problem—interpreting your A1c by itself without also maximizing your nutrient density and carbohydrate tolerance is a common (and very costly) mistake in the long term. If you assume that a lower A1c value indicates improved metabolic health without also maximizing your nutrient density and insulin sensitivity, your risk for future diabetes complications may still be high.

**A diet low in nutrient density is a breeding ground for chronic disease, *even if your blood glucose is controlled within a tight range and your A1c is low*. A diet high in nutrient density protects you against chronic disease, even if your blood glucose control and A1c are elevated during your transition.**

What this means is simple. In order to interpret your A1c properly, first determine the nutrient density of your diet and your carbohydrate tolerance. If you eat foods with a low nutrient density containing small quantities of vitamins, minerals, fiber, water, antioxidants, and phytochemicals, or you find that your carbohydrate tolerance is low, then you are at a high risk for chronic disease and long-term complications of diabetes. If, on the other hand, your diet is high in nutrient density and your carbohydate tolerance is also high, then you can slightly relax your blood glucose control and A1c range during your transition and still achieve excellent long-term metabolic health.

## Take the Time to Set SMART Goals

As you begin this process, take a moment to ask yourself a simple question: "Why am I changing my nutrition habits to maximize my insulin sensitivity?" We like to call this your *why,* and it's important to think hard about what that is before embarking on what can be a challenging journey. Clarity is the key to finding strength and dedication to make this transition effectively. Maybe it's because you want to feel less numbness and tingling in your feet; maybe it's so you'll have more energy to spend time doing the things you enjoy with the people you love most; maybe it's to reduce the side effects of multiple medications; or maybe it's to save your own life. Whatever it is, connect with your *why* and commit to understanding it inside and out.

Reinforcing your *why* on a daily basis is absolutely critical to your success when following the Mastering Diabetes Method. It's easy to get distracted in our modern environment, and when you run into obstacles and experience tough times, having clarity about your motivation to master your nutrition habits can truly be a game-changer. That's why we also recommend setting compelling, reachable goals for yourself that are in line with your *why*. We recommend creating SMART goals that are *specific, measurable, attainable, relevant,* and *timely.* Each of these attributes makes the difference between a goal that feels large and vague and one that feels realistic, specific, and achievable.

**Step 1:** Take a few minutes to write down your SMART goals on a piece of paper. Write down what you are trying to accomplish in this program; be very specific in your language. Rather than saying, "I want to lose weight," write "I want to lose 45 pounds over the next 9 months so that I can return to running every day." Give yourself reasonable specifics within a reasonable time frame. And don't be surprised if you achieve your goal earlier than anticipated!

**Step 2:** Making your goals readily and regularly visible is one of the keys to successfully working toward them. That's why we recommend posting your goals in at least THREE separate locations where you'll have no choice but to see them on a daily basis. These can include:

- Your refrigerator
- Your bathroom mirror
- Your desk
- Your computer monitor
- The back of your front door

**Step 3:** Resume your normal life and connect with your *why* every day. When you see it written down, read your *why* out loud at least once a day to further reinforce your determination to reverse insulin resistance using your food as medicine.

# Your New Diet: Green Light, Yellow Light, and Red Light Foods

To make your transition to a low-fat plant-based whole-food diet as straightforward as possible, we created a three-part system to help you easily identify which foods to eat in abundance, which foods to minimize, and which foods to eliminate altogether. As for what to eat, it's a simple, easy-to-follow *green light, yellow light, red light* system, which is summarized in the table below:

| Green Light Foods (Unprocessed whole plant foods naturally low in fat; can be fresh or frozen) | Yellow Light Foods (Minimally processed or whole plant foods containing a higher fat content) | Red Light Foods (Animal products and highly processed foods) |
|---|---|---|
| • Fruits *(e.g., bananas, mangoes, oranges)*<br>• Starchy vegetables *(e.g., potatoes, butternut squash, corn)*<br>• Legumes *(e.g., beans, lentils, peas)*<br>• Intact whole grains *(e.g., brown rice, quinoa, farro)*<br>• Non-starchy vegetables *(e.g., tomatoes, cucumbers, broccoli)*<br>• Leafy greens *(e.g., lettuce, arugula, spinach)*<br>• Herbs and spices *(fresh or dried)*<br>• Mushrooms *(e.g., shiitake, cremini, portobello)* | • Avocados<br>• Nuts and seeds<br>• Nut and seed butters<br>• Plant-based milks<br>• Coconut meat<br>• Soy products *(e.g., edamame, tofu, tempeh)*<br>• Olives<br>• Pasta alternatives *(e.g., lentil, bean, brown rice)*<br>• Sprouted bread<br>• Dried fruits *(e.g., dates, raisins, dried apricots)*<br>• Fermented foods *(e.g., sauerkraut, kimchi, coconut kefir)* | • Red meat<br>• White meat<br>• Eggs<br>• All dairy products<br>• Oils of any kind<br>• Fish and shellfish<br>• Processed baked goods *(e.g., croissants, muffins, cookies)*<br>• Sweeteners *(e.g., HFCS, sorbitol, maltodextrin)*<br>• Refined "white" foods *(e.g., white pasta, white bread, white sugar, white flour)*<br>• Coconut products *(processed, high-calorie products excluding coconut kefir and aminos, e.g., yogurt, ice cream)*<br>• Processed vegan foods *(e.g., processed veggie burgers, vegan cheeses, nut milk ice creams)* |

## Green Light Foods

Perhaps the most important aspect of the Mastering Diabetes Method is that *carbohydrate-rich foods are easy to metabolize when your total fat intake is kept low (especially saturated fat).* In fact, unless you are injecting fast-acting insulin, when you eat a low-fat plant-based whole-food diet, it's not necessary to micromanage your carbohydrate intake. When you're consistently eating a maximum of 15 percent of your total calories as fat, your body's ability to metabolize whole carbohydrate-rich foods will increase over time, allowing you to eat larger quantities of carbohydrate-rich foods while maintaining excellent blood glucose control.

The foods in the green light category are to be eaten *ad libitum*, which means that you can eat as much of these foods as you want. Collectively, green light foods are the most nutrient-dense foods on the planet, complete with all three macronutrients, as well as vitamins, minerals, fiber, water, antioxidants, and phytochemicals. Green light foods are fiber-rich and contain between 60 and 90 percent water, which means that when they make up the bulk of your meal, they will make you *mechanically full and nutritionally full* before you become *calorically full.* This means that when your stomach begins to distend, it will send a neurological impulse to your brain that says "Slow down!" or "Stop eating!" Your brain responds by curbing your appetite, which decreases the number of calories you eat while remaining satisfied. Green light foods contain only a fraction of the calorie density of red light and yellow light foods, meaning that you won't even have to think about overconsuming calories. We'll cover calorie density in greater detail in chapter 11.

## Yellow Light Foods

The foods listed in the yellow light category are plant-based foods that can certainly be part of your diet in small amounts. Avocados, nuts, seeds, olives, coconut meat, and soy products are all whole foods high in fat, and even though they contain predominantly unsaturated fat, when eaten in large quantities they, too, can cause insulin resistance and high blood glucose. As we covered in chapter 4, substituting foods containing unsaturated fat for foods high in saturated fat and trans fat dramatically improves your insulin sensitivity within weeks. That said, it's still very important to be mindful of your *total* fat intake, even if the majority of your fat comes from unsaturated sources. This will ensure that your liver and muscles have the greatest chance of maximizing their sensitivity to insulin.

Non-wheat pasta alternatives, such as products made from lentils, quinoa, beans, and brown rice, are also in the yellow light category because they are often highly processed, and we advocate eating foods in their most intact whole form whenever possible. Conventional pastas are made from wheat and require many processing steps before making it into the package that you recognize at the grocery store, including grinding, sifting, extruding, and drying. At each step in the process, the micronutrients originally present in the wheat are lost, resulting in a micronutrient-depleted end product that is low in nutrient density.

As a result, many companies now make pasta alternatives using non-wheat sources including chickpeas, quinoa, black beans, mung beans, soybeans, brown rice, and lentils. While these pasta alternatives generally have a higher nutrient density than conventional pastas, they are still more processed than the intact food from which they originated. As a general rule of thumb, when choosing between two foods like brown rice and brown rice pasta, choose the brown rice because it requires less processing and has a higher micronutrient content than the brown rice pasta.

---

## The Truth About Soy

Understanding whether soy products are healthy has become a very controversial topic in our nutrition world today. Many health experts condemn soy and soy products altogether, claiming that they increase estrogen levels and act as endocrine disrupters, both of which have been linked to developmental disorders and various cancers. As a result, eating and drinking soy products has recently waned in popularity, even though the evidence in support of these claims is questionable. If you're like most people, you may be asking yourself, *What is the truth about soy?*

It turns out that many evidence-based investigations have not only found soy to be safe, it's actually *protective* against a host of chronic diseases, including breast cancer, prostate cancer, and cardiovascular disease. Studies comparing adults who ate the most soy compared with the least showed a 59 percent risk reduction in breast cancer and a 31 percent risk reduction in prostate cancer. A meta-analysis published in *The New England Journal of Medicine* found that the consumption of soy protein versus animal protein significantly decreases total cholesterol, LDL cholesterol, and triglycerides. A study published in the *Journal of Nutrition* in 2010 analyzed twenty years of research on soy consumption and found that soy reduces breast cancer risk, prostate cancer risk, coronary heart disease risk, and bone fracture risk. The authors conclude: "There is almost no credible evidence to suggest traditional soyfoods exert clinically relevant adverse effects in healthy individuals when consumed in amounts consistent with Asian intake." And most recently, a 2018 meta-analysis of thirty studies published in the journal *Nutrients* found a statistically significant association between soy consumption and decreased prostate cancer risk.

Given the protective nature of soy and the weight of the scientific evidence above, we support including some soy in your diet. Because some soy products are highly processed and soybeans themselves contain more fat than other beans, we consider soy a yellow light food. We recommend adding soy to your diet in small quantities to add texture and flavor to your dishes. You'll now find a plethora of soy-based items at the grocery store, ranging from whole-food options like edamame and tempeh to more processed items like ice cream and yogurts. If you choose to include soy in your diet, here are the best options:

Edamame is a whole food and does not require any special processing other than cooking to eat. Add edamame to soups, stews, and salads, or eat them as a snack.

Tempeh is a fermented soy product with a high nutrient density and minimal processing, which is beneficial for maintaining optimal gut

health. Tempeh can be sautéed or baked and used as a satisfying
meat substitute.

Tofu is made from soybean pulp that is separated from the soy milk,
and the remaining curds are processed into solid white blocks. Tofu
is a highly processed food and a far cry from eating edamame, but
certainly a great alternative to eating meat, poultry, fish, or eggs.

Soy milk is highly processed and lacks the micronutrient density
of unprocessed whole soybeans, but is a good alternative to
dairy milk.

---

## Red Light Foods

The red light category includes two main groups of foods: animal products
and processed foods. As we've discussed earlier, red light foods increase your
risk of chronic diseases and hinder glucose absorption into tissues. We've also
included oil in this category because oil is the most refined and calorie-dense
food in the grocery store. Some oils contain trace amounts of vitamins and
minerals, but oils are devoid of carbohydrate, protein, fiber, and water, and the
vast majority of vitamins, minerals, antioxidants, and phytochemicals have
been removed in the extraction process. So what you're left with is the single
most calorie-dense food in existence, containing minimal micronutrient value.

The good news is that once you start to build your meals around green
light foods, you are likely to become nutritionally satisfied, and cravings for
processed foods will likely fade away. Countless clients have told us how satisfied they are eating green light foods, and how much they enjoy eating large
quantities of fruits and starchy vegetables, guilt-free.

---

### Oil Is Not a Health Food!

Practically all health professionals agree that processed and refined foods
are problematic for human health and increase your risk for chronic
disease. Despite this, oil has been marketed as a health food even though
it is as refined as white table sugar. What started as an olive, coconut,

walnut, or avocado has been pressed into a liquid and separated from the flesh, resulting in a liquid that is 100 percent fat, devoid of carbohydrate, protein, fiber, and water.

**Think of oil as the fatty equivalent of table sugar. Both products contain only a single macronutrient, and both are highly refined products that will significantly impair your metabolic health.**

### Oils Have Low Nutrient Density

No matter how you slice it, all oils contain only one macronutrient—fat. Whether you are talking about olive oil, coconut oil, MCT oil, walnut oil, grapeseed oil, avocado oil, corn oil, canola oil, or rice bran oil (to name a few), all oils have been stripped of carbohydrate and protein energy, resulting in a liquid that contains 100 percent fat.

In addition, oils are also stripped of fiber—one of the most valuable and metabolically protective nutrients in whole foods. Fiber helps slow the entrance of carbohydrates, protein, and fat into your blood, and protects tissues from rapid surges in glucose, amino acids, and fatty acids that trigger inflammatory processes. As we covered in chapter 6, fascinating science is now uncovering that fiber is actually food for your microbiome, a collection of trillions of bacteria that colonize the lining of your large intestine. Fiber is considered a *prebiotic*—food that your gut bacteria metabolize—and this prebiotic is vitally important in helping these bacteria manufacture short-chain fatty acids that boost immune function, fight infections, improve insulin signaling, and promote insulin sensitivity.

The manufacturing process used to separate oil from its original whole food also decreases the nutrient density of the end liquid. As the fiber leaves, so do vitamins, minerals, antioxidants, and phytochemicals, resulting in a refined liquid that has significantly less micronutrient content than the original whole food from which it came. To illustrate this point, you may have heard that olive oil is a great source of *polyphenols*—powerful antioxidants that are found in a wide variety of green light foods. For example, you can get the same amount of polyphenols from 12 calories of lettuce as you would from 120 calories of oil—that's ten times the number of calories!

## Oils Contribute to Insulin Resistance

As we discussed in chapter 4, saturated fat—the primary component of coconut oil and most vegetable oils—is the most common trigger for insulin resistance because even small amounts can impair the function of insulin receptors in your muscle and liver within hours of a single high-fat meal. People living with insulin-dependent diabetes following the Mastering Diabetes Method find that even small amounts of oil in a single meal significantly increase their blood glucose starting about two to six hours after the meal, which then increases their need for exogenous insulin between one and four *days* after that meal. The same biological phenomenon occurs in people living with prediabetes, type 2 diabetes, and gestational diabetes, resulting in higher blood glucose values than expected. If you're not convinced, follow the Mastering Diabetes Method for two to four weeks, then eat a single meal containing 2 or more tablespoons of oil. We're willing to bet you'll be convinced to drop oil from your diet after you feel the difference and see what it does to your postprandial (post-meal) blood glucose.

## Oils Can Increase Your Omega-6 to Omega-3 Ratio

Oils such as sunflower, corn, soybean, and cottonseed oil contain more than 30 percent of calories from pro-inflammatory omega-6 linoleic acid (LA). Even small amounts of LA in your diet increase your overall omega-6 to omega-3 ratio, resulting in an increase in whole body inflammation. In addition, increased flow through the omega-6 pathway results in reduced flow through the omega-3 pathway, resulting in a reduced production of EPA and DHA, two important anti-inflammatory fatty acids that are critical for optimal brain function and eye health.

# Green, Yellow, and Red Light Beverages

In the same way that we categorize foods using a green, yellow, and red light system, we have developed a similar methodology to help you understand how to think about various beverages on the market today.

## Green Light Beverages

We encourage you to enjoy these beverages without concern. These include green juice made from primarily leafy greens, water, carbonated water, and unsweetened herbal teas, all of which contain zero calories.

Water: When you eat green light foods, your intake of water will naturally increase, but despite that, it's still important to drink water throughout the day. Feel free to squeeze juice from a lemon or lime into your water, or add pieces of fruits or vegetables for a subtle but delicious flavor and negligible impact on your blood glucose values.

Staying well hydrated is very important for physical and cognitive performance; gastrointestinal, kidney, and heart function; skin health; and the prevention of headaches. The amount of water to drink on a daily basis varies significantly from person to person, so we recommend observing the color of your urine to determine when it's time to hydrate. A light yellow color indicates that you are well hydrated, and a dark yellow color indicates that you are dehydrated.

Carbonated Water: The term *carbonated water* includes seltzer water, club soda, sparkling mineral water, and tonic water, and all of these can be a fun way to drink more water on a daily basis. If you prefer bubbles in your water, feel free to drink carbonated water to your heart's delight. Oftentimes, food manufacturers add "natural flavors," or sweeteners, so look out for these ingredients and do your best to avoid them.

Green Tea: Green tea is one of the healthiest beverages on Earth. Evidence-based research has consistently demonstrated that green tea

helps reduce your risk for cancer, improves artery function, and protects against cardiovascular disease. That said, research has also
shown that adding small amounts of milk to green tea can block its
protective action, so be sure to enjoy your tea plain or with a squeeze
of lemon juice.

**Herbal Teas:** Herbal teas can be an excellent addition to a low-fat plant-
based whole-food diet because they are packed with valuable antioxidants. A true herbal tea is caffeine-free, but some herbal blends can
contain tea leaves with caffeine, so read the packaging carefully if
you're caffeine-sensitive. (And check out page 227 for our evidence-
based suggestions about caffeine.) Feel free to drink multiple glasses
of herbal tea per day, and enjoy the flavor and metabolic benefit that
they bring.

**Green Juices:** Green juices are made from leafy greens and non-starchy
vegetables such as cucumber, celery, lettuce, and tomato. These juices
can be extremely nutrient-dense additions to your diet and do not
contain enough carbohydrate energy to have a significant impact on
your blood glucose. If you're using fast-acting insulin, your body may
require a small amount when drinking a green juice. Using decision
trees will help you learn exactly how much insulin your body requires
(if any).

## Yellow Light Beverages

When you drink yellow light beverages, your blood glucose may begin to
rise rapidly. If you're seeking optimal diabetes health, we recommend no
more than one cup of a yellow light beverage per day.

**Coconut Water:** When talking about coconut water, we are referring to
coconut water from a fresh coconut, free of refined sugars and syn-
thetic flavor enhancers. Fresh coconut water provides important nutrients such as B vitamins, vitamin C, and sodium, and the cytokinins
found in coconut water may contain potent anti-cancer properties.
Believe it or not, coconut water also includes small amounts of fiber.

However, it still contains liquid calories that are not nearly as satiating as eating whole foods. If you are trying to lose weight, drinking coconut water can easily add unnecessary calories, which can stall your weight-loss efforts.

**Plant-Based Milks:** Plant-based milks include almond, cashew, coconut, hemp, oat, rice, soy, and quinoa milk. The reason plant milks are yellow light beverages is that they are liquids that can add unnecessary calories, and the benefits of chewing whole foods are unmatched. It's worth pointing out, however, that milks made from high-fat ingredients such as almonds or cashews are not high in total fat content because the final product contains predominantly water. Do your best to avoid plant milks with added sugar or other unnecessary additives.

**Starch-Based Vegetable Juices:** Juices made from starchy foods like carrots, parsnips, or sweet potatoes can lead to blood glucose spikes because they contain a significant amount of glucose and little to no fiber. Minimize your intake of starch-based vegetable juices for best results.

**Kombucha:** Kombucha is a fermented tea beverage that has recently become very popular. Research has shown that kombucha is a good source of B vitamins and vitamin C, as well as disease-fighting polyphenols. Kombucha has been shown to improve resistance against cancer, prevent cardiovascular diseases, promote digestive functions, stimulate the immune system, reduce inflammation, and aid in liver detoxification. However, kombucha is a yellow light beverage because it often contains residual table sugar in the final product because refined sugar is added in order to "feed" the bacteria and yeast, and because the acidity can damage your teeth in the long term.

**Fresh Fruit Juices:** Fresh-squeezed orange juice is an example of a beverage that contains a high quantity of vitamins, minerals, antioxidants, and phytochemicals, but is low or devoid of fiber and can therefore increase your blood glucose rapidly. Limit your intake of fruit juice for best results.

## Red Light Beverages

Beverages in the red light category have the largest number of liquid calories of any category and have been well documented to raise your blood glucose and cholesterol while promoting full-body inflammation. We recommend minimizing or completely avoiding these beverages.

**Alcohol:** All alcoholic beverages such as beer, liquor, and wine are included in this category. While there are several meta-analyses that suggest low to moderate levels of alcohol consumption can be beneficial for cardiovascular health and reduced mortality, compelling research has shown that drinking even small amounts of alcohol is harmful. A study published in 2018 reviewed over 1,250 articles that included prospective and retrospective studies on the risk of alcohol use. The authors concluded that the safest level of alcohol consumption is none.

Steven Bell is a genetic epidemiologist at the University of Cambridge and the lead author of a *British Medical Journal* paper about the effects of alcohol on the human body. His interpretation of his own research is compelling: Alcohol carries a risk of liver disease, and the most powerful ways to improve your metabolic health include quitting smoking, exercising regularly, and eating a healthy diet.

**Sodas:** Regular sodas are a perfect example of a sugar-sweetened beverage that is high in calories and completely devoid of nutrition. Sodas often contain between 10 and 20 tablespoons of sugar per can, while diet sodas include refined sweeteners, which have been documented to damage your metabolic health, as we covered in chapter 6. We recommend removing both regular and diet sodas from your diet in order to control your blood glucose with more precision and decrease or eliminate your medication and insulin requirements.

**Sweetened Tea, Energy Drinks, and Sports Drinks:** Each of these beverages contains refined sugars, artificial sweeteners, and potentially dangerous additives. It's best to avoid them in favor of the green light beverages listed above.

# How Much Food Can You Eat?

The beauty of the Mastering Diabetes Method is that as long as you're following the green, yellow, and red light suggestions, you can eat food in large quantities. We'll go into more detail in the following chapters about how you can structure your meals to maximize your insulin sensitivity, but for now let's keep it simple. Our guidelines follow five basic rules.

## Rule 1: Don't Count Your Calories; Just Eat Until You're Satisfied

The Mastering Diabetes Method does not ask you to count calories. That's partially because we think that counting calories is a huge pain and a waste of time, but it's mostly because research has shown that eating fiber-rich foods is a great way to feel full without having to worry about how many calories you are eating. While it's true that when you eat foods high in calorie density the easiest way to prevent yourself from eating too many calories is to control your portion size, the beauty of eating low-fat plant-based whole foods is that they are naturally low in calorie density and high in fiber content, both of which are very effective at protecting you against eating excess calories. Therefore, contrary to what you may have been told in the past, it is not actually necessary to count your calorie intake in order to achieve your ideal body weight. At the same time, we do encourage you to track some elements of what you're eating. We recommend being aware of the total grams of fat you are eating; the percentage of your diet coming from carbohydrates, fat, and protein; and your total carbohydrate intake.

Since recording your food intake can be tedious and extremely time-consuming, we encourage you to simplify your life by using nutrition-logging software. We recommend using Cronometer (www.cronometer.com) because the app is simple to use and extremely informative, but feel free to use whichever app you like best. Just ignore the calorie data and focus on the useful information that will lead to making beneficial changes to your health and body.

In chapter 10, we will do a deep dive into the science of satiation—the feeling of being satisfied after eating a meal—and explain exactly how your digestive system and brain talk to each other to determine when you're full. It may be hard to believe that you can eat green light foods without counting calories or restricting your portion sizes (and this may be contrary to what you have learned from other experts in the past), but the science about calorie density is crystal clear. As long as you have an open mind, we promise you'll be happy maximizing your metabolic health by eating *more* food. We'd much rather that you get in touch with your body's innate hunger cues and not concern yourself with the calories or nutrients, especially at the beginning of your transition.

## Rule 2: Pay Attention to Your Total Fat Consumption

As a general guideline, we suggest eating between 15 and 30 grams of fat per day, which is a simple guideline to target your total fat intake to a maximum of 15 percent of calories from fat. As you will see in the following table, your total fat intake for maximum insulin sensitivity depends on your body's energy needs, which are highly influenced by your activity level. To determine your ideal daily maximum fat intake, find the appropriate row in the table:

| General Activity Level | Suggested Maximum Fat Intake (grams per day) |
|---|---|
| Sedentary (0 minutes of physical activity per day—see chapter 14) | 15 |
| Low Activity Level (~15 minutes of physical activity per day) | 20 |
| Medium Activity Level (~30 minutes of physical activity per day) | 25 |
| High Activity Level (~60 minutes of physical activity per day) | 30 |

Take a look at the image on the next page. In the top half of the image, you'll see a full day of eating, containing more than 5 pounds of food and a total of 15 grams of fat, specifically designed to maximize your insulin sensitivity. In the bottom half of the picture, you'll see a collection of nine common foods that each contain 15 grams of total fat, none of which will keep you full for an entire day. In this way, eating large quantities of food to stay satisfied while minimizing your total fat intake is easily achievable.

## Rule 3: Remember That All Whole Foods Contain Carbohydrate, Protein, and Fat

All whole-plant foods contain fat, and some contain more than others. Foods like nuts, seeds, avocados, coconuts, and olives contain more fat than foods like bananas, broccoli, beans, arugula, and rice. Even though you may think of a banana as pure carbohydrate, the truth is that a banana contains carbohydrate, fat, and protein. It may seem strange that fruits and vegetables contain fat and protein, but they do, and the small amounts that you eat in fruits and vegetables contribute to your daily fat and protein total. If you eat a variety of green light foods, approximately 5 to 10 percent of your calories will come from fat before you eat any higher-fat yellow light foods such as nuts, seeds, avocados, soy-based foods, or coconut products. Take a look at the table on page 168 to understand the macronutrient content of a collection of whole plant foods.

Based on this information, if you had a standard Mastering Diabetes breakfast of 2 large bananas, 2 cups of papaya, and 1 tablespoon of ground flaxseeds, you would eat 4.0 grams of fat and 6.7 grams of protein. Even though the amount of fat and protein in each individual food is a small number, combining multiple foods together over the course of a 24-hour period results in a larger fat and protein count than most people predict. In addition, notice the difference in fat content of foods like avocado, walnuts, almonds, and edamame in comparison with the other foods in this table. No matter how you combine individual foods, for best results maximize your intake of green light foods and include only small amounts of yellow light foods to stay at or below your daily target.

# Eat All of These Foods to Consume 15 Grams of Fat

5 lb 6 oz
15 g fat

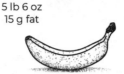

### Apple
6.5 oz
0.3 g fat

### Banana
4 oz
0.4 g fat

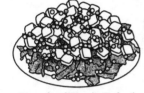

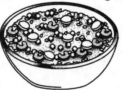

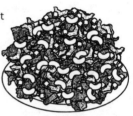

### Tropical Fruit Salad
1 lb 9 oz
9 g fat

### Curried Red Lentils
Over Fluffy Quinoa
1 lb 10 oz
3.8 g fat

### Greens and Beans
1 lb 8 oz
1.8 g fat

——————— **OR Eat One of These Foods Below** ———————

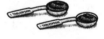

### Olive Oil
1 tbsp
15 g fat

### Sesame Seeds
0.9 oz
15 g fat

### Peanut Butter
1.8 tbsp
15 g fat

### Almonds
1.1 oz
15 g fat

### Coconut Meat
1.6 oz
15 g fat

### Swiss Cheese
1.7 oz
15 g fat

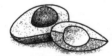

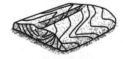

### Avocado
3.5 oz
15 g fat

### Eggs
5 oz
15 g fat

### Salmon
6.5 oz
15 g fat

When controlling your total fat intake to maximize insulin sensitivity, you can either eat a full day's worth of green light foods (top panel) or a single serving of various yellow or red light foods (bottom panel).

| Whole Food | Carbohydrate (grams) | Fat (grams) | Protein (grams) |
|---|---|---|---|
| Banana (large) | 31 | 0.4 | 1.5 |
| Papaya (1 cup) | 28 | 0.7 | 1.2 |
| Butternut squash (1 cup) | 21.5 | 0.2 | 1.8 |
| Sweet potato (large) | 31 | 0.2 | 2.4 |
| Zucchini (1 cup) | 4.6 | 0.5 | 1.8 |
| Tomatoes (1 large) | 7.1 | 0.4 | 1.6 |
| Romaine lettuce (1 cup) | 1.5 | 0.1 | 0.6 |
| Lentils (1 cup) | 40 | 0.8 | 18 |
| Brown rice (1 cup) | 52 | 2.0 | 5.5 |
| Black beans (1 cup) | 41 | 0.9 | 15.2 |
| Quinoa (1 cup) | 34.2 | 3.6 | 8.1 |
| Avocado (medium) | 11.8 | 21 | 2.7 |
| Walnut halves (3 tbsp) | 1.3 | 12.2 | 2.9 |
| Chopped almonds (3 tbsp) | 2.2 | 12.2 | 5.2 |
| Edamame (1 cup) | 5.8 | 8.1 | 18.5 |
| Ground flaxseeds (1 tbsp) | 0.5 | 1.8 | 1.5 |
| Ground chia seeds (1 tbsp) | 0.6 | 1.8 | 1.0 |

## Rule 4: Treat Fruit Like Your New Best Friend

Most people with diabetes are taught to avoid fruit from the moment they're diagnosed. They're told that eating a banana or mango is nutritionally equivalent to a piece of cake—containing nothing but "sugar" and likely to lead to weight gain and worsened health. If you're like millions of people living with diabetes around the world, you may have tried eating fruit, only to see your blood glucose spike.

As we covered in chapter 7 when discussing the ketogenic diet, most people who eat a high-fat diet find that they have excellent blood glucose control most of the time, and experience high blood glucose the moment they eat carbohydrate-rich foods such as fruits, starchy vegetables, legumes, or intact whole grains. From a biological perspective, this makes perfect sense, because the more fat you eat, the less *tolerant* of carbohydrates your muscles and liver become, regardless of whether your dietary fat comes from animal products like meat, cheese, fish, or eggs, or from plants like avocados, nuts, seeds, olive oil, or coconut oil.

**Fruit is not to blame for elevated blood glucose; it's the high-fat foods you ate *before* eating fruit that makes it difficult for your muscles and liver to metabolize glucose effectively.**

Even though fruits have been relentlessly marketed as *simple sugars,* they are in fact complex nutritional packets containing an exceptionally high density of micronutrients, including vitamins, minerals, fiber, water, antioxidants, and phytochemicals. Micronutrients are some of the most powerful components of whole foods, and when you minimize your fruit intake, you limit the opportunity for all the tissues in your body to absorb valuable anti-inflammatory compounds required for optimal physiological function and tissue longevity.

### Your Foolproof Strategy for Increasing Your Fruit Intake Living with Diabetes

Now that you know how beneficial fruits are for your metabolic health, it's time to develop a plan for increasing your fruit intake without spiking your blood glucose. Here's how:

**Step 1:** During your first week on the program, focus on decreasing your total fat intake.

**Step 2:** Simultaneously increase your intake of legumes (beans, lentils, and peas) in *substitution* for the fat-rich foods you previously ate. Legumes are really satisfying, so pay attention to how you feel at each meal. If you feel hungry frequently, then eat larger portions. Aim to have a minimum of 1 to 2 cups of beans, lentils, and/or peas every day for best results. If for any reason you choose not to eat beans, the same effect can be achieved by *adding* (not substituting) non-starchy vegetables or leafy greens to your new calorie-dense meals made of fruit, starchy vegetables, and intact whole grains. Otherwise you are likely to eat an insufficient number of calories and remain very hungry. We'll cover this in more detail in chapter 10.

**Step 3:** After four to seven days, begin increasing your intake of fruit and monitor your two-hour postprandial blood glucose to ensure that it is well controlled. Reducing your total fat intake will maximize your chances of maintaining stable blood glucose while enjoying multiple pieces of fruit per meal.

**Step 4:** Over the course of two to four weeks, steadily increase your intake of fruit to between 5 and 15 servings per day in order to maximize your energy levels and micronutrient intake. We know this is a pretty exciting prescription, but don't be in a rush to increase your fruit intake too quickly—take your time and increase your fruit intake only as your total fat intake plateaus around your daily target.

**Step 5:** Be consistent! Your blood glucose reflects the *consistency* in your approach to food. Do your best to resist "cheat days" or high-fat meals, because they are likely to cause high blood glucose within two to six hours after that meal, especially if that high-fat meal also contains carbohydrate energy. If you do eat a high-fat meal, simply return to eating green light foods as soon as possible and do your best to remain as consistent as possible as your insulin sensitivity increases once again.

## Rule 5: Log Your Food

Creating a daily habit of entering your food into nutrition logging software will pay dividends down the road. Almost without exception, clients who believe they are eating a low-fat diet still discover that their total fat intake is too high to truly maximize their insulin sensitivity, lose weight, gain energy, and minimize or eliminate their need for oral medications and insulin. Nutrition logging software makes your life easy by doing complicated math that would otherwise take you many painstaking hours.

Logging your meals is especially beneficial if you inject fast-acting insulin to manage your blood glucose. In this case, it's important to quantify (but not necessarily limit) the total carbohydrate content of your meals and snacks because that will allow you to accurately predict how much insulin to inject at mealtime.

There are many different online nutrition logging tools available, making it easier than ever to gain insight into the composition of your food. In order to get the most accurate data from your app, it's important that you set your macronutrient targets to approximately 70 to 80 percent of calories from carbohydrates, 10 to 15 percent of calories from fat, and 10 to 15 percent of calories from protein. It's not necessary to hit these values exactly, but consider them guidelines for tracking your food intake.

To analyze your own personal data, view the 24-hour summary to determine if your fat intake is less than 15 percent of total calories or under your target intake in grams. If there are any yellow light or red light foods in your diet, do your best to track those carefully and honestly, because small amounts of those foods can dramatically change your macronutrient profile. It's important to visualize how the information you gather from logging your diet is related to your blood glucose, oral medication, and insulin requirements. By doing so, you can gain tremendous insight into the true impact of the food you eat on your health and use that information to optimize your lifestyle.

## Before You Start, Establish Your Baseline Diet

**We recommend tracking your** pre-program diet for three days in a row so that you can get a rough idea of your baseline food intake prior to beginning the Mastering Diabetes Method. While you might have a general understanding of your diet, visualizing your baseline diet in a food-logging app such as Cronometer will give you even more insight into your blood glucose levels. It will also help you see, in no uncertain terms, the difference between what you were eating before and what you're eating now.

To do this, start with breakfast and include all meals, snacks, and drinks that you have in a day. If you usually eat prepared foods or dine out at restaurants, try entering the brand name or restaurant into the app. Most nutrition-logging software includes hundreds of thousands of name-brand products and restaurant foods, so there's a good chance that you'll find what you're looking for. If not, try to find an item with a similar nutritional profile. Don't worry about entering your sample day perfectly; you are just looking for a bird's-eye view of your baseline diet at this point in the process.

## Understanding Essential Fatty Acids

Understanding the basics of essential fatty acids (EFAs) and fat-soluble vitamins is important and has become unnecessarily confusing over the past twenty years. There are only two EFAs that your body cannot manufacture for itself—alpha-linolenic acid (ALA, omega-3) and linoleic acid (LA, omega-6). ALA and LA are considered *essential* because the human body does not possess the enzymatic machinery to manufacture these two fatty acids, and as a result it's essential to get them from your diet. When you eat ALA and LA, cells in many tissues convert them into longer chain fatty acids that are either anti-inflammatory or pro-inflammatory. Eicosapentaenoic acid (EPA) and docosahexaenoic acid (DHA) are both anti-inflammatory omega-3 fatty acids, whereas arachidonic acid (AA) is a pro-inflammatory omega-6 fatty acid. While the omega-6 pathway produces essential compounds known as *leukotrienes* and *prostaglandins,* which are manufactured in response to injury, persistent activation of the omega-6 pathway induces a state of chronic inflammation, which negatively affects your metabolic health.

As you can probably guess, it's beneficial to increase production of anti-inflammatory compounds and decrease production of pro-inflammatory compounds, and a simple way to do that is to decrease your intake of omega-6 fatty acids and increase your intake of omega-3 fatty acids so that your omega-6 to omega-3 ratio improves. For reference, the standard American diet (SAD) has an omega-6 to omega-3 ratio of approximately 20:1. A better ratio for optimal metabolic health is between 4:1 and 1:1.

There are two primary reasons why eating too many omega-6 EFAs is problematic. The first, as we've pointed out, is that your body converts LA into an omega-6 fatty acid, AA, which is significantly pro-inflammatory. Research shows that excessive omega-6 intake is associated with chronic inflammatory diseases, including fatty liver disease, cardiovascular disease, obesity, inflammatory bowel disease, rheumatoid arthritis, and Alzheimer's disease. The second is that the elongation and desaturation reactions in both the omega-3 and omega-6 pathways use the same set of enzymes, which means that when your omega-6 to omega-3 ratio increases, these enzymes become more active in the omega-6 pathway, likewise increasing the synthesis of the pro-inflammatory compound AA and decreasing the synthesis of anti-inflammatory compounds (EPA and DHA).

Flooding the omega-6 pathway limits the ability of tissues to produce two important omega-3 compounds known as eicosapentaenoic acid (EPA) and docosahexaenoic acid (DHA). EPA has been shown to be effective at preventing and reversing depression, and DHA is critical for optimal brain and eye function. Together, both EPA and DHA promote the formation of new neurons in your brain, improve memory, and may help prevent against dementia and Alzheimer's disease.

It's very important to eat sufficient ALA in order to make sufficient quantities of EPA and DHA. The good news is that this is very easy to do when following the Mastering Diabetes Method, because all whole foods have small amounts of ALA. Men should eat 1.6 grams of ALA per day and women should eat 1.1 grams of ALA per day. To be extra safe, we provide you with an EFA insurance policy—eat one tablespoon of freshly ground flaxseeds (containing 1.6 grams ALA) or one tablespoon of freshly ground chia seeds (containing 2.5 grams ALA) per day to ensure that you have met your omega-3 daily requirement. Do your best to grind them up immediately prior to eating them so that the EFAs are easy to absorb and have the highest chance of increasing your omega-3 status.

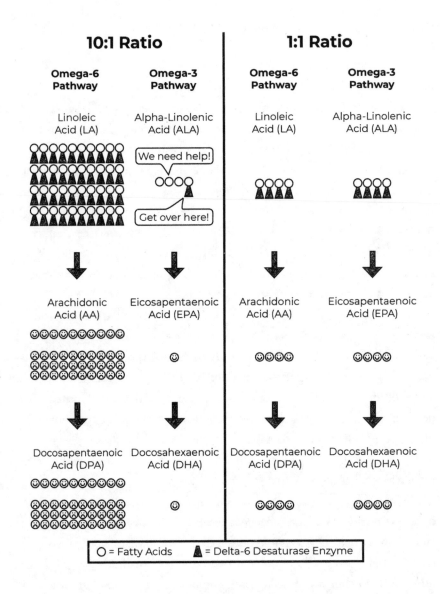

It's optimal to maintain a low omega-3 to omega-6 ratio in order to maximize your insulin sensitivity and reduce your level of total-body inflammation. This is a big reason why we recommend completely eliminating oils in your diet.

## Is Essential Fatty Acid Supplementation Necessary?

EPA and DHA supplementation has been shown to be beneficial for reducing Alzheimer's disease risk; improving language skills, concentration, and motor skills; reducing depressive symptoms; reducing suicidal thoughts and behaviors; reducing schizophrenic symptoms; reducing aggressive impulse behavior; and reducing anxiety. Scientists agree that a healthy fatty acid profile is incredibly important for overall health, and the truth is that eating a low-fat plant-based whole-food diet is a very reliable way to obtain an excellent fatty acid profile for most people.

Obtaining omega-3 EFAs from whole foods is a very effective way to improve your overall fatty acid status, because it solves both problems at once—it decreases your exposure to the inflammatory fatty acid AA (omega-6) and increases your exposure to the anti-inflammatory fatty acids EPA and DHA (omega-3s) simultaneously. Cells in tissues all over your body possess the machinery to convert ALA into EPA and DHA efficiently, but it's your job to ensure that this can happen effectively by decreasing your omega-6 intake.

The scientific literature contains many articles that measure how the EFA status of people improves when they supplement with EPA and DHA. These studies, however, are performed on people with varying omega-6 to omega-3 ratios, not in people who eat a *truly* low-fat plant-based whole-food diet with a more optimal omega-6 to omega-3 ratio. Therefore, the speculation that vegetarians and vegans are unable to convert ALA to EPA and DHA effectively is not well validated by scientific research.

The only way to conclusively know your omega-3 status is to test it routinely. By doing so, you can determine whether your diet is providing you with an optimal fatty acid profile and how your diet is affecting your omega-6 to omega-3 ratio. You can measure your fatty acid profile simply and accurately using an at-home blood test via OmegaQuant.com. By testing your omega-3 status approximately every four months, you'll have the knowledge to optimize your diet with precision and determine whether omega-3 supplementation is necessary in addition to eating one tablespoon of freshly ground flaxseeds or chia seeds per day. If you choose to supplement because your omega-3 status is low, we recommend choosing an algae-based EFA supplement and working with a plant-based physician to determine the proper dose.

---

### Results of an N-of-2 Experiment

Even though we are proponents of large-scale studies, experiments performed with small numbers of people can be very powerful. In 2017 and 2018, we each tested our omega-3 index and were pleased by the results we achieved from following the Mastering Diabetes Method.

| Person | Years Following the Mastering Diabetes Method | Omega-3 Index | Omega-6: Omega-3 Ratio |
|---|---|---|---|
| Robby Barbaro | 11 | 8.28% | 2.2:1 |
| Cyrus Khambatta | 15 | 7.11% | 3.3:1 |

As you can see in the table above, our omega-3 indices were both greater than the 4 percent threshold for excellent health, and our omega-6 to omega-3 ratios were both between the 1:1 and 4:1 ratio as described earlier. We accomplished these values eating only very small amounts of nuts, seeds, and avocados, and without the use of EPA and DHA supplements. Medical professionals have told us that our omega-3 indices are higher than either those who eat significant quantities of nuts and seeds or those who use daily EPA and DHA supplements.

---

## What About Fat-Soluble Vitamins?

Fat-soluble vitamins are a class of vitamins that are essential for optimal tissue function, and include vitamins A, D, E, and K. These vitamins are fat-soluble because they are stored in fatty environments in your body and are more absorbable in a fat-rich environment. Eating green light foods can ensure that your intake of all fat-soluble vitamins meets or exceeds nutritional requirements.

## Vitamin A

Vitamin A plays important roles in cell differentiation, eye health, skin integrity, mucous membranes, bone growth, teeth health, reproduction, and hormone synthesis. There are two forms of vitamin A—preformed vitamin A from animal foods and provitamin A carotenoids from plant foods. Preformed vitamin A has zero antioxidant activity, whereas carotenoid compounds found in plants are potent anti-inflammatory antioxidant pigments that give many fruits and vegetables their characteristic red, orange, and yellow colors.

Plant-based diets can easily provide more than enough vitamin A; there is no need to micromanage your food intake to ensure sufficient vitamin A. Deficiency symptoms such as nighttime blindness are virtually nonexistent in our world today. Eat enough green light foods to meet your calorie needs and you'll be more than covered. With that said, common plant foods with high carotenoid content include apricots, cantaloupes, carrots, mangoes, nectarines, papayas, peppers, persimmons, pumpkins, squash, sweet potatoes, tomatoes, yams, broccoli, turnips, leafy greens, seaweeds, plantains, and prunes. You can exceed your daily requirement for vitamin A by eating 1 baked sweet potato, 1.5 cups of cooked spinach, 1.5 cups of cooked butternut squash, or 1 medium carrot.

## Vitamin D

Vitamin D is required for normal bone growth and remodeling, and a lack of vitamin D can set the stage for osteopenia and osteoporosis. Research has demonstrated the importance of vitamin D for fighting infections and building a strong immune system. In addition, vitamin D deficiency has been linked to impaired glucose metabolism, insulin resistance, an increased risk of developing type 1 diabetes, and an increased risk for developing type 2 diabetes.

The amount of vitamin D necessary for optimal health is a controversial topic, with a lot of conflicting perspectives. In a 2010 report, the Institute of Medicine analyzed over 1,000 studies addressing vitamin D metabolism and found that a 25-OH vitamin D level of 20 ng/ml is sufficient for excellent bone health. Over time, this report has been extensively debated, with many studies and experts suggesting that the optimal vitamin D level is 2.5 to 5 times as high, between 50 ng/ml and 100 ng/ml.

While it has been recognized that obtaining vitamin D from sun exposure is optimal—and studies have shown it's best to expose as much of your body to the sun as possible between the hours of ten A.M. and three P.M., at least three times per week, for fifteen to thirty minutes per session—this often isn't possible or even sufficient for people who live in places that don't get as much sunlight, such as the northern latitudes.

We suggest you maintain a 25-OH vitamin D level of 20 ng/ml or higher. Based on routine lab tests, your health history, and your current state of health, we recommend working together with a plant-based physician to decide how to optimize your vitamin D level using a combination of sun exposure and supplementation if necessary.

## Vitamin E

Vitamin E refers to a group of compounds with potent antioxidant activity that fight free radicals, boost your immune system, and prevent blood clots. Vitamin E donates electrons to neutralize free radicals, and its antioxidant activity can be regenerated in the presence of vitamin C. Foods rich in vitamin E include avocados, broccoli, carrots, kiwis, blackberries, leafy greens, nuts, peanuts, seeds, and intact whole grains. Eating abundant quantities of green light foods is a simple way to ensure that your vitamin E intake meets or exceeds the RDA of 15 mg per day.

## Vitamin K

Vitamin K plays an essential role in blood clotting in response to injury, stimulating bone growth, depositing minerals into bone tissue, and maintaining optimum calcium levels in your blood. The good news is that it's very easy to meet your vitamin K requirements by eating leafy greens including spinach, kale, collard greens, dandelion greens, Swiss chard, turnip greens, and parsley, as well as other plant-based foods like broccoli, Brussels sprouts, cabbage, cauliflower, grapes, kiwis, lentils, pumpkins, and green peas. As little as 2 tablespoons of parsley, 1/8 cup of cooked kale, or 1/4 cup of cooked spinach is sufficient to meet your daily requirement for vitamin K.

### Can You Absorb Enough Fat-Soluble Vitamins?

Now that you know the basic functions of fat-soluble vitamins and how to obtain them from your diet and sun exposure, still an important question remains: Can your body absorb enough fat-soluble vitamins when eating a low-fat plant-based whole-food diet containing a maximum of 15 percent calories from fat?

First, let's review the (flawed) research that makes people believe they have to eat fat-rich foods like avocados, nuts, seeds, coconut meat, or oils in order to absorb fat-soluble vitamins. One study published in the *American Journal of Clinical Nutrition* found that taking a beta-carotene supplement with no food after 12 hours of fasting resulted in no detectable change in beta-carotene levels in the blood. When patients took the same beta-carotene supplement with two-thirds of a pint of almond ice cream containing 200 grams of fat, the amount of beta-carotene in their blood increased 2.5-fold. While it is true that adding fat to a meal increases beta-carotene absorption in comparison with a zero-fat meal, keep in mind that when you eat meals containing green light foods, your fat intake is usually between 3 and 10 grams per meal, which significantly improves the absorption of beta-carotene and other fat-soluble vitamins.

A famous study published by researchers at Ohio State University in 2013 and funded by the California Avocado Commission showed that eating either salsa or a small salad with either avocado or avocado oil enhanced the absorption of alpha-carotene, beta-carotene, lutein, and lycopene, in comparison with low-fat and zero-fat meals. In this study, the first control meal contained a total of zero grams of fat from a fat-free salsa and fat-free bread.

The second control meal contained a small salad with a total of 0.7 grams of fat. In comparison with both control diets, eating avocado or avocado oil significantly enhanced fat-soluble vitamin absorption. However, both control meals contained unrealistically low amounts of fat, making it challenging to interpret their results. Another design flaw of this study was the two-week washout period in which participants were instructed to avoid carotenoid-rich foods, which put the subjects in an unrealistic state of carotenoid deficiency. Without this unrealistic deficiency, which does not apply to those eating a nutrient-dense diet, the results might have been much less dramatic. This type of research is designed to get a specific result to benefit industry and is not applicable to those who maximize their nutrient density with every bite.

Some research suggests that optimal beta-carotene absorption occurs with as little as 5 grams of fat per day in children. Another study in children found that either 2.4 grams of fat per meal or 21 grams of fat per day is sufficient for optimal utilization of vitamin A. Research conducted in adults suggests that eating as little as 3 to 5 grams of fat per meal results in optimal absorption of alpha-carotene, beta-carotene, and vitamin E, and that higher-fat meals improve only lutein absorption. We have worked hard to ensure that meals in the Mastering Diabetes Method contain between 3 and 10 grams of fat, so that you can rest easy knowing that your ability to absorb fat-soluble vitamins has been considered in great detail.

Besides the fact that the naturally occurring fat content in whole plants is more than enough to absorb carotenoids, it's also important to understand that if a particular meal or snack does not have sufficient quantities of fat to absorb carotenoids into chylomicron particles, carotenoids can be temporarily stored in epithelial cells until an adequate amount of fat present in a subsequent meal becomes available.

Research has identified at least nine different factors that affect the absorption of carotenoids. The mnemonic SLAMENGHI describes these factors: species of carotenoids, linkages at molecular level, amount of carotenoid, matrix, effectors, nutrient status, genetics, host-related factors, and interactions among these variables. As you may predict, the absorption of carotenoid compounds from your diet is incredibly complex and depends on a number of factors that scientists may never fully understand. Despite this, the research suggests that the naturally occurring fat in whole-plant foods is adequate for the optimal absorption of carotenoids, and this can easily be obtained on a low-fat plant-based whole-food diet. If you are concerned with your fat-soluble vitamin status, we suggest asking your doctor for routine blood tests.

## Vitamin B$_{12}$

B$_{12}$ is a water-soluble vitamin that is necessary for the formation of red blood cells, neurological function, and DNA synthesis. Symptoms of B$_{12}$ deficiency include anemia, peripheral neuropathy, concentration loss, memory loss, insomnia, impaired bowel and bladder control, appetite loss, flatulence, and constipation.

If your vitamin B$_{12}$ level drops, then two other compounds begin to rise in your blood—methylmalonic acid (MMA) and homocysteine (HC). It is possible to have a normal vitamin B$_{12}$ level but still have elevated MMA and HC, but this condition is quite rare. For these reasons, measuring both MMA and HC can help detect early vitamin B$_{12}$ deficiency. If you are experiencing any of the symptoms listed above, we recommend working with your physician to have your vitamin B$_{12}$, MMA, and HC levels tested. All three values will provide information that you and your physician can use to decide the best course of action.

Here's the problem: You don't make vitamin B$_{12}$. Animals don't make it either. Vitamin B$_{12}$ is made by bacteria found in the soil, which accumulates in land-grazing animals that eat grass and plants close to the ground. When you eat animal products, you receive vitamin B$_{12}$ from them, even though they received it from soil-borne bacteria in the first place. Now that you understand why minimizing or avoiding animal products optimizes your insulin sensitivity and reduces your risk for a wide range of chronic diseases, supplementing vitamin B$_{12}$ becomes necessary when eating a plant-based diet.

While you can get some $B_{12}$ from foods such as brewer's yeast and nutritional yeast (which is a green light condiment, by the way), we still recommend taking a supplement. Just about any oral supplement will work because all forms are broken down into cobalamin, which your body then converts into active forms in tissues. Your body requires between 4 and 7 micrograms of vitamin $B_{12}$ per day, and is capable of absorbing only about 1.5 and 2 micrograms at any given time. The good news is that about 1 percent of vitamin $B_{12}$ is passively absorbed into your blood, which means that you can easily meet your vitamin $B_{12}$ requirement by supplementing with a single 2,500-microgram dose once per week. We personally use a liquid vitamin $B_{12}$ containing 2,500 micrograms (mcg) of methylcobalamin and adenosylcobalamin per day.

## Focus on the Big Picture

When you are beginning to change your diet, it can be easy to get lost in the details, study graphs, analyze tables of micronutrient data, and worry about becoming deficient in omega-3 EFAs and fat-soluble vitamins. Instead, we encourage you to focus mainly on your macronutrient intake and don't let the details of your micronutrients get in the way. Eat as many of the green light foods as possible, limit your intake of yellow light foods, and avoid red light foods to the best of your ability. Start slowly and improve your nutrition habits every day by making small and sustainable changes.

Micromanaging your intake of vitamins, minerals, antioxidants, and phytochemicals can be exhausting, and the truth is that scientists are only scratching the surface when it comes to understanding the complex interactions between the human body and nutrients in food. Don't forget, your body is composed of trillions of cells performing thousands of metabolic reactions every second of every day, and getting lost in the details of a few specific reactions may actually get in the way of making substantial progress. So instead focus on the big picture and allow your body to do what it does best: metabolize the most nutrient-dense high-quality ingredients that nature has to offer.

## How to Find a Plant-Based Doctor

If your doctor is not supportive of your choice to follow the Mastering Diabetes Method, then we strongly recommend finding a physician who is. In order to do this, you can search for a plant-based doctor online using the resources listed on our website (www.masteringdiabetes.org/bookresources/). When choosing a doctor, ask whether they require in-person appointments, or whether they are licensed to practice telemedicine using videoconferencing (a great option that reduces the amount of time you spend commuting to their office). We work closely with a number of trusted plant-based physicians who can help you either in person or via the internet.

## Take-Home Messages

- The speed at which you transition to a low-fat plant-based whole-food diet is less important than developing sustainable daily habits and becoming as consistent as possible.
- Before beginning the program, take some time to write down your *why* so that you become crystal clear on what you are trying to achieve.
- Before beginning the program, log your diet for three days to get a clear picture of your baseline food intake.
- For best results, eat green light foods in abundance (including fruit!), limit your intake of yellow light foods, and do your best to completely eliminate red light foods from your diet (especially animal products and oils!).
- All whole foods contain carbohydrate, protein, and fat, without exception.
- We recommend eating 1 tablespoon of freshly ground flaxseeds or chia seeds per day to ensure that you are meeting your omega-3 EFA requirements.
- The Mastering Diabetes Method is likely to reduce your omega-6 to omega-3 ratio to between 4:1 and 1:1, to reduce chronic inflammation and increase your production of EPA and DHA.

- To maximize your vitamin D status, expose as much of your body to the sun as possible between the hours of ten A.M. and three P.M., at least three times per week, for fifteen to thirty minutes per session. Work with a plant-based physician to determine if supplementation is necessary.
- Eating a wide variety of green light foods provides sufficient dietary fat to efficiently absorb fat-soluble vitamins from your food.
- Working with a doctor who supports a plant-based diet will increase your chances of success.

To view the 85+ scientific references cited in this chapter, please visit us online at www.masteringdiabetes.org/bookinfo.

# Chapter 9

# Getting to Know Your New Needs: Diagnostic Blood Tests and Managing Oral Medications

## Reversing 57 Years of Diabetes Complications in 3 Months: Chris

Chris was diagnosed with type 1 diabetes when he was 2 years old. Having received his diagnosis in the early 1960s, he has since witnessed the evolution of blood glucose testing meters, syringes and needles, insulin, insulin pumps, and continuous glucose monitors. Despite advances in diabetes technology, one thing that never changed was the food that he was told to put in his mouth. For 57 years, Chris followed his medical team's advice to eat a low-carbohydrate diet that was high in protein and fat. But when he watched a video featuring the Mastering Diabetes team and learned about the presence of insulin resistance in people with type 1 diabetes, he felt that that could finally explain the diabetes complications he had been experiencing for years, including atherosclerosis, hypertension, high cholesterol, rheumatoid arthritis, neuropathy, retinopathy, and erectile dysfunction, in addition to being overweight. Chris had been prescribed a total of twelve medications to treat these conditions and suffered from both the symptoms of each condition and the side effects of taking multiple oral medications for many years. To make matters worse, despite eating a low-carbohydrate diet, he had an A1c a littler higher than his target 6.5%.

Within a day of watching this video, Chris began following the Mastering Diabetes Method, hopeful that his diabetes health would begin to improve. Chris began to notice rapid decreases in his need for insulin, so he reduced his basal and bolus injections to prevent hypoglycemia. Soon he began feeling more energy and was able to exercise for significantly longer periods of time.

Over the course of ten months, Chris changed his life completely. He lost a total of 76 pounds, he cut his basal and bolus insulin use by 50 percent, he dropped his A1c from 6.5% to 4.9%, his blood pressure is 118/68, and his total cholesterol is 108 mg/dL. With the help of his doctor, he stopped taking eleven medications (at this point using only insulin) and no longer suffers from hypertension, high cholesterol, atherosclerosis, neuropathy, retinopathy, erectile dysfunction, or rheumatoid arthritis.

Chris was able to reverse multiple chronic diseases by focusing on the *root cause* of chronic inflammation in his body—insulin resistance. He didn't even know that these multiple conditions were connected to one another, but by maximizing his insulin sensitivity by using his food as medicine, he not only improved his health in relation to diabetes but was also able to reverse multiple chronic diseases (including rheumatoid arthritis, which is considered "incurable"). He considers himself a completely new man!

---

By now we hope you have a good sense of the philosophy and effectiveness of the Mastering Diabetes Method and are ready to significantly improve your health while living with any form of diabetes. For most people, applying the principles outlined in this book provides tremendous benefits, but for some people, producing insufficient insulin prevents improved blood glucose control. One of the main reasons for this difference is that the latter group has been mistakenly diagnosed with the wrong form of diabetes and therefore has been prescribed ineffective (and often unnecessary) medications. In this chapter, we'll teach you how to become more confident in identifying the *exact* form of diabetes you're living with, give you insight into how various oral and injectable diabetes medications work, and equip you with the tools to become confident in reducing your use of all diabetes medications as you gain insulin sensitivity. We suggest familiarizing yourself with this information and then teaming up with your healthcare provider to effectively and *safely* make any changes to your lifestyle and medication regimen.

## Diagnostic Blood Tests

When you are attempting to maximize your insulin sensitivity, we strongly recommend measuring multiple biomarkers routinely in order to get a more complete picture of your overall metabolic health. Your A1c value is important, but it is an incomplete indicator of your diabetes health when interpreted in isolation. Simply remember the mnemonic PILAF, which describes five important biomarkers that you can use to monitor your metabolic health. These biomarkers are listed in the following table, along with reference ranges and the frequency with which we recommend measuring each. To learn more about how to track your level of insulin resistance over time, visit the Insulin Resistance Checklist at www.masteringdiabetes.org/bookresources/. You will be able to download a handy PDF to help you track the biomarkers listed.

| Biomarker | Reference Range | Recommended Frequency |
|---|---|---|
| P: Blood Pressure | 120/80 mmHg or less | **If you are hypertensive:** Daily <br> **If you are not hypertensive:** Every 6 to 12 months |
| I: Ideal Body Weight | **Women:** 105 + 4 pounds per inch over 5 feet of height <br> **Men:** 115 + 5 pounds per inch over 5 feet of height | Between once per week and once per month |
| L: Lipid Panel | **Total Cholesterol:** Less than 150 mg/dL <br> **LDL Cholesterol:** Less than 100 mg/dL <br> **Triglycerides:** Less than 150 mg/dL <br> **HDL Cholesterol:** 40 mg/dL or greater (men) <br> 50 mg/dL or greater (women) | Every 3 months |
| A: A1c | **Non-Insulin-Dependent:** 5.6% or less <br> **Insulin-Dependent:** 5.5-6.5% | Every 3 months |
| F: Fasting Blood Glucose | **Non-Insulin-Dependent:** 80-100 mg/dL <br> **Insulin-Dependent:** 80-99 mg/dL | Daily |

If you have been diagnosed with prediabetes or type 2 diabetes and are unable to control your blood glucose after 1 to 3 months following our recommendations, we suggest getting two blood tests, which give you and your doctor a much clearer picture of what's going on in your body. These include the C-peptide blood test and the diabetes antibody panel.

## C-peptide Blood Test

The C-peptide test is one of the most important diabetes blood tests, and it's a test that many physicians are not trained to administer upon initial diagnosis. A C-peptide test indicates how much endogenous (self-produced) insulin your beta cells are capable of making in order to control your blood glucose. Although it is possible for medical professionals to make an accurate educated guess about what type of diabetes you are living with without directly measuring your C-peptide value, having a quantitative indicator of how much insulin your beta cells are able to manufacture and secrete into your blood gives you and your doctor tremendous insight into your diabetes health.

In fact, the C-peptide test is so important, it can determine the entire course of your diabetes treatment and allow you to understand whether lifestyle change is enough to fully transform your diabetes health or whether it's necessary to use oral medication or insulin to help control your blood glucose in addition to lifestyle change. Researchers believe it to be the most suitable measurement for assessing your endogenous insulin secretion. Since type 1 diabetes, type 1.5 diabetes, type 2 diabetes, prediabetes, and gestational diabetes each requires a different treatment plan, being diagnosed with the correct type of diabetes can completely alter the course of your treatment and save you years of frustration and thousands of dollars.

The range of fasting C-peptide varies between labs, but the reference range is usually between 0.8 and 4.0 ng/mL. If your fasting C-peptide value exceeds 4.0, this can indicate that the beta cells in your pancreas are working in overdrive to secrete excess insulin in response to a high degree of insulin resistance, and that increasing your insulin sensitivity can prevent against beta cell burnout. A fasting C-peptide value of between 3.0 and 4.0 ng/mL indicates that your beta cells are capable of manufacturing sufficient insulin, and that it's possible to completely reverse insulin resistance and eliminate your need for diabetes medications by maximizing your insulin sensitivity. A fasting C-peptide value of between 1.5 and 3.0 ng/mL indicates that you likely have adequate insulin production to fully reverse prediabetes or type 2 diabetes, but that it's imperative to maximize your insulin sensitivity in order to prevent beta cells from becoming exhausted over time. A fasting C-peptide value of less than 1.5 ng/mL means that your beta cells have been significantly impaired. We have found that most people in this category eventually require insulin to control their blood glucose.

Although optimal beta cell function may never be completely restored, adopting the Mastering Diabetes Method is one of the most powerful things you can do to prevent further damage and even restore beta cell function. For more information about C-peptide and antibody testing and how to interpret your results, see Appendix A.

## Diabetes Antibody Panel

The second blood test that provides useful information about the type of diabetes you are living with is called a *diabetes antibody panel*. This series of tests will help you determine whether you are living with an autoimmune form of diabetes (type 1 or type 1.5) or a lifestyle-related form of diabetes (type 2 diabetes, prediabetes, or gestational diabetes). The diabetes antibody panel measures whether your immune system is actively manufacturing proteins called *antibodies* (also called *autoantibodies*) that target beta cells for destruction or that target insulin itself. There are five antibodies that are mainly responsible for the destruction of beta cells and insulin, listed in the table below.

| Antibody Name | Abbreviation(s) | Function |
|---|---|---|
| Glutamic acid decarboxylase | GAD, GADD, GADA, GAD-65 | Targets a specific enzyme in pancreatic beta cells |
| Islet cell antibody | ICA | Targets specific proteins in pancreatic beta cells |
| Insulin antibody | IAA | Targets insulin |
| Islet antigen-2, insulinoma-2 associated antibody | IA-2A | Targets a specific protein in pancreatic beta cells |
| Zinc transporter antibody | Zn-T8A | Targets a specific protein in pancreatic beta cells |

Even though these antibodies each have different targets, testing positive for at least one of these antibodies is a strong indicator that you may be living with a form of autoimmune diabetes, either type 1 or type 1.5 diabetes. One notable exception is the GAD antibody—some people test positive but do not display any symptoms of blood glucose instability or autoimmune diabetes.

Type 1 diabetes generally occurs in individuals younger than 30 years of age who test positive for one or more antibodies and have a fasting C-peptide of 0.2 nmol/L or less. The majority of people diagnosed with type 1 diabetes experience a state called *diabetic ketoacidosis* (DKA), characterized by extremely high blood glucose values (greater than 300 mg/dL), excessive thirst, unexplained weight loss, frequent urination, muscle cramping, and low energy. Because type 1 diabetes is caused by the autoimmune destruction of beta cells or insulin, usually due to multiple antibodies, people diagnosed with type 1 diabetes often transition to full insulin dependence within twelve to eighteen months after diagnosis. This is considered a fast-progressing, strong autoimmune reaction.

Type 1.5 diabetes, also known as latent autoimmune diabetes in adults (LADA), generally occurs in individuals older than 30 years of age who test positive for only one antibody and have a fasting C-peptide above 0.2 nmol/L. Even though this classification is less known, researchers believe that type 1.5 diabetes affects more people than type 1 diabetes around the world. Think of LADA as an adult-onset slow-progressing version of type 1 diabetes in which your pancreas is still capable of manufacturing and secreting insulin, but the presence of one antibody (in most cases) leads to a slow decline in insulin production. Unlike people living with type 1 diabetes who progress to full insulin dependence very quickly, people living with type 1.5 diabetes may transition to full insulin dependence over the course of five to ten years or may never become fully insulin dependent at all.

As the name implies, type 1.5 diabetes has characteristics of both type 1 and type 2 diabetes and is often misdiagnosed as type 2 diabetes. As a result, many people living with type 1.5 diabetes are treated with ineffective oral medications to control their blood glucose even though the most effective course of treatment involves the use of basal and/or bolus insulin to substitute for insufficient endogenous insulin production. Type 1.5 diabetes is also common in patients diagnosed with type 2 diabetes who are lean and do not have the metabolic syndrome (high blood pressure, high cholesterol or triglycerides, and excess fat around their waist), especially if they eat well and are physically active.

# Understanding the Ins and Outs of Diabetes Medications

As you begin to follow the Mastering Diabetes Method and gain insulin sensitivity, you'll likely notice that your basal and bolus insulin needs may drop quickly. That's why we want you to be prepared to calculate your new insulin needs so that you don't over-inject insulin and experience low blood glucose. As you make changes to your diet, remember to keep one thing in mind:

**As you reverse insulin resistance using your food as medicine, your blood glucose may fluctuate. Focus on your overall blood glucose trend rather than micromanaging individual blood glucose values.**

The truth is that managing your blood glucose while transitioning to a low-fat plant-based whole-food diet is often quite straightforward, but at times it can become confusing and noisy. We both live with insulin-dependent diabetes, and we use basal and bolus insulin to manage our blood glucose in combination with impeccable nutrition habits. When the going gets tough, just remember that your body weight, energy levels, blood glucose, cholesterol levels, blood pressure, exercise tolerance, digestive health, skin condition, and mental clarity are changing simultaneously *because* you are improving your insulin sensitivity. Do your best to pay attention to each of these variables without losing sight of the bigger picture. Set yourself up for long-term success and observe the day-to-day changes, but make sure to keep your long-term vision in full focus.

## Monitor Your Blood Glucose Patterns Like the Stock Market

**A simple way to** think about this transition process is to visualize how the stock market moves. Rather than watch hour-by-hour or even day-to-day fluctuations in price, monitoring the overall trend over the course of weeks, months, and years helps you understand how your investments are changing over time. Some people choose to be day traders, buying and selling securities quickly, which comes with more stress and the need to watch the market constantly. This is not the approach we recommend when it comes to making significant lifestyle changes. While it's true that people living with insulin-dependent diabetes generally benefit from watching their blood glucose on an hour-by-hour basis, people living with non-insulin-dependent diabetes can take a more relaxed bird's-eye-view approach. Regardless of the type of diabetes you are living with, monitoring your overall blood glucose patterns is a powerful practice that will help you relax the need to micromanage your readings 24 hours a day. It will also allow you to see how your lifestyle changes are making a true difference in your overall health.

## Calculating Your New Basal Insulin Needs (Insulin-Dependent Diabetes)

Within the first few days of the program, and certainly within the first few months, your basal insulin needs are likely to drop between 10 and 60 percent. The most accurate way to recalculate your basal insulin needs is to perform a series of 24-hour intermittent fasts. We recognize that the prospect of not eating for 24 hours may feel daunting, but if you want to optimize your blood glucose control, understanding your basal insulin injection dose (if you use syringes or pens) or your basal rate (if you use an insulin pump) is absolutely essential.

## Pro Tip: Adjust Your
## Basal Insulin Strategy Early!

**When people first start** observing lower blood glucose values, they often begin adjusting their mealtime carbohydrate-to-insulin ratios without first reducing their basal insulin. Our approach is different. We suggest making changes to your basal insulin strategy within the first few weeks of the program in addition to changing your bolus insulin strategy.

We have found that those who adjust their basal insulin strategy early in this process are able to prevent their blood glucose from becoming dangerously low. You will likely want to adjust your basal and bolus strategies frequently, and this ongoing balancing act may last for many weeks or months, depending on how your body responds. That's okay, because this process is still the most efficient method to keep your blood glucose under control in the beginning stages of your transition, when you are likely to experience the most rapid change in your insulin sensitivity.

We will discuss intermittent fasting in much more detail in chapter 13—including how to find the most ideal fasting option for you—but here are our basic recommendations for performing a 24-hour intermittent fast to adjust your basal insulin strategy:

- Start your 24-hour fast at least 3 hours after the last time you injected bolus insulin. We actually recommend starting your 24-hour fast in the evening after you have eaten dinner to avoid low blood glucose values while sleeping. It's also wise to plan for when you are less active, since you will need to wake up several times during the night.
- Begin your intermittent fast only if your blood glucose is between 80 and 130 mg/dL.
- Check and record your blood glucose every 2 hours using the decision tree during the day, and approximately every 3 hours during the night. (See pages 197–200.) Yes, we recommend setting multiple alarms to record accurate data.

- We recommend avoiding exercise during your 24-hour fast in order to prevent exercise-induced hypoglycemia that may confuse your basal injection strategy.
- Postpone your 24-hour fast if you are sick or stressed because you may end up with erroneous measurements resulting from adrenaline, cortisol, or a compromised immune system.
- For menstruating women, if you know your period is approaching, be aware that your basal rate may be significantly higher in the days leading up to the beginning of your period. For most women, this window is short and begins about 3 days before their period begins and can last up to 3 days after their period starts. We recommend tracking your menstrual cycles carefully to know when to expect a higher degree of insulin resistance so that you can adjust your basal and bolus settings accordingly.

## Troubleshooting Your "Basal Testing" Intermittent Fast (Insulin-Dependent Diabetes)

- You will know that your basal injection strategy is set properly when your blood glucose stays between approximately 80 and 130 mg/dL (4.2–6.8 mmol) for the entire 24-hour period. If your blood glucose climbs above this range, record the value and continue the fast. If your blood glucose increases beyond 250 mg/dL and you use fast-acting insulin, consider stopping the fast and correcting your high blood glucose. If you don't use fast-acting insulin, continue your fast until 24 hours are complete.
- If your blood glucose drops below this range, eat approximately 15 grams of carbohydrate, record the value, and discontinue your fast for the day. This is an indication that your basal insulin is too high, and continuing fasting could lead to more hypoglycemic events.
- If you are using an insulin pump, we suggest establishing a *maximum* of two or three basal rates. Many people using insulin

pumps often have between four and ten programmed basal rates to cover a 24-hour period, which can significantly complicate your blood glucose control.

## How to Calculate Your New Bolus Insulin Needs (Insulin-Dependent Diabetes)

Mastering your bolus insulin strategy is an exciting game when you are able to eat more carbohydrate-rich foods using less fast-acting insulin. There are many variables that control how much bolus insulin you'll need at any moment in time, including the amount of exercise you performed recently, your current stress level, (for women) your menstrual cycle, the injection site you choose to use, deliverability issues with your insulin pump, your insulin timing strategy, the altitude of your current location, and the macronutrient content of your diet, to name a few. Understanding the effect of each of these variables can be challenging, but who doesn't love a good challenge?

As we'll discuss more in the next chapter, we recommend that you change your habits over a period of three to six weeks (one to two weeks per meal—breakfast, lunch, and dinner). This means that during the transition, your fat intake will likely remain above our recommended guidelines at first, but will decrease as you integrate more green light meals. Getting into the habit of using the steps below during your transition is going to make it much easier to optimize your bolus dosing strategy down the road. To calculate your new bolus insulin needs, follow this simple strategy:

**Step 1:** Become very good at counting your carbohydrate intake. Do your best to assess how many grams of carbohydrates you are eating at every meal so that you can carefully monitor how much insulin is required. A simple method of doing this is to eat *go-to meals,* meals containing a known amount of carbohydrate energy that you can eat repeatedly to test your bolus insulin needs. Do your best to make your go-to meals thoroughly enjoyable, simple to prepare, and very satisfying. See chapter 15 for some of our favorite recipes and meal suggestions.

**Step 2:** Fill out a decision tree *every day*. In the next section, we'll teach you how to use a decision tree to record and interpret important information, which is designed to teach you the cause-and-effect relationship between your carbohydrate intake, fat intake, exercise, insulin dosing, and blood glucose values.

## The Decision Tree

Most people don't enjoy writing down how much food they have eaten, what they have eaten, what their blood glucose values are, how much medication they took, how much insulin they injected, or how much exercise they performed. Why? Because it's time-consuming. Because it's easy to forget. Because it's inconvenient.

We completely understand this because we used to take painstakingly detailed notes ourselves, and it *was* very time-consuming. The reason we were so detail oriented at the beginning of the process was because the mere act of documenting diabetes decisions significantly improved our chances of learning from our experiences. In fact, we took notes for years, scribbling down every last detail that could help piece together a complex picture with many moving parts. And what we both found (independently of each other) is that the more we wrote, the more we learned, and the more we learned, the less we needed to write.

So, in the spirit of learning how your glucose metabolism relates to your new daily habits, we created our decision tree to simplify the process of tracking many variables in a single location. It will enable you to make moment-by-moment decisions that improve your blood glucose control using relevant information. The decision tree is specifically designed to help you understand how to reduce your basal and bolus insulin in real time, how to reduce your oral medications (with the help of your doctor), and how to keep your blood glucose in range as you rapidly gain insulin sensitivity during your transition.

We recommend that you fill out a new decision tree every day to document each of your daily activities in chronological order. See Appendix C for sample completed decision trees, and visit our website to download and print copies of the decision tree (www.masteringdiabetes.org/bookresources/). Every day make new entries for each of the following activities:

- Blood glucose measurements
- Consumption of a meal or snack
- Oral medication or other injectable medications
- Basal insulin injections
- Bolus insulin injections
- Feelings of hunger or satiety
- Exercise

Every time you eat, do your best to be as descriptive as possible about what you had and how much. Refrain from writing things like "I ate lunch," and instead write detailed entries like *Lunch: 1 sweet potato, ½ cup quinoa, 2 medium tomatoes, 1 cup of steamed broccoli.* The more descriptive you are, the easier it will be to troubleshoot your blood glucose when it comes time to analyze your decision trees. When you eat a meal, use nutrition logging software to document the carbohydrate and fat content (in grams) to understand how your food choices are affecting your insulin sensitivity.

## The Decision Tree for Insulin-Dependent Diabetes

The goal of using the decision tree is to fully understand how much basal and bolus insulin to use every day. In this way you can become an intuitive eater and feel confident in dosing insulin with precision while keeping your blood glucose under control. Most important, the decision tree is the tool that allows you to understand how to reduce your insulin use to minimize your risk for hypoglycemia.

One of the reasons why the decision tree is so valuable for those with insulin-dependent diabetes is because it enables you to make predictions about how much insulin to inject based on your previous records, and then check whether that prediction was correct after your meal. The decision tree is designed to help you recognize patterns in your blood glucose and understand how your food, medication use, and exercise are affecting your blood glucose control. Think of it as a *metabolic guess-and-check* that you can use to make moment-by-moment decisions that will ultimately improve your blood glucose control as you begin to recognize repeating patterns.

## The Decision Tree for Non-Insulin-Dependent Diabetes

For those living with non-insulin-dependent diabetes, use the decision tree to help you understand how the Mastering Diabetes Method is affecting your insulin sensitivity. The decision tree will provide you with insight into how your oral medication, injectable medication, food, movement patterns, and stress levels are influencing your blood glucose. Having this information at your fingertips is truly eye-opening and can provide you with insight into blood glucose patterns that may have been previously invisible.

## How Long Is It Necessary to Use a Decision Tree?

We have been following the Mastering Diabetes Method for a combined total of twenty-nine years, and we have filled out hundreds of decision trees over the course of time. We understand that the process of documenting every decision throughout the day can be time-consuming and tedious, but the value of the information far outweighs the effort it takes to complete.

We strongly encourage you to use the decision tree to learn as much as you can. In the beginning of the process of changing your lifestyle, recording daily events is incredibly important because it allows you to see the cause-and-effect relationship between seemingly confusing variables. We suggest filling out a decision tree every day for the first twenty-eight days when you begin the program so that you can fully understand how your insulin sensitivity is changing. After that, use decision trees as you see fit, whenever you're keen to learn more information about what's affecting your blood glucose control, body weight, digestion, or energy levels.

For those living with insulin-dependent diabetes, decision trees will help you become confident in your insulin dosing strategy and will enable you to make real-time adjustments smoothly and predictably. For those living with non-insulin-dependent diabetes, decision trees will help you become less reliant on pharmaceutical medication, teach you how to predictably reduce your A1c to a nondiabetic level of 5.6% or below, and maximize your chances of fully reversing insulin resistance.

Filling out decision trees is an involved process and an activity that takes time to develop a clear picture of your blood glucose patterns. Despite this, it is a necessary first step in achieving *full* control of an otherwise elusive and confusing process. We have found that people who don't fill out decision trees consistently at the beginning of their transition find themselves confused and frustrated with various aspects of their blood glucose control. In these situations, we always suggest documenting hour-by-hour decisions, which inevitably helps you uncover the cause(s) of confusing blood glucose patterns, usually within a few days. To see sample decision trees for both insulin-dependent diabetes and non-insulin-dependent diabetes, refer to Appendix C.

## Bolus Insulin Timing

If you are using bolus insulin to manage your blood glucose, learning how to properly time your insulin injections is a game-changer and one of the most important lessons in the Mastering Diabetes Method. In order to eat a meal or snack of carbohydrate-rich foods, we recommend that your blood glucose be below 120 mg/dL and trending down.

The glucose from carbohydrate-rich foods can enter your blood quickly, so it's important that insulin is already in your blood and ready to act at the time you begin eating. This is particularly important to know because *rapid-acting insulin does not work immediately after it is injected*. Rapid-acting insulins usually take between 15 and 60 minutes to begin working, and the more insulin resistant you are, the longer it will take for insulin to begin lowering your blood glucose. Eating immediately after injecting insulin can be problematic, so do your best to ensure that your blood glucose is less than 120 mg/dL and trending down before digging into your meal.

In some cases, your blood glucose may be trending up before you want to eat a meal. When this happens, our most successful clients take their time, calculate the amount of insulin they predict will be appropriate, inject insulin, and wait to eat their meal. Let's run through a simple example:

9:00 A.M.—Your blood glucose is 120 mg/dL. You inject 5 units to eat your breakfast meal.

9:15 A.M.—Your blood glucose is 140 mg/dL and has risen over the past 15 minutes.

9:30 A.M.—Your blood glucose is 130 mg/dL and is now on a downward trend.

9:45 A.M.—Your blood glucose is 107 mg/dL and continuing on a downward trend. Time to start eating breakfast!

In this example, your blood glucose was trending up at the time you injected insulin, and 15 minutes later had increased by 20 mg/dL. Because you waited another 30 minutes, your blood glucose eventually dropped below 120 mg/dL, at which point it was smart to begin eating. Depending on how high your glucose climbs before you eat, you may consider adding a correction bolus to ensure that you have enough insulin to drop your blood glucose and fully metabolize your upcoming meal.

It's also important to note that continuous glucose monitor (CGM) data is delayed by approximately 15 minutes. If you waited until your CGM read "120 mg/dL and trending down," you may be on your way to a low blood glucose value. As you become more in tune with your body, you'll know how long to wait before eating and won't require additional finger sticks to know if you have timed your insulin injection properly. With that said, we cannot overemphasize the importance of checking your blood glucose frequently at the beginning of your transition to gain firsthand experience managing your insulin timing strategy.

Improper insulin timing is a common practice that frustrates insulin-dependent individuals. Many people eat a high-carbohydrate meal immediately after injecting insulin and get frustrated when their blood glucose rapidly increases. Properly timing your insulin dosing and systematically checking your blood glucose can help you prevent this problem and enable you to control your blood glucose with precision.

---

# An Overview of Oral and Injectable Diabetes Medications

Controlling your blood glucose using oral medications is usually the first line of defense after you have been diagnosed with non-insulin-dependent diabetes. As you know, we suggest using your food as medicine first and resorting to pharmaceutical medication only if your new lifestyle requires more assistance. Understanding exactly what physiological mechanisms pharmaceutical medications are designed to alter can have a tremendous impact on your diabetes health. If you are already taking oral medications for diabetes or other chronic conditions, we recommend that you continue your treatment as prescribed and work closely with your physician to adjust your medication strategy as your health improves.

Every year, it seems as though the list of "state-of-the-art" medications to treat conditions like diabetes, high blood pressure, high cholesterol, rheumatoid arthritis, fibromyalgia, and chronic kidney disease gets longer. In addition, recalls and "black box" warnings alert the public of dangerous side effects. Prime-time television is littered with commercials featuring chronic disease sufferers playing tennis, rowing canoes, running through the sprinklers with their grandkids, and shopping for groceries, urging you to "ask your doctor if [medication name] is right for you" before the list of common side effects is intoned: "nausea, constipation, diarrhea, genital yeast infections, bone fractures, high cholesterol, urinary tract infections, swelling, difficulty breathing or swallowing, allergic reactions, joint and muscle pain or weakness, rash, hives, upper respiratory infections, sore throat, headache, stomach pain, pancreatitis, ketoacidosis, or death."

Oftentimes the side effects of pharmaceutical medications are more severe than the condition they're attempting to control, which makes the cost-benefit analysis not work in your favor. What's worse is that doctors who treat chronic diseases rely heavily upon pharmaceutical medications instead of on lifestyle change. Again, doctors are not to blame for their lack of education about the power of lifestyle change in reversing and not simply managing conditions like diabetes. Instead, many doctors have been educated about how to use pharmaceutical medications as their primary strategy, with a general suggestion to improve diet and exercise.

**Pharmaceutical companies spend billions of dollars every year designing medications that improve your laboratory blood work but don't reverse the underlying physiological mechanisms that cause insulin resistance and chronic disease.**

In this section, we'll explain the actions and side effects of commonly prescribed diabetes medications so that you stay informed of their actual function in your body. The medications below are listed in order of their risk for causing hypoglycemia during your transition.

### Bolus Insulin

Bolus insulin, also known as *rapid-acting* or *short-acting* insulin, is designed to be injected before you eat food in order to control the blood glucose elevation that occurs after your meal. Depending on the exact brand name, bolus insulin begins working in your blood within 10 to 60 minutes after you inject, and directly interacts with all tissues in your body to help transport glucose out of your blood.

Bolus insulin is extremely effective at reducing your blood glucose and is considerably more powerful than basal insulin. It is therefore imperative to accurately measure your carbohydrate-to-insulin ratios at breakfast, lunch, and dinner so that you know the exact amount to inject in order to prevent both high and low blood glucose in the hours following a meal.

**Commonly prescribed brand names:** Humalog, NovoLog, Apidra

**Side effects:** The most notable side effects of bolus insulin therapy include mild or severe hypoglycemia. Mild hypoglycemia results in weakness, sweating, tremors, slurred speech, trouble concentrating, rapid heartbeat, fainting, and increased appetite, and severe hypoglycemia results in seizure or death. Some people are allergic to specific formulations of insulin, causing skin inflammation and itchiness.

## Basal Insulin

Basal insulin is also called background insulin or long-acting insulin. Basal insulin can be delivered via a drip feed with an insulin pump or injected once or twice per day via syringe or pen. Injections of basal insulin are designed to act over a period of 16 to 24 hours.

Beta cells continually secrete small amounts of insulin in order to keep your blood glucose controlled at all times, and basal insulin is designed to mimic this action. Basal insulin is required only in patients with a low C-peptide level, as a result of damage to beta cells (prediabetes and type 2 diabetes) or autoimmune destruction of beta cells (type 1 and type 1.5 diabetes).

Your insulin pump uses only one type of insulin, and it's usually fast-acting or rapid-acting insulin. Your pump has two functions: (1) to drip feed basal insulin to mimic the basal action of your pancreas and (2) to allow you to inject a bolus injection at mealtime.

Basal insulin can be quite powerful at reducing blood glucose. Thus, it's very important to work with your physician to determine the exact dosage required to meet your body's background insulin requirement, and use periodic intermittent fasts to become extra confident.

**Commonly prescribed brand names of injectable basal insulin:** Lantus, Basaglar, Levemir, Toujeo, and Tresiba

**Side effects:** The most notable side effects of basal insulin therapy occur when you inject too much or your basal rate on a pump is too high, resulting in either mild or severe hypoglycemia.

## Sulfonylureas (*sulf-on-ul-ureas*)

Sulfonylureas stimulate beta cells in your pancreas to secrete insulin and are extensively used for the treatment of type 2 diabetes. Over the past fifty years, sulfonylureas have been the most widely prescribed antidiabetic medications in the world because of their low cost and effectiveness at reducing blood glucose.

**Common medications include:** Glipizide, Glyburide, Glucotrol, Glucotrol XL, Micronase, Glynase, Diabeta, Glimiperide, Amaryl, Diabinese, and Tolinase

**Side effects:** Although scientists do not know the exact mechanism of action, sulfonylureas are known to stimulate beta cells in the manufacture and secretion of insulin, to increase liver glucose output, and to moderately increase insulin sensitivity. Because they directly stimulate insulin production, sulfonylureas can cause serious side effects that cannot be overlooked, including hypoglycemia, weight gain, nausea, skin reactions, jaundice, hepatitis, liver failure, and heart attacks.

In addition, sulfonylureas impair the function of existing beta cells, leading to declining insulin production over time. What this means is very important—sulfonylureas may stimulate your beta cells to make more insulin today, but over the course of time they cause beta cell damage, eventually resulting in impaired insulin production. Worst of all, a study involving more than 5,000 participants showed that use of sulfonylureas for an average of 4.8 years led to a 70 percent increase in the risk of death as compared with metformin. Given these serious risks, please talk to your doctor about these side effects before using sulfonylureas.

## Meglitinides (*meg-lit-in-ides*)

Meglitinides are a class of diabetes medication that acts similarly to sulfonylureas, by stimulating beta cells to secrete insulin. The main difference between the two types of medications is that meglitinides stimulate beta cells to secrete insulin for shorter periods of time than sulfonylureas, which means that they are slightly less effective at reducing blood glucose but come with very similar side effects.

**Commonly prescribed brand names:** Starlix, Prandin, and GlucoNorm

**Side effects:** Given that meglitinides directly stimulate insulin production by the beta cells in your pancreas, the most notable side effects include hypoglycemia and weight gain, followed by gastrointestinal inflammation.

## GLP-1 Receptor Agonists (Injectable Medications)

Glucagon-like peptide 1 (GLP-1) receptor agonists are a class of pharmaceutical medication that stimulates the function of GLP-1 receptors located in your intestine, stomach, pancreas, and brain. When you eat food, your small intestine and colon release GLP-1, a powerful hormone with many actions, which include activating smooth muscles to assist in moving food through your intestines, inhibiting the secretion of glucagon to prevent your liver from dumping glucose into your blood, communicating with your brain to turn off hunger signals, and stimulating your beta cells to make more beta cells and secrete more insulin.

**Commonly prescribed brand names:** Tanzeum, Trulicity, Byetta, Bydureon, Victoza, Xultophy, Adlyxin, and Soliqua

**Side effects:** Because GLP-1 agonists act on hormones in your digestive system that assist in insulin production, they cause extensive damage to your digestive organs. GLP-1 agonists are known to cause gastrointestinal problems including gas, bloating, diarrhea, and flatulence, and have been shown to also increase your risk for pancreatitis and gallbladder disease. They are considered safer alternatives to sulfonylureas because they target multiple tissues simultaneously, but exercise caution when evaluating whether using a GLP-1 receptor agonist makes sense for you.

## DPP-4 Inhibitors

DPP-4 inhibitors are a class of diabetes medication that helps to prolong the action of GLP-1, a hormone that assists insulin in lowering blood glucose. Think of DPP-4 inhibitors as helping to preserve the function of a powerful hormone that promotes insulin secretion in beta cells, slows the rate at which food exits your stomach, and reduces your appetite.

**Commonly prescribed brand names:** Januvia, Janumet, Janumet XR, Onglyza, Kombiglyze XR, Tradjenta, and Jentadueto

**Side effects:** There are numerous ugly side effects of DPP-4 inhibitors, including increased risk for pancreatitis and severe joint pain. DPP-4 inhibitors have also been linked with a significantly increased risk of heart failure.

## SGLT-2 Inhibitors

A nondiabetic kidney filters about 180 grams of glucose out of your blood per day, and some of that glucose is then reintroduced to your blood. Given that your kidneys are a simple way for glucose to exit your blood and enter the toilet, pharmaceutical companies found a way to prevent your kidneys from reintroducing glucose back into your blood once it has been pulled out. SGLT-2 inhibitors do just that—they alter the way your kidney functions so that it becomes very good at "wasting" glucose into the toilet, allowing the amount of glucose in your blood to drop 24 hours a day.

While this may seem logical at first, the list of side effects is daunting, affecting your bladder, your genitalia, your bones, your cholesterol, and your blood pressure. Most important, SGLT-2 inhibitors have been associated with kidney damage. Even though they are effective at reducing your blood glucose, they cause extensive tissue damage.

**Commonly prescribed brand names:** Invokana, Invokamet, Farxiga, Jardiance, Glyxambi, and Synjardy

**Side effects:** The list of side effects of SGLT-2 inhibitors is not only long but downright scary. To begin, SGLT-2 inhibitors can cause genital yeast infections in both men and women, can also cause urinary tract infections (UTIs), and may increase your risk for bladder cancer. In addition, they can cause dizziness and low blood pressure, and can raise your LDL cholesterol. SGLT-2 inhibitors can also cause low blood potassium levels (especially in people with compromised kidney function), bone fractures, and reduced bone mineral density. They may also increase your risk for limb amputation.

Because SGLT-2 inhibitors target your kidney, SGLT-2 inhibitors are known to cause acute kidney injury, which can be treated only with dialysis. In 2016, the FDA issued alerts about this dangerous side effect, and yet they continue to be frequently prescribed to patients with type 2 diabetes. In more than 50 percent of the cases reported to the FDA, "the events of acute kidney injury occurred within 1 month of starting the medication, and most patients improved after stopping it."

## Thiazolidinediones (*thi-a-zol-a-deen-die-own*)

Thiazolidinediones (TZDs) are a commonly prescribed class of diabetes medication that increases the storage of fatty acids in adipose tissue as well as increases adipose tissue mass, and spares your muscles, liver, and beta cells from the harmful metabolic effects of excess fatty acids. Think of TZDs as medications that "keeps fat where it belongs." In addition, TZDs increase the insulin sensitivity of your muscle and liver, allowing both of these tissues to uptake glucose from your blood and therefore lower your blood glucose. TZDs are also known to increase your appetite by acting directly on receptors in your brain that make you hungry.

**Commonly prescribed brand names:** Actos, Actoplus MET, Actoplus MET XR, Avandia, Avandamet, and Avandaryl

**Side effects:** TZDs come with their fair share of side effects, including weight gain, fluid retention, increased appetite, increased LDL cholesterol, liver dysfunction, and increased risk for stroke and congestive heart failure. The risk of heart failure from TZDs is so drastic that in 2010 the European Medicines Agency suspended sales of drugs containing rosiglitazone, and in 2011 the French and German medicines agencies suspended sales of pioglitazone. The United States and United Kingdom soon followed by banning sales of troglitazone because it caused liver dysfunction and liver failure in some patients.

## Alpha-Glucosidase Inhibitors
### (*al-fa-glue-ko-side-ase inhibitors*)

Alpha-glucosidase inhibitors are a type of oral medication that blocks your ability to digest carbohydrates in the food you eat. Carbohydrates are digested and absorbed through the walls of your intestine using a series of enzymes called glucosidases, and alpha-glucosidase inhibitors are specifically designed to inhibit the action of these enzymes to block your intestine from absorbing carbohydrates. Patients are instructed to take this class of medications with meals.

**Commonly prescribed brand names:** Precose and Glyset

**Side effects:** Because alpha-glucosidase inhibitors disrupt your ability to digest food, they may cause gastrointestinal problems including gas, bloating, diarrhea, and flatulence. Human clinical trials are currently under way to evaluate cardiovascular risks associated with this class of medication.

## Amylin Analogues

Amylin is a protein that is secreted from pancreatic beta cells along with insulin. Beta cells secrete approximately a hundred times as much amylin as they do insulin, and amylin's job is to prevent your blood glucose from rising too high when you eat by slowing the rate at which food exits your stomach and making you less hungry. Amylin analogues are designed to mimic the action of amylin.

**Commonly prescribed brand names:** Symlin

**Side effects:** Because amylin analogues act on specific regions of your digestive system, they cause the same side effects as alpha-glucosidase inhibitors, including gas, bloating, diarrhea, and flatulence.

## Biguanides (*bih-gwan-ides*)

Biguanides are a class of diabetes medication that have effects on many tissues in your body, including your liver, intestines, and muscle. Metformin is the most widely prescribed biguanide and is the first line of treatment for patients with type 2 diabetes, prediabetes, PCOS, and gestational diabetes.

In your liver, metformin reduces liver glucose export; in your intestine, metformin reduces glucose absorption; and in your muscle, metformin increases glucose uptake. The net effect is that metformin can lower your A1c value by as much as 1.0% to 1.5% when used in isolation, without causing weight gain. One of the most interesting aspects of metformin use is that research indicates that it may actually reduce your risk for cardiovascular disease, especially in obese patients. For this reason, metformin is considered the safest and most effective first line of treatment.

**Commonly prescribed brand names:** metformin, Glucophage, Glucophage XR (metformin is also available in combination with other oral medications)

**Side effects:** The most common side effects include abdominal pain, nausea, diarrhea, cramping, vitamin $B_{12}$ deficiency, and lactic acidosis.

# How to Reduce Oral and Injectable Medications Safely

For the best and safest results, we recommend that you and your doctor take a proactive approach to reducing your oral medication use, because as your insulin sensitivity increases, you are likely to find that you quickly need fewer medications. Overmedicating yourself can lead to life-threatening hypoglycemia, so it is actually safer to keep your blood glucose slightly elevated than it is to become frequently hypoglycemic. Our guidelines for reducing your oral medication use are as follows:

- At the beginning of the program, notify your doctor that you are changing your lifestyle and may need to reduce your oral medications quickly.
- If your fasting blood glucose is between 80 and 100 mg/dL for 3 to 7 days in a row or if your blood glucose falls below 80 mg/dL at any time, call your doctor and ask for a medication reduction immediately.
- If your fasting blood glucose consistently reads above 100, continue optimizing your lifestyle and approach your doctor when your fasting blood glucose is between 80 and 100 mg/dL for 3 to 7 days in a row or falls below 80 mg/dL at any time.

# Choosing Lifestyle Change Over Medication

The take-home message is that your body is an incredibly complex biological system that functions like a puzzle with countless moving parts, many interdependent relationships, and many redundant feedback mechanisms. Pharmaceutical medications function by attempting to alter a few biological reactions inside of an incredibly complex biological system, leading to a ripple effect that causes unwanted side effects in tissues all over your body.

That's exactly why every medication listed above comes with a list of side effects—because even though scientists think they know how to develop "safe" medications, many medications act like runaway trains, causing one side effect after another, eventually decreasing your quality of life and increasing your risk for other unwanted chronic health conditions.

Remember that improving biomarkers of your diabetes health on paper *does not* translate to better long-term health. Don't be fooled—pharmaceutical medications may help to control your blood glucose, improve insulin secretion, reduce your blood pressure, reduce your cholesterol, and reduce pain, but intensive treatment of blood glucose with medications can increase your risk for heart failure, liver failure, kidney failure, stroke, and even death, and that's certainly nothing to take lightly.

**Pharmaceutical medications are not designed to treat the underlying cause of diabetes, heart disease, and many other chronic conditions. They are designed to help you manage the symptoms rather than reverse the underlying cause.**

For these reasons, we strongly encourage you to exhaust every lifestyle change option you have available before making the decision to use pharmaceutical medications, including a nutrient-dense low-fat plant-based whole-food diet, various medicinal plants (you'll learn more about them in chapter 10), a daily exercise regimen, periodic intermittent fasting, and frequent decision trees. In the long term, minimizing your use of oral medications and injectable medications can dramatically increase your overall health and quality of life. And who doesn't want that?

To view the 50+ scientific references cited in this chapter, please visit us online at www.masteringdiabetes.org/bookinfo.

# Chapter 10

# Starting Strong: Breakfast

## Meals over Medication: Adam

Adam was diagnosed with attention deficit hyperactivity disorder (ADHD) at the age of 12 and used Ritalin to manage ADHD throughout his teenage years. In high school, Adam switched from Ritalin to Adderall, and soon he found himself addicted to the effects of the medication. At the age of 20, Adam became a criminal drug addict. He bought and sold Adderall on the street and secretly worked with multiple doctors, each of whom prescribed him more without the knowledge of the others.

When Adam temporarily ran out of Adderall, he began eating large amounts of fast food to soothe his feelings of low self-worth. At the age of 29, Adam became severely depressed and began experiencing erectile dysfunction. He took an average of 450 mg of Adderall per day, fifteen times the typical daily dose of 30 mg. He felt terrible, his self-esteem was nonexistent, and at the age of 30 he weighed 320 pounds. Frustrated with the way he looked and felt and plagued with a diminishing desire to live, he tried to commit suicide by intentionally overdosing on painkillers. After passing out on the floor of his apartment, he woke up a few hours later to the smell of his own vomit surrounded by empty fast-food containers and pill bottles. He picked up the phone, called his parents, and said the words "I need help." Immediately his parents jumped into action, rescued him from his apartment, and checked him into rehab. There a doctor diagnosed him with hypertension and type 2 diabetes—his fasting blood glucose had climbed to more than 300 mg/dL and his A1c was greater than 9.0%.

Adam's dad, Jim, reminded him of an event they attended about a year prior in which Rip Esselstyn (creator of the Engine 2 Diet) taught him how to reverse chronic Western diseases using a plant-based whole-food diet. Motivated to take action, Adam began eating this way, and within six months his fasting blood glucose dropped from over 300 mg/dL to between 60 and 70 mg/dL. Within one year, he discontinued the use of medications for type 2 diabetes, high blood pressure, insomnia, ADHD, depression, and an unstable mood.

What enabled Adam to transition to a plant-based diet with great success was eating simple meals using only a few ingredients. The transition to a low-fat plant-based whole-food diet was admittedly uncomfortable at first, but Adam taught himself how to "be comfortable being uncomfortable." Soon the thought of eating the standard American diet (SAD) became unimaginable. He left nothing to chance and planned his simple meals well in advance. He remembers telling himself that "preparation beats motivation any day of the week," and he used that mantra to resist impulsive behavior.

He often says, "the simplest change on your fork can make the most profound change of your life," a statement that helped him lose 170 pounds (more than half of his body weight), reverse type 2 diabetes, reverse high blood pressure, reverse erectile dysfunction, and overcome insomnia and depression. Today Adam has devoted his life to helping others transform their life using the Mastering Diabetes Method, and is an incredibly influential health coach for the Total Health Immersion Program of Whole Foods Market and for the Mastering Diabetes Coaching Program. He has helped thousands of people reverse various chronic diseases by providing them with the knowledge, passion, and confidence required to succeed with flying colors.

You've probably heard that breakfast is the most important meal of the day. The truth is that each meal is important for different reasons. But breakfast is the *first* meal of the day, which makes it very important for establishing excellent blood glucose control in preparation for the rest of the day. The foods you choose to eat at breakfast are crucial for giving your muscles and brain the energy they require to perform optimally. Whole carbohydrate-rich foods are excellent choices to rev up your physical and mental stamina, because they are extremely nutrient dense and contain easily available energy. Especially if you enjoy exercising in the morning hours—or want to start enjoying exercise in the morning—eating a generous portion of foods rich in whole carbohydrate energy is a simple way to stay energized during your workout.

For many people, breakfast usually contains foods that are packed with *refined* carbohydrates—breads, cereals, and processed grains like instant oatmeal and grits. As you learned in chapter 6, these refined carbohydrates can cause unwanted glucose fluctuations, especially if the fat content of your diet remains high. In this chapter, we'll show you how to replace those foods with other options that will kick-start the process of increasing your insulin sensitivity and help you feel energized.

## Take the Insulin Resistance Quiz

In order to determine your ideal breakfast, it's important to first understand your baseline level of insulin resistance. Start by taking the quiz below. For each question, choose the most appropriate answer, then calculate your final score by adding up your total points.

**How many pounds overweight do you consider yourself?**

❑   I'm underweight, or I weigh my ideal weight = 0 points

❑   I'm 1–10 pounds overweight = 5 points

❑   I'm 10–30 pounds overweight = 10 points

❑  I'm 30–50 pounds overweight = 15 points

❑  I'm 50–100 pounds overweight = 20 points

❑  I'm 100+ pounds overweight = 25 points

**How many minutes of medium- or high-intensity exercise do you perform per week?**

Medium-intensity exercise elevates your heart rate significantly, is moderately challenging, and can be performed continuously for at least 30 minutes. High-intensity exercise also elevates your heart rate significantly, is extremely challenging, and can only be performed in 1- to 5-minute intervals.

❑  I don't exercise = 25 points

❑  I perform medium- or high-intensity exercise for 1–30 minutes per week = 20 points

❑  I perform medium- or high-intensity exercise for 30–60 minutes per week = 15 points

❑  I perform medium- or high-intensity exercise for 1–1.5 hours per week = 10 points

❑  I perform medium- or high-intensity exercise for 1.5–3 hours per week = 5 points

❑  I perform medium- or high-intensity exercise for 3 or more hours per week = 0 points

**How many servings of oils and fat-rich plant foods do you eat in your baseline diet per day on average?**

1 serving is approximately 1 tablespoon of oil of any kind, 1/2 avocado, 1.5 ounce nuts or seeds, 1 tablespoon nut or seed butter, 1/4 cup coconut meat, or 5 medium olives.

❑  My baseline diet contains 0 servings of oil and fat-rich plant foods per day = 0 points

❑  My baseline diet contains 1 serving of oil and fat-rich plant foods per day = 5 points

❑   My baseline diet contains 2 servings of oil and fat-rich plant foods per day = 10 points

❑   My baseline diet contains 3 servings of oil and fat-rich plant foods per day = 15 points

❑   My baseline diet contains 4 servings of oil and fat-rich plant foods per day = 20 points

❑   My baseline diet contains 5 or more servings of oil and fat-rich plant foods per day = 25 points

**How many servings of refined carbohydrate foods do you eat in your baseline diet per day on average?**

1 serving is approximately 1 slice of bread, 1½ cups of processed grains or cereal, 5 crackers, 2 cookies, or 1 cup of conventional pasta.

❑   I don't eat any refined carbohydrate foods! = 0 points

❑   My baseline diet contains 1 serving of refined carbohydrate foods per day = 5 points

❑   My baseline diet contains 2 servings of refined carbohydrate foods per day = 10 points

❑   My baseline diet contains 3 servings of refined carbohydrate foods per day = 15 points

❑   My baseline diet contains 4 servings of refined carbohydrate foods per day = 20 points

❑   My baseline diet contains 5 or more servings of refined carbohydrate foods per day = 25 points

**On average, how many total servings of red meat, chicken, fish, shellfish, and eggs do you eat in your baseline diet per day?**

1 serving is approximately 4 ounces of red meat, 4 ounces of chicken, 3 ounces of fish, 3 ounces of shellfish, or 1 egg.

❑   I don't eat red meat, chicken, fish, shellfish, or eggs! = 0 points

- ❏  My baseline diet contains 1 serving of red meat, chicken, fish, shellfish, and eggs per day = 5 points
- ❏  My baseline diet contains 2 servings of red meat, chicken, fish, shellfish, and eggs per day = 10 points
- ❏  My baseline diet contains 3 servings of red meat, chicken, fish, shellfish, and eggs per day = 15 points
- ❏  My baseline diet contains 4 servings of red meat, chicken, fish, shellfish, and eggs per day = 20 points
- ❏  My baseline diet contains 5 or more servings of red meat, chicken, fish, shellfish, and eggs per day = 25 points

**How many servings of dairy products do you eat in your baseline diet per day on average?**
1 serving is approximately 1 glass of milk, 1 slice of cheese, 1 tablespoon of butter, or ½ cup of ice cream.

- ❏  I don't eat dairy products! = 0 points
- ❏  My baseline diet contains 1 serving of dairy products per day = 5 points
- ❏  My baseline diet contains 2 servings of dairy products per day = 10 points
- ❏  My baseline diet contains 3 servings of dairy products per day = 15 points
- ❏  My baseline diet contains 4 servings of dairy products per day = 20 points
- ❏  My baseline diet contains 5 servings or more of dairy products per day = 25 points

To determine which of the two breakfast strategies is best for you, calculate your total score by adding together the points you earned from each question, then follow the instructions in the box below:

| Your Score | Your Baseline Insulin Resistance | How to Begin the Mastering Diabetes Method |
|---|---|---|
| 0–20 | Low | Begin eating Breakfast Option 1 |
| 25–45 | Medium | Eat Breakfast Option 2 for approximately 1 week, then switch to Breakfast Option 1 |
| 50–70 | High | Eat Breakfast Option 2 for approximately 2 weeks, then switch to Breakfast Option 1 |
| 75+ | Very High | Eat Breakfast Option 2 for approximately 4 weeks, then switch to Breakfast Option 1 |

# The Perfect Breakfast Option 1: Fruit Bowl Topped with Ground Chia or Flax

One of the best ways to start your morning off right is to eat a generous serving of fresh fruit because it provides your body with easily digestible carbohydrate energy that lasts for hours and provides your brain with exactly the fuel it's designed to run on: glucose.

As you learned in chapter 6, carbohydrate-rich whole foods require large amounts of insulin *only* if the total amount of fat in your diet is high, and especially if the amount of saturated fat in your diet is high. Remember, when you eat fat-rich foods, your ability to metabolize carbohydrate-rich foods declines immediately. Eating a low-fat fruit-centric meal first thing in the morning substitutes for fat-rich and protein-rich foods. Fresh fruits contain a complex collection of macronutrients including carbohydrate, fat, and protein, as well as micronutrients, including vitamins, minerals, fiber, water, antioxidants, and phytochemicals. It's the presence of a vast array of behind-the-scenes micronutrients that increases the nutrient density of your fruit-centric meal and helps protect your blood glucose from rising rapidly.

Sweeteners like table sugar, high-fructose corn syrup, and agave nectar, on the other hand, are much more likely to spike your blood glucose because they have been processed into potent concentrated sweeteners and are devoid of protective nutrients, including vitamins, minerals, fiber, water, antioxidants, and phytochemicals. When you eat foods containing these added and refined sugars, your blood glucose may spike because the glucose inside is *unprotected* by fiber and other valuable micronutrients.

We understand that it may be difficult to unlearn years of avoiding fruits, so if you find yourself struggling with the concept of eating a fruit bowl first thing in the morning, then take a deep breath and learn from thousands of others who have successfully transitioned their diets. Most of our clients are pleasantly surprised that eating a carbohydrate-rich breakfast containing fruits does not cause blood glucose spikes, even after they have avoided fruit for years. Though it may seem like a scary task, when you are ready to eat a fruit-centric breakfast, do so for seven consecutive days and be sure to document any changes you discover in your blood glucose in the 1 to 3 hours after your meal.

## Start constructing a fresh fruit bowl by combining the following ingredients:

- 3 to 4 servings of fruit (or more if you're highly active). A serving of fruit is one of the following:
  1 whole fruit (banana, apple, orange, pear, mango, etc.)
  1 cup of berries (strawberries, blueberries, blackberries, etc.)
  1 cup of grapes
  1 cup of small fruits (figs, kumquats, etc.)
- 1 tablespoon freshly ground chia seeds or 1 tablespoon freshly ground flaxseeds
- Spices like cinnamon, cloves, nutmeg, cardamom, or cumin to sprinkle on top for added flavor and antioxidant power

## Understanding the Glycemic Index and Glycemic Load

The glycemic index (GI) measures how quickly a food raises your blood glucose level. The food with the highest GI is pure glucose, at 100. Foods can be listed as low glycemic (55 or less), medium glycemic (56–69) or high glycemic (70–100). The glycemic index of a given food varies by the temperature at which the food is eaten, the cooking method, the ripeness, and the variety (e.g., sweet potato vs. white potato).

The GI is moderately useful because green light foods that are particularly low on the GI (leafy greens, non-starchy vegetables, and legumes) will help prevent blood glucose spikes and result in a steadier blood glucose profile throughout the day. Eating significant quantities of a higher GI food like pineapple could result in a larger blood glucose spike than would eating a food like blueberries. This is quite helpful during your transition, especially if your baseline level of insulin resistance is high or very high, and is useful if you inject bolus insulin and want to adjust your insulin dosing strategy accordingly.

Despite its utility in these specific situations, the GI can also be misleading, because it does not factor in the nutrient density of a given food. For example, a Snickers bar has a GI of 43 and peanut butter has a GI of 33, both of which are low. But as you now know, both will increase your level of baseline insulin resistance and result in elevated post-meal blood glucose the next time you attempt to eat carbohydrate-rich foods.

Even though all green light foods fall in the low or medium category (except watermelon, with a GI of 72), we suggest disregarding the glycemic index. The glycemic index does not take into account the quantity or type of macronutrients in your food, the presence of other foods in the same meal, the nutrient density of your food, the status of your gut microbiome, or your level of insulin sensitivity. For these reasons, the glycemic index is not very useful.

The glycemic load (GL) is based on the glycemic index but also factors in the total amount of carbohydrate in a given food. The more carbohydrate you eat, the higher the GL. The glycemic load range is categorized as low (1–10), medium (11–19), or high (20+).

The GL can also be misleading. For example, a banana has a low GI of 47. If you ate two medium bananas, the GL would be high at 29. If instead you ate only one banana, the GL would be medium at 15. Unfortunately the GL is a flawed system that does not take into account your insulin sensitivity and your ability to tolerate high-carbohydrate meals.

Both of these glycemic rating systems are incomplete and provide useful information only when you are living in an insulin-resistant state. As you gain insulin sensitivity, both the glycemic index and the glycemic load become somewhat irrelevant. Eat green light foods including greens, non-starchy vegetables, and legumes because they are rich in whole carbohydrate energy and have a high nutrient density, and refrain from choosing foods based on their glycemic index or glycemic load.

---

# The Perfect Breakfast Option 2: Focus on Fiber and Nutrient Density

If you fall in the medium, high, or very high categories of baseline insulin resistance, pay attention to how many green light foods you eat every day. The more green light foods you eat, the more fiber can help slow the absorption of glucose into your blood, which in turn will help to reduce unwanted blood glucose elevations. Here are our tips for eating a breakfast meal that is optimized for fiber and nutrient density:

**Eat fruit with greens and/or non-starchy vegetables.** When you're living with a higher level of insulin resistance, include foods that slow the absorption of glucose into your bloodstream while still meeting your calorie needs. This can be accomplished by eating 3 to 4+ servings of fruit with significant portions of leafy greens (lettuce, spinach, kale, arugula, etc.) or non-starchy vegetables (cucumber, celery, zucchini, etc.). See Appendix B for a full list of leafy greens and non-starchy vegetables.

**Eat intact whole grains with fruit.** An intact whole-grain fruit bowl is another great option for breakfast. This breakfast meal contains an intact whole grain such as quinoa, wild rice, or millet as the base, topped with fruits like berries, apples, peaches, or pears. We have found that eating oatmeal can cause unwanted blood glucose elevations in people living with a medium, high, or very high level of baseline insulin resistance. The presence of intact whole grains also delays the rate at which glucose enters your blood, which protects against unwanted blood glucose elevations when you are living with high levels of insulin resistance.

**Add beans, lentils, and peas.** Legumes are great foods to enjoy for breakfast, especially when you are beginning your transition from a highly insulin-resistant state. They include large amounts of resistant starch, which help prevent unwanted blood glucose spikes. Additionally, beans, lentils, and peas have a slightly higher protein content than other green light foods, and because of this you are likely to stay full for a longer period of time. Legumes are also incredibly nutrient dense, and not only help keep your blood glucose flat after the meal in which they're eaten but also reduce blood glucose elevations at your next meal. This "second-meal" effect has been observed by many researchers, and results from happy gut bacteria that release short-chain fatty acids into circulation that moderate your post-meal blood glucose values brilliantly. Including legumes in your breakfast meal is a great way to control your blood glucose for many hours in the beginning of the day.

**Add freshly ground chia, flaxseeds, and spices.** We suggest adding 1 tablespoon of freshly ground flaxseeds or freshly ground chia seeds to any of the options presented above to ensure that you eat sufficient EFAs every day. Also including spices like cinnamon, cloves, nutmeg, cardamom, or cumin can enhance the flavor and antioxidant power of your breakfast meal.

## Add Medicinal Plants to Your Breakfast

Beyond green light foods, there are specific medicinal plants with measurable glucose-lowering and insulin-mimicking effects. Including these plants in your daily regimen can make a big difference in your blood glucose control; they also possess potent antioxidant cholesterol- and lipid-lowering activity. The most well-known glucose-lowering plants include Gymnema sylvestre, bitter melon, berberine, sea buckthorn, fenugreek, and amla.

Amla (also known as Indian gooseberry) is a particularly potent plant that we've incorporated into the Mastering Diabetes Method. It is the world's most powerful antioxidant-rich food, boasting 75 times the antioxidant power of goji berries, 50 times the antioxidant power of blueberries, and 2 times the antioxidant power of fresh turmeric. Amla has been shown to be more effective than some pharmaceutical medications in reducing blood glucose, cholesterol, and blood pressure, and is considered to be the most powerful cholesterol-reducing food on the planet and one of the most powerful antidiabetic foods on the planet.

In a 2011 study published in the *International Journal of Food Sciences and Nutrition*, scientists investigated the effect of consuming 1, 2, or 3 grams of amla powder per day on blood glucose and cholesterol levels vs. glimepiride, a commonly prescribed diabetes medication. They investigated the effect of both daily amla powder and glimepiride in subjects with and without type 2 diabetes. In comparison with baseline values, daily consumption of amla fruit powder led to a significant decrease in blood glucose values after 21 days across all subjects.

All doses significantly reduced blood glucose values—and using only 1 gram of amla per day was just as effective as glimepiride. Both fasting and postprandial (post-meal) blood glucose values were significantly reduced within 3 weeks.

They also observed significant decreases in total cholesterol and triglyceride values in subjects with and without type 2 diabetes given either 2 grams per day or 3 grams per day. LDL cholesterol was reduced by more than 40 percent in 3 weeks, triglycerides were reduced by more than 45 percent, and HDL cholesterol increased by more than 25 percent.

In 2012, researchers in the *Indian Journal of Pharmacology* compared the effects of a 500 mg daily amla capsule in a head-to-head competition with 20 mg of simvastatin, one of the leading statin medications. They investigated the effect of amla and simvastatin in sixty patients with total cholesterol greater than 240 mg/dL and LDL cholesterol greater than 130 mg/dL. Forty of the sixty patients were treated with a 500 mg capsule containing pure amla powder, and the remaining twenty patients were treated with 20 mg simvastatin. All patients were followed for 6 weeks, to determine the effect of each treatment on lipids and blood pressure. Amla was found to be just as effective as simvastatin at reducing total cholesterol, reducing LDL cholesterol, and increasing HDL cholesterol. Simvastatin treatment was found to be more effective than amla at reducing VLDL cholesterol and triglycerides.

Given that statin medications increase your risk for type 2 diabetes, finding natural alternatives to statin medication is an excellent long-term decision. A meta-analysis published in 2010 in *The Lancet* that evaluated fourteen clinical trials involving more than 91,000 people found that using statin medication to control cholesterol increases the risk for type 2 diabetes by approximately 9 percent, and another meta-analysis published in *JAMA: The Journal of the American Medical Association* in 2011, including more than 32,000 people, found that statin medication increased the risk of developing type 2 diabetes by approximately 12 percent.

Raw amla tastes very bitter when eaten, so we created an extremely antioxidant-rich tea called Amla Green, which has been helping thousands of people improve their metabolic health. If you choose to incorporate Amla Green into your daily regimen, know that we have observed excellent results from people who drink one or two glasses per day in addition to a low-fat plant-based whole-food diet. Visit www.amlagreen.com for more details.

## What About Gluten?

In the past twenty years, the word *gluten* has become part of our vernacular because of celiac disease, an autoimmune condition that causes severe gastrointestinal problems in people who have a genetic gluten intolerance. Celiac disease affects roughly one in a hundred people (1 percent), and roughly one in a thousand (0.1 percent) may suffer from a condition known as non-celiac gluten sensitivity (NCGS), a mild intolerance to gluten that is not autoimmune by nature.

In the case of type 1 diabetes, research is now connecting the dots between gluten intolerance and beta cell destruction. The lining of your small intestine is composed of a single-cell layer known as your *gut epithelium,* and the job of these cells is to absorb fully digested nutrients and pass them to your blood so that they can be transported to their target tissues for use or storage. These cells are designed to form a protective barrier and are connected by a collection of proteins called *tight junctions.* Think of tight junctions as cellular glue that keeps these cells tightly connected to prevent nutrients from gaining free access to your blood without passing through the epithelial cells first.

Gluten refers to a class of proteins containing *gliadin* and *glutenin* found in wheat, barley, and rye. In individuals with a genetic predisposition toward autoimmunity, the gliadin fraction of gluten can trigger a series of reactions that eventually lead to the degradation of these critically important tight junctions, creating microscopic holes between the cells in your gut lining. When these small holes appear, partially digested protein from your food gains the ability to escape into your blood before it is fully digested. Cells in your blood recognize these protein fragments as nonhuman (or non-self), which then triggers your immune system to degrade them by manufacturing antibodies.

As you learned in chapter 5, the process of *molecular mimicry* is a sneaky tactic that bacteria and viruses use to avoid being detected by the human immune system. When you develop a leaky gut containing thousands of microscopic holes in your gut epithelium, undigested food proteins can trigger your immune system to mistakenly target similar proteins on human cells. In some individuals, the gliadin fraction of gluten triggers an autoimmune reaction that can result in the destruction of insulin-producing beta cells in your pancreas.

If you have a compromised intestinal barrier, then every time you eat food partially digested proteins leak into circulation, resulting in a chronic state of inflammation that either raises your risk for autoimmune disease or exacerbates your preexisting autoimmune disease. Researchers have discovered that a large proportion of people with type 1 diabetes also have impaired gut function, suggesting that an impaired intestinal barrier may actually be a *prerequisite* for the development of type 1 diabetes. Take a look at the illustration on the next page to get a better understanding of the interaction between gliadin and intestinal cell tight junctions.

**Normal Gluten Metabolism** | **Abnormal Gluten Metabolism**

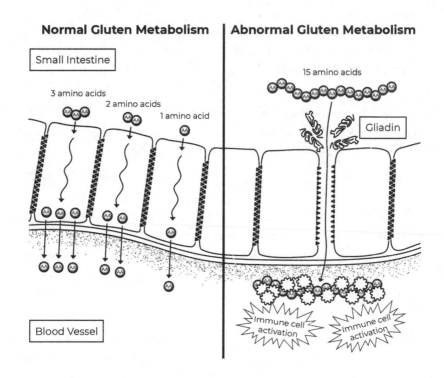

Your gut epithelium is designed to absorb chains of amino acids that are either one, two, or three units long. In people who have a sensitivity to gluten, the gliadin fraction of the gluten protein can irritate these cells, resulting in the breakage of "tight junctions." When this happens, large protein fragments can enter your blood, triggering an immune response.

By increasing their intake of fresh fruits, starchy vegetables, non-starchy vegetables, legumes, and intact non-gluten whole grains like oat groats, quinoa, or millet, many of our clients have inadvertently eliminated inflammation triggered by gluten, resulting in dramatically less bloating, gas, diarrhea, brain fog, and abdominal pain usually caused by gluten sensitivity.

You can perform a simple experiment to determine the effect of gluten on your body, using an elimination-reintegration protocol. Start by eliminating all wheat, barley, rye, and spelt products from your diet for a total of 30 days, and increase your intake of fresh fruits, starchy vegetables, and legumes as a substitute. After 30 days, eat a single serving of a wheat, barley, rye, or spelt, and monitor your symptoms over the course of the next 24 hours. Because the breakdown products of wheat have been out of your digestive system and blood for 30 days, if you experience bloating, gas, diarrhea, brain fog, or abdominal pain, it will likely be a very strong reaction. Pay attention to the immediate effects (0–3 hours), medium-term effects (3–12 hours), and long-term effects (12–24 hours). Repeat this test approximately three times with one or two days in between each test. Use this information to determine whether you choose to keep or eliminate wheat, barley, rye, or spelt products in your diet. If you believe that you are someone who will benefit from avoiding gluten, then feel free to include gluten-free intact whole grains such as quinoa, brown rice, oat groats, wild rice, sorghum, farro, buckwheat, amaranth, bulgur, or millet.

## What About Caffeinated Beverages?

Understanding how caffeine affects your metabolic health can be a complicated topic, but it's worth understanding. Much like carbohydrates, fat, and protein, you don't drink or eat caffeine by itself. Caffeine is found in a wide variety of beverages—including many different kinds of tea, coffee, energy drinks, and soda—and the way in which caffeinated beverages are prepared dramatically affects how they behave in your body.

We recommend that you completely eliminate sodas and energy drinks not necessarily because of the caffeine but because they are highly processed products that often contain refined sweeteners, flavor additives, and electrolyte salts. Sodas are highly sweetened beverages that impair the function of your liver, stimulate excess insulin production and weight gain, and worsen your cardiovascular health. Data published in *Diabetes Care* from more than 300,000 participants show that people who consume the most soda are 26 percent more likely to develop type 2 diabetes than those who drink the least. Data from the Nurses' Health Study and Health Professionals Follow-Up Study published in the *American Journal of Clinical Nutrition* demonstrate that regular consumption of sugar-sweetened sodas increased the risk of cancers such as non-Hodgkin's lymphoma and multiple myeloma. By simply eliminating both sodas and energy drinks from your diet, you can dramatically improve your blood glucose control, lose weight, and improve your cardiovascular health quickly.

As for coffee, some research suggests that it has negative metabolic effects. In a study published in *Clinical Science,* a single cup of coffee containing 80 mg of caffeine has been shown to dramatically reduce the ability of blood vessels to dilate by as much as 72 percent, depending on how many cups you drink. It was also recently discovered that drinking caffeinated coffee reduced insulin and C-peptide in the same subjects. Both of these findings suggest that caffeinated coffee can impair both cardiovascular health and glucose metabolism.

In direct opposition to this, some research shows that drinking coffee has positive metabolic effects. Researchers have found that drinking caffeinated coffee improves fasting blood glucose and blood glucose control and reduces hyperinsulinemia in both men and women. Another research group found that those who drank 5 cups of caffeinated coffee or more per day experienced 1.5 percent lower fasting blood glucose and 4.3 percent lower postmeal blood glucose in comparison with those who did not drink coffee on a daily basis. Other research published in the *Journal of Internal Medicine* shows that men who drank 5 or more cups of caffeinated coffee per day experienced a 55 percent reduced risk of developing type 2 diabetes, and women who drank 5 or more cups of caffeinated coffee per day experienced a 73 percent reduced risk, in comparison with those who drank 2 or fewer cups of coffee per day. In addition, subjects who drank more caffeinated coffee were more insulin sensitive. A study of Dutch men and women found that those who drank 7 or more cups of caffeinated coffee per day had a 31 percent reduced risk of developing type 2 diabetes compared to those who drank 2 or less cups per day.

Aside from coffee, both green tea and black tea have been extensively studied, and researchers consistently demonstrate that caffeinated green and black tea improve cardiovascular health and increase the ability of blood vessels to dilate. An overwhelming amount of evidence shows that—more than any other tea—adding green tea to your diet is a simple and excellent way to increase your intake of antioxidants, keep your blood vessels flexible, and prevent the development of atherosclerosis.

Based on this research and our coaching experience, our recommendations for caffeinated beverages are as follows:

- If you currently do not drink coffee or other caffeinated beverages, we suggest remaining caffeine-free. Adding caffeine to your diet to improve your blood glucose control or lower your A1c is unnecessary. Instead, eat a nutrient-dense diet with an abundant quantity of green light foods.
- If you currently drink caffeinated green or black tea, or if you drink non-caffeinated herbal tea, feel free to continue.
- If you currently drink black coffee on a regular basis, do your best to prepare your coffee in a way that retains the highest antioxidant and polyphenol content to maximize its positive metabolic effects. To do so, store your beans in an airtight container, grind your beans just before brewing, and refrain from adding milk and other dairy creamers.

## What About Smoothies?

Many people enjoy drinking smoothies in the morning instead of eating a bowl of fruit, because it can often be quicker, more convenient, and easy to purchase from a café or smoothie bar. Technically speaking, you can combine the ingredients from the fruit bowl topped with chia or flaxseeds into a blender and process them into a smoothie for breakfast. However, we do not recommend drinking your breakfast for two main reasons.

First, the carbohydrate energy is digested and absorbed by your small intestine much more rapidly than if you eat the fruit in its whole state. Blending fruit also partially breaks the long-chain fiber molecules of the fruit into smaller pieces, which means that when you drink a smoothie, your stomach and small intestine can access the carbohydrate chains quicker, resulting in rapid absorption of glucose into your blood.

Second, long-chain fiber molecules are food for trillions of bacteria that live in the microbiome of your large intestine and gut. Every time you eat fiber-rich foods, you feed those bacteria, which in turn secrete immune-boosting short-chain fatty acids into your blood. Processing long-chain fiber molecules into short-chain fiber molecules—through blending—reduces the amount of food that your microbiome receives.

We have found that people living with diabetes have a difficult time drinking smoothies because they often experience a rapid rise in their blood glucose in the 1 to 3 hours following the meal. We recommend drinking smoothies in moderation, adding greens before blending, or eating fresh greens in addition to your smoothie. If you choose to drink a smoothie, do your best to drink it slowly to limit the chances of unwanted high blood glucose.

# Troubleshooting High Blood Glucose Before and After Breakfast

### If Your Fasting Blood Glucose Is High

Be patient and monitor your fasting blood glucose trend over the next few weeks. As you make changes to your lunch and dinner menus, your fasting blood glucose is likely to come down steadily. Alternatively, you can speed up the rate at which you make changes to your diet if you want quicker results. Start by reducing the total fat content of your diet to a maximum of 15 percent of total calories for 14 days in a row, and monitor what effect this has on your fasting blood glucose before breakfast.

### If You Experience High Blood Glucose After Breakfast

Consider adjusting the rate at which glucose gets into your bloodstream at your breakfast meal temporarily by focusing on Breakfast Option 2 described above. Additionally, limiting your fat intake to no more than 15 percent of calories will also help lower your blood glucose after breakfast. This will ensure that the foods you eat at lunch and dinner don't negatively affect your blood glucose the next morning.

Try elevating your heart rate for about 10 to 15 minutes before or after your next breakfast meal by walking, jogging, cycling, strength training, or swimming to accelerate the rate at which glucose is burned for energy and utilized by tissues. Small exercise sessions are a very effective way to reduce your post-meal blood glucose. For more information on managing your blood glucose before, during, and after exercise, see chapter 14.

If you are using fast-acting bolus insulin, also pay attention to the timing of your insulin injection (covered in depth in chapter 9) to ensure insulin is available and active in your blood. Paying attention to your insulin timing strategy is a simple and powerful way to limit postprandial blood glucose elevations.

## If You Experience Low Blood Glucose After Breakfast

If you experience low blood glucose within 3 hours of eating the perfect breakfast, this is a strong indicator that you are gaining insulin sensitivity and carbohydrate tolerance. Low blood glucose is also referred to as *hypoglycemia,* and is often accompanied by sweating, slurred speech, blurry vision, difficulty concentrating, and dizziness. Hypoglycemia occurs when your blood glucose drops below 70 mg/dL and can be life-threatening, so it's important to pay close attention to how you feel to minimize your risk for an emergency.

If you are insulin-dependent, consider using the decision tree to reduce the amount of insulin you administer at breakfast, and if you are on a glucose-lowering oral medication, ask your doctor to help you reduce your dosage so you remain safe.

## If You Get Hungry After 1 to 2 Hours

Because fruits are processed by your digestive system quickly, you may feel hungry after a few hours—and that's okay. Increase the size of your breakfast bowl or eat a second breakfast in the middle of the morning. Usually, increasing the size of your bowl by adding more fruits, beans, peas, lentils, or intact whole grains solves the problem quickly.

Many people who adopt a plant-based diet are often quite hungry as they adjust to eating larger volumes of foods with lower calorie density. Feel free to eat green light foods generously in order to feel full throughout the day. Some people choose to eat fresh whole fruit every 2 to 3 hours or just snack on whole fruit when they feel hungry between meals. Enjoy as much as you like to stay satisfied!

# How to Know When to Move On

By focusing on changing only one meal at a time, you are allowing your muscles, liver, and cardiovascular system time to adjust to the changes you're making, which keeps you from feeling overwhelmed. However, when you feel satisfied with the results you're seeing from changing your breakfast, then refer to the list below to confirm you are ready to change your lunch. In general, we recommend moving on to lunch once you feel as though you have accomplished the following:

- You have eaten either of the two breakfast options for a minimum of 7 consecutive days.
- You understand how much food to eat in order to stay full for 3 to 4 hours, or until it's time to eat lunch.
- You have mastered the logistics of the morning hours and understand how and when to prepare your meal as part of your daily morning routine.
- If you are insulin-dependent, you understand how much bolus insulin to inject in order to maintain a post-meal (2 to 3 hours after you finish eating) blood glucose of between 80 and 140 mg/dL.

If you have accomplished these four tasks, then it's time to move on to lunch, our favorite meal of the day!

To view the 45+ scientific references cited in this chapter, please visit us online at www.masteringdiabetes.org/bookinfo.

# Chapter 11

# Gaining Momentum: Lunch

## Fatty Liver Disease, Obesity, and Type 2 Diabetes Reversed: Raj

Raj, a lifelong vegetarian, felt that he was in peak health in 2008, when his career on Wall Street was well underway. However, after he chose to prioritize his career and put his health on the back burner, the stress of his fast-paced job began to wear him down. After leaving Wall Street, he became an entrepreneur, which made it difficult to establish a comfortable work-life balance and caused significant amounts of stress. He found himself working long hours and indulged in fat-rich and refined comfort foods to cope with the increased stress. Over the course of time, Raj's weight steadily increased from 170 pounds to 265 pounds, and he began to feel himself slowing down. Then, one day at a routine doctor's appointment, his doctor diagnosed him with fatty liver disease. That's when Raj realized that it was time to change his lifestyle immediately.

He had tried a vegan diet, a low-carbohydrate diet, and juice fasts to lose weight, but nothing seemed to work. Despite his best efforts, Raj was ultimately diagnosed with type 2 diabetes in December of 2016. Then one day Raj overheard his two sons talking about him while playing basketball.

His younger son said, "Forget asking Dad to join us. He's lazy and too overweight to play basketball with us anymore." Hearing this comment broke Raj's heart, because at the age of 39, he was not only losing his health but also his family.

Raj began researching how he could reverse type 2 diabetes and an enlarged liver through lifestyle change, even though he had been told that each condition was irreversible and that managing both conditions with medications was the best he could hope for. Intuitively, Raj knew that he could reverse both fatty liver disease and type 2 diabetes using his food as medicine, so he began researching how to accomplish this as soon as possible. After watching the documentary *What the Health,* which features a segment with Neal Barnard, MD, explaining how to reverse type 2 diabetes using a low-fat plant-based whole-food diet, Raj immediately typed the words "diabetes reversal" into YouTube and found the Mastering Diabetes Coaching Program.

In March 2018, Raj committed to the program and eliminated foods from his diet that he had previously considered healthy—primarily ghee, cheese, avocados, and olive oil. In substitution for these foods, he began eating more plants and started moving his body every day. He was amazed at how simple it was to do these things, even with a hectic schedule and incredibly demanding job. After only 6 months, Raj successfully shed 64 pounds and reduced his A1c to a nondiabetic level of 5.2%, normalized his fasting blood glucose, reduced his cholesterol to 149 mg/dL, and reversed fatty liver disease. After 16 months following the Mastering Diabetes Method, he is back at 170 pounds, and now has more muscle than ever before. He enjoys eating 4 to 5 pieces of fruit for breakfast and a salad with either potatoes or beans for lunch; he thoroughly enjoys re-creating popular Indian dishes using only whole foods. Today, Raj has reconnected with his family and is able to play with his kids to his heart's content. Most important, Raj reports that his self-esteem, happiness, and satisfaction are higher than they've been in years, and for that he is eternally grateful.

ongratulations! You're ready to take the next step in the Mastering Diabetes Method: constructing your perfect lunch. It might sound straightforward—and ultimately it really is—but planning for your midday meal requires more nuanced considerations than we've previously given you. Up until now, we've kept the guidelines very simple: Eat as much green light foods as you want, minimize yellow light foods, and eliminate red light foods to the best of your ability. These recommendations are still in place for lunch, but we're going to home in on the details a bit more and give you an even deeper understanding of how to construct the "perfect" midday meal for maximum insulin sensitivity.

It's important to optimize your lunch for many reasons, but mainly because you eat it in the middle of the day, which is when you are most cognitively and physically active. In this chapter we'll talk about exactly which types of meals will provide you with long-lasting energy, no matter what's going on in your day. When you eat the perfect lunch, we hope you will experience the following:

1. You will feel energized and remain satisfied for a minimum of 3 to 4 hours.
2. You will remain alert, focused, and full of energy throughout the afternoon, and you don't experience a post-lunch food coma.
3. You will feel more energized in the middle of the day.

What's the secret to achieving all of the things listed above? The key to having ample energy and maintaining control of your blood glucose is to choose green light foods that are *calorie dense*.

## The Ins and Outs of Calorie Density: A Lifestyle of Abundance

A key benefit of the Mastering Diabetes Method is that you don't have to be hungry in order to maximize your insulin sensitivity. You don't have to count calories or control your portion sizes in order to gain full control of your health and reach your ideal body weight. We know this may sound crazy, but we sincerely mean it when we say that you can eat carbohydrate-rich foods to satisfaction. And when you understand the principles of calorie density, feeling satisfied becomes virtually effortless.

Before we go any further, let's first define calorie density. *Calorie density* is a term that refers to the *number of calories in a given weight of food*. It's also commonly framed as *the number of calories per pound of edible food.* The calorie density of commonly eaten foods spans a wide range, from as few as 50 calories per pound to 4,010 calories per pound. Below is a table to further illustrate the large span in calorie density among foods you routinely encounter:

| Green Light Foods (calories per pound) | Yellow Light Foods (calories per pound) | Red Light Foods (calories per pound) |
|---|---|---|
| Watercress: 50 | Brown rice pasta: 550 | Shrimp: 540 |
| Broccoli: 150 | Avocados: 730 | Steak: 730 |
| Bananas: 400 | Dates: 1,050 | Chicken: 790 |
| Sweet potatoes: 410 | Gluten-free bread: 1,100 | Salmon: 830 |
| Brown rice: 560 | Dried figs: 1,130 | Oreos: 2,140 |
| Black beans: 600 | Almonds: 2,630 | Olive oil: 4,010 |

When you eat predominantly from the green light category, not only will you maximize your ability to lose weight, reverse insulin resistance, stay satisfied, and improve your athletic performance and recovery, but green light foods also happen to have the lowest calorie density. When it comes to our recommendations of *how many* of these green light foods to eat, we have extended from the research of Barbara Rolls, PhD, professor of nutritional sciences at Pennsylvania State University—a leader in the field of calorie density.

**When assembling your lunch, we recommend you freely eat green light foods containing 700 calories per pound or less, eat yellow light foods sparingly, and minimize or completely eliminate red light foods.**

Through our own experience and our experience with clients, the experience of our colleagues, and research into the healthiest long-lived populations in the world, we know that long-term success on a low-fat plant-based whole-food diet is dependent on building meals around calorie-dense whole-plant foods.

Now, let's revisit the table above. You'll notice that there's some overlap in the ranges of calorie density between green, yellow, and red light foods, as you can see in the illustration below.

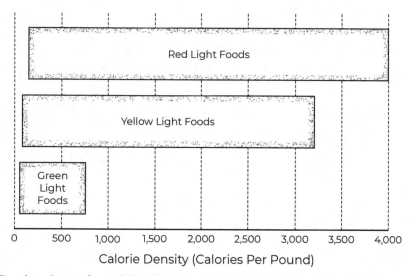

The calorie density of green light, yellow light, and red light foods has a considerable overlap. We recommend eating as many green light foods from the high end of the green light category as possible in order to stay energized, full, and insulin sensitive.

Technically speaking, if you're eating foods in the upper levels of the green light category, you could also eat the equivalent amount of energy from foods in the middle of the yellow light category or from the bottom of the red light category. From a calorie density perspective, this strategy may be safe, but based on what you know about how yellow and red light foods increase insulin resistance, this strategy is not an optimal choice for your overall health. When it comes to weight loss, it's possible to lose weight even when small amounts of red light foods are present in your diet. However, when it comes to maximizing your insulin sensitivity, even small quantities of red light foods have a drastic negative impact on your blood glucose values and medication needs. Eating the majority of your food from the green light category maximizes your chances of losing weight and reversing insulin resistance *simultaneously*.

As long as you eat a wide selection of fruits, starchy vegetables, beans, lentils, peas, intact whole grains, non-starchy vegetables, leafy greens, and mushrooms, you can confidently eat large portions knowing that they will maximize your metabolic health and help you attain your ideal body weight. And in addition to being lowest on the calorie density scale, as you learned in chapter 6, green light foods are also the most nutrient-dense because they contain a wide variety of vitamins, minerals, antioxidants, and phytochemicals with potent anti-inflammatory properties. That's great news for you, because the more of them you eat in substitution for yellow and red light foods, the more likely you are to maximize your metabolic health by providing high-quality micronutrients to all tissues.

## Eat More, Weigh Less

Research has shown that most people eat approximately the same weight of food on a daily basis, with very small day-to-day variations. Studies have shown that people eat about 3 to 5 pounds of food per day, regardless of whether it contains foods with a low, medium, or high calorie density. Therefore, if you strategically eat green light foods with a low calorie density, by the time you're full you will have eaten substantially fewer total calories than if you ate foods in the yellow or red light categories.

Simply stated, if your digestive system accepts the same weight of food per day, then filling it with foods low on the calorie density scale will maximize your ability to lose weight and gain insulin sensitivity simultaneously. If instead you're trying to maintain your current body weight or gain weight, eat the majority of your diet from the most calorie-dense foods in the green light category, including sweet fruits, starchy vegetables, legumes, and intact whole grains.

**The implications of this extensive body of research may be hard to believe—if you eat foods with a low calorie density, you can eat more and weigh less.**

This research shows that you can cut out as many as 2,000 calories per day by eating foods low in calorie density, and you're likely to feel just as satisfied as if you were eating foods with a high calorie density. How is this possible? It's simple—as long as you eat approximately the same *weight* of food per day, your digestive system won't know the difference between a diet with a low calorie density and one with a high calorie density, but eating fiber-rich high-quality plant-based foods will make a tremendous difference in your metabolic health.

## What *Actually* Makes You Feel Full?

If you've ever asked yourself the question "What components of my food actually make me feel full?" then join the club. The human digestive system is incredibly complex and is in constant communication with your brain to control your appetite as well as how quickly food moves through your stomach, your small intestine, and your large intestine. Your digestive system is intricately designed with a sophisticated collection of nerves that sense carbohydrates, fats, protein, nutrients, salt, changes in pH, and the amount of mechanical stretch at various locations.

When you eat food, these neurons are in constant communication with your brain to make minute-by-minute decisions about when to start eating, when to slow down, and when to stop eating altogether. Nerves in your stomach and small intestine secrete *serotonin,* which not only makes you feel happy but also propels partially digested food through your small intestine and tells your stomach to wait before releasing more food downstream. Think of serotonin as a traffic light that constantly switches from green to red in order to control how and when your stomach empties.

One of the most important components in your food that tells your brain when to slow or completely shut off your hunger signal is known as *bulk*. Bulk is a term given to the combination of water and fiber, which occupies space in your digestive system and mechanically stretches your stomach, your small intestine, and your large intestine. Scientists believe that because bulk is the most effective satiety signal, the amount of bulk in your food is the most important determinant of how satisfied you feel after a meal.

Not only does bulk stretch your stomach and small intestine in the upper part of your digestive system, but scientists have also discovered something fascinating about the way that fiber interacts with your large intestine and brain. When you eat fiber-rich foods, bacteria in your microbiome ferment it into short-chain fatty acids, as we discussed in chapters 5 and 7. Not only do these short-chain fatty acids boost immune function, fight infections, improve insulin signaling, and promote insulin sensitivity, they also communicate with your brain to control how much food you eat. What's amazing is that your digestive system can talk to your brain using a combination of electrical signals from nerves, hormones manufactured by your digestive organs, and short-chain fatty acids created in your large intestine as a result of eating fiber.

Many people who eat a low-carbohydrate or ketogenic diet that is low in fiber find themselves quite hungry. It can be hard to predict how eating a low-fiber diet will affect your appetite, but a growing body of research shows that diets low in fiber can interrupt the communication between your digestive system and your brain, resulting in a larger appetite and weight gain. Perhaps you've experienced the sensation of feeling constantly hungry no matter how much food you eat. If so, you may be in this subset of the population. Researchers have found that adding fiber-rich foods to your meals and significantly increasing your total fiber intake can make a dramatic difference in how full you (and your gut bacteria) feel at all times.

In contrast to those mentioned above, there are many people who report that eating a low-carbohydrate diet actually *suppresses* their appetite. Many people who adopt a low-carbohydrate or ketogenic diet find that they are less hungry than before, and as a result, they eat fewer total calories, which can promote rapid weight loss.

Drinking water before a meal does not have the same effect on satiety as eating foods with a high water content. Eating foods that come prepackaged with water and fiber together is your ticket to feeling well fed. The good news is that all green light foods contain both fiber and water, so you don't have to worry about drinking extra water to get a bulking effect. For a table of the water content of select plant foods, refer to chapter 6.

Although this concept may be challenging at first, understanding how bulk affects your digestive system and brain is actually quite straightforward. The following images illustrate the dramatic weight difference between foods that are low and high on the calorie density scale. As you read the comparisons below, ask yourself a simple question: *Which foods do you think will leave you feeling more satisfied?*

### Olive Oil vs. Hearty Sweet Potato and Squash Soup

In this comparison, 3.5 tablespoons of olive oil have an equivalent number of calories as one serving of Hearty Sweet Potato and Squash Soup (see chapter 15 for the soup recipe). The olive oil has zero water and zero fiber, whereas

## Both of the Foods Below Contain About 420 Calories

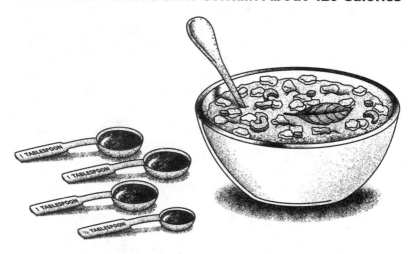

3½ Tablespoons
of Olive Oil

**OR**

1 Serving of Hearty
Sweet Potato
and Squash Soup

the soup has 23 grams of fiber per serving and a high water content. Even though these foods have an equal calorie value, the soup is much more likely to keep you satiated than is a small amount of olive oil.

### Oreos vs. Cantaloupe

Which do you think will leave you feeling more satiated, two Oreos or two cups of cubed cantaloupe? Both contain approximately 110 calories. Very few people will feel full from eating only two Oreos, so if you chose the cantaloupe, then you're correct. In this case, both foods are low in fat, but the cantaloupe is considerably more satiating than the Oreos and contains more water and fiber than the equivalent calories in Oreos.

**Both of the Foods Below Contain About 110 Calories**

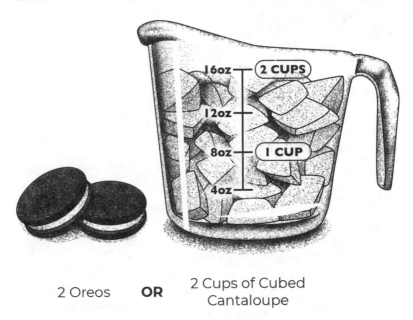

2 Oreos        **OR**        2 Cups of Cubed Cantaloupe

### Peanut Butter vs. Baked Potatoes

Do you think you'd feel more satisfied eating three tablespoons of peanut butter or one large baked potato? Both contain approximately 110 calories.

Peanut butter is more calorie dense and has much less water content in an equal calorie comparison, as shown below. The baked potato contains 224 grams of water and 6.5 grams of fiber, whereas the peanut butter has less than 1 gram of water and 2.5 grams of fiber. Both are nutrient dense, although the baked potato will allow you to eat a larger volume of food, feel satisfied, and optimize your insulin sensitivity simultaneously.

## Both of the Foods Below Contain About 110 Calories

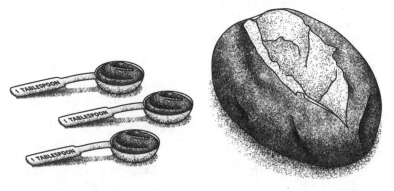

3 Tablespoons     **OR**     1 Large Baked Potato
of Peanut Butter

### Dried Apricots vs. Whole Apricots

Which do you think would keep you feeling more full—½ cup of dried apricots or nine whole apricots? Both contain approximately 150 calories. Dried apricots and whole apricots both originate from apricots; the only difference is that dried apricots contain substantially less water than their whole counterparts. Dried fruits are a common afternoon snack for many people who want to stay full between lunch and dinner. But eating the equivalent calories in whole apricots will actually keep you fuller for a longer period of time because the increased water content occupies more space in your digestive system, sending a stronger signal to your brain to stop eating.

**Both of the Foods Below Contain About 150 Calories**

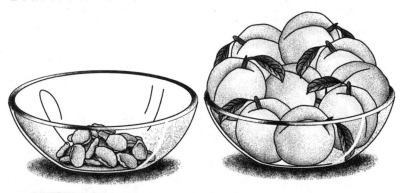

½ Cup of Dried Apricots    **OR**    9 Whole Apricots

## Constructing the Perfect Lunch

For best results, choose a few calorie-dense green light ingredients as the foundation of your lunch, then add a few less calorie-dense non-starchy vegetables for flavor and texture. Excellent choices for calorie-dense foods at lunch include:

- **Fruits:** plantains, bananas, persimmons, figs, papaya, or mangoes
- **Starchy vegetables:** potatoes, sweet potatoes, butternut squash, yams, or corn
- **Legumes:** any variety of beans, lentils, or peas
- **Intact whole grains:** brown rice, quinoa, millet, amaranth, farro, or barley
- **Minimally processed pasta alternatives:** pasta made with chickpeas, quinoa, black beans, mung beans, brown rice, or lentils

The great news is that almost any recipe that you enjoyed eating for lunch in the past can be re-created with primarily green light foods, including sandwiches, burgers, tacos, stews, sushi, lasagna, and even ice cream. For examples of some of our favorite lunch makeovers, refer to chapter 15. You can also find more recipes on our website by visiting www.masteringdiabetes.org/recipes.

## How to Construct No-Recipe Lunch Meals

While we have a large collection of time-tested, appetite-approved recipes at your disposal in chapter 15, we've also worked hard to perfect the art of the no-recipe meal. These meals may seem overly simplistic at first, but constructing a meal without the use of a recipe is something that will save you large amounts of time in the future because it simplifies the process of preparing food while also keeping you insulin sensitive. For a combined total of more than twenty-nine years, no-recipe meals have been our midday meal go-tos—because they're satisfying, delicious, and very energizing. We have also received feedback from thousands of people online saying that they love no-recipe meals because they're efficient and require almost no thought to execute.

The first step is to ask yourself, "Am I in the mood for sweet or savory?" If you want to go with a fruit-based meal, choose 2 to 5 fruits, peel them as needed, and add them to a bowl. Feel free to include leafy greens like lettuce, arugula, or spinach because they slow the absorption of glucose and can help keep your post-meal blood glucose well controlled. Grab a fork and dig in, or if you're feeling extra fancy, add spices like cinnamon, cardamom, carob powder, or cloves to take the flavor of your fruit bowl to the next level.

If you prefer a savory meal at lunch, then first choose a calorie-dense option as the base, including potatoes (any type or color), squash (any variety), yams, corn, beans (all varieties), lentils (all varieties), green peas, or intact whole grains like rice (all varieties), quinoa, or millet. Next, garnish your base with less calorie-dense vegetables such as artichokes, cauliflower, onions, mushrooms, eggplants, tomatoes, okra, asparagus, cucumber, zucchini, radishes, jicama, mushrooms, cauliflower, broccoli, or beets. Again, if you're feeling fancy, add savory spices or herbs like cumin, paprika, curry powder, black pepper, red pepper, thyme, oregano, or sage to flavor the dish just the way you like.

## Minimally Processed Pasta Alternatives

As you know by now, we are big fans of eating intact whole grains instead of refined grains. Intact whole grains are significantly better for your overall health because they are nutrient-dense and contain valuable vitamins, minerals, fiber, antioxidants, and phytochemicals that aid in nutrient absorption and transport. And remember, the term *whole grain* unfortunately doesn't actually mean much for packaged products, which is why we recommend eating minimally processed pasta alternatives instead.

One of the primary reasons that pasta alternatives are listed as yellow light foods (as opposed to red light foods) is that when they are cooked, they absorb water, which lowers their calorie density while still delivering vitamins, minerals, fiber, water, antioxidants, and phytochemicals. Luckily, there are now many pasta alternatives in the grocery store that are made from chickpeas, quinoa, black beans, mung beans, soybeans, brown rice, and lentils. Technically speaking, they are still processed foods, but much less processed than conventional pastas made from wheat.

## Dressings, Sauces, and Condiments

You can also include dressings, sauces, and condiments to add flavor to a meal made of green light foods. Often, sauces are made using yellow light ingredients like nuts, seeds, coconut meat, and avocados, but as long as you use them sparingly, you can feel free to add these sauces to your meals. Also, don't forget that oil is a red light food; we strongly suggest that you avoid it completely in order to maximize your insulin sensitivity. You can make many delicious sauce recipes without adding any oil, and once you get used to eating food without oil, sauces or dressings that do contain oil may taste overwhelmingly heavy. Examples of condiments that we enjoy include coconut aminos, hot sauce, mustard, apple cider vinegar, balsamic vinegar, nutritional yeast, and oil-free hummus. You may notice that processed coconut products are red light items and yet we're recommending coconut aminos here. That's because this highly flavorful condiment is used in small quantities and does not contribute a large amount of fat or calories to your meal.

When it comes to sourcing condiments, you have two primary options:

- Make them at home with clean ingredients. Homemade condiments can last for many days in the fridge and for months in the freezer.

- Buy select packaged condiments that are made of green light and yellow light ingredients, free of added sugar, oil, and salt.
- You can see a list of approved condiments on our website (www.masteringdiabetes.org/bookresources).

In either case, you'll be avoiding added sodium, refined sugars, oil, and harmful additives found in many packaged condiments.

# Making Meals Easily: Batch Cooking, Meal Planning, and Grocery Shopping

Over the course of time, we guarantee that following the Mastering Diabetes Method can eventually become second nature and will likely become fully integrated into your everyday life. There is no doubt that this process takes time, but feeling comfortable without spending excessive amounts of effort thinking and planning ahead may come sooner than you might think.

In particular, learning how to *batch prep* food can save you a lot of time and frustration. Think of batch prepping as a way to simplify your life in the short term. Specifically, it's cooking large amounts of food in a short period of time, storing it in the fridge or freezer, and grabbing it on the go when you are looking for a Mastering Diabetes–friendly meal and don't have much time.

## Benefits of Batch Prepping

- **It saves you money.** You can purchase large bags of uncooked intact whole grains, beans, or lentils in the bulk section of the grocery store, or you can purchase these same ingredients precooked in the freezer section. They cost significantly less than they would at a restaurant, café, or meal delivery service.
- **It means you'll always have something to eat.** Prepped meals containing foods like rice, beans, and potatoes can last for about a

week in your fridge and for months in your freezer. That means that eating a home-prepared meal is only minutes away, especially when you haven't had a chance to get to the grocery store or are pinched for time. It's especially great for tossing into travel-friendly containers, so you can take healthy meals with you, whether it's to work or when you're traveling.

- **It makes it easy to prepare healthy meals.** Not only will you always have something to eat, you'll always have something *healthy* available. Batch prepping your favorite green light foods ensures that you'll never run into the problem of relying on a refined snack food when you're hungry and have limited options. Bring a premade lunch to work in a plastic or glass container, and easily prevent against eating less healthy food in the workplace. With a little advance preparation, grabbing a premade meal from the fridge is just as easy as using a vending machine. And that's exactly the point.

- **It saves you time.** We know that dedicating time to grocery shop and batch prep may sound overwhelming. But the truth is that batch prepping actually saves you time in the kitchen. By preparing everything at once, you eliminate the need to cook and clean multiple times a week. If you're a busy individual, then batch prepping can dramatically reduce the amount of time you spend in the kitchen, especially as your skills improve and you become more efficient.

## What to Batch Prep

- **Fruits:** Most fruits are best eaten fresh and do not require batch prepping. However, there are a few fruits that you can cut and store in the fridge that will stay fresh for days, including jackfruit, pomegranate, pineapple, papaya, cantaloupe, honeydew, and watermelon.

- **Starchy vegetables:** Essentially all starchy vegetables can be cooked in advance and stored in your refrigerator or freezer. These include potatoes, yams, and butternut squash.

- **Beans, peas, and lentils:** Legumes are perfect foods to batch prep because cooking them from scratch can take a long time. We recommend preparing legumes starting from dry ingredients. If you are strapped for time, you can always purchase low-sodium canned beans with no oil, prepared vacuum-sealed lentils with no oil, or frozen peas.

- **Intact whole grains:** Cooking intact whole grains like brown rice, quinoa, millet, or farro each time you want to prepare a meal can be time-consuming, but if you cook them in large quantities at the beginning of the week, this can save you a tremendous amount of time down the road.

- **Non-starchy vegetables:** At the beginning of the week, cut up non-starchy vegetables like onions, bell peppers, carrots, broccoli, cauliflower, cucumbers, and zucchini and store them in the fridge in separate containers. When it comes time to eat, add them uncooked to salads, sauté them in water, or boil, steam, broil, or bake them as you wish.

- **Greens:** Clean large batches of greens such as lettuce, arugula, Swiss chard, and kale and store them in bags in your fridge containing a dry paper towel to soak up any excess moisture. Many grocery stores also sell prewashed greens in plastic containers or bags, so feel free to purchase these if they save you time. Either way, when it comes time to eat, grab your prewashed greens and enjoy raw or cooked.

- **Herbs and spices:** If you plan to use fresh herbs, we recommend cutting the stems off while batch prepping and store the de-stemmed herbs and spices in a bag or container in your refrigerator. And be sure to use them quickly, because fresh herbs have a short shelf life. You can also purchase garlic that has already been removed from the bulb and peeled, which can save you a lot of time.

- **Make-ahead meals, sauces, and condiments:** In addition to preparing staple ingredients that you use often, batch prepping recipes like hummus, tomato sauce, dressings, or homemade broth or soups can add a lot of convenience to your life. These homemade options are likely to be more flavorful than their store-bought counterparts.

### How to Batch Prep

The key to successful batch prepping is to find a time that works well in your schedule. Make a list of all the meals you'd like to eat for the next 5 to 7 days (hint: keep it simple and aim to prepare about 3 to 5 dishes in total). Next, make a list of all the ingredients you'll need to prepare those meals, and purchase them from the grocery store or grocery delivery service.

When preparing your food, do your best to multitask. At the same time that you're steaming broccoli and cauliflower in the same pot, boil sweet potatoes in another pot. In a third pot, cook your beans, quinoa, or brown rice, and set a timer for each individual pot. While those are cooking, cut up non-starchy vegetables and fruit and pack them in separate plastic bags. You'll be surprised at how much you can accomplish in 60 to 90 minutes, especially as you become more practiced.

You can also cook food while you're sleeping. If you own a slow cooker, add rice, beans, squash, potatoes, or a full recipe (like soup or chili) to your slow cooker before you go to bed. When you wake up, store the prepared food in the fridge or freezer.

Do your best to refrigerate or freeze batch-prepped food in equal meal-sized portions to make life easy at the time you're ready to eat. If you are using fast-acting insulin, putting the food into equal portions makes it easy to calculate the carbohydrate value of each meal. Divide the total carbohydrate count of a recipe by the number of equal-sized containers to determine the carbohydrate count of each portion.

# Meal Planning

Now that you know exactly what foods are best to eat for breakfast and lunch, it's time to commit to the Mastering Diabetes Method. Meal planning is a great way to get started. In fact, it could also be referred to as meal *committing*. In addition to helping you organize your life and shop for groceries, meal planning is extremely useful because it assists you in committing to eating with your health in mind. There are many different ways to meal plan (with varying levels of complexity), but the purpose is to help you answer two questions:

1. Do you know which ingredients to buy for the week ahead?
2. Do you have a general idea of what you want to eat for each meal over the next seven days (including which restaurants or cafés you plan to visit)?

Take a moment to consider how much thought you put into meal planning right now. You probably don't overthink what you are going to eat or where you're going to eat it. Maybe you have a few favorite dishes and a few favorite restaurants, and the combination of those covers the majority of your meals. While meal planning and batch prepping can seem quite intimidating at first, we are committed to helping you become comfortable with this new lifestyle, so that you don't have to overthink any aspect of your food ecosystem. Becoming comfortable won't happen overnight, but over the course of a few weeks to months, you'll likely find dishes and food combinations that you really enjoy, and you may find yourself eating the same foods often.

Like any new habit, meal planning takes time to become second nature. Until it does, we highly recommend writing down your meal plan for each week on a piece of paper. Create spaces for breakfast and lunch next to each day (and eventually dinner, when you get there) and then pencil in what you plan to eat for those meals. Your meals don't have to be complicated—they can be as simple as "bananas, mangoes, and freshly ground chia seeds" or "quinoa, tomatoes, cucumbers, and lime juice." Remember also to write down any meals that you eat at a restaurant or café, including things like breakfast dates, lunch meetings, or dinners with friends. The process of writing down what you are going to eat will help you execute your meal plan, no matter how busy your days are. This exercise allows you to think through any challenging obstacles that may throw you off course, and prepares you to know exactly what to buy from the grocery store.

## How to Grocery Shop Like a Pro

Just a few shopping tips and tricks can make your transition to the Mastering Diabetes Method quite smooth. We know this process can become overwhelming and that looking for new items in the grocery store can be a pain. The information below will help you learn how to shop efficiently and save time and money. Trust us when we say that learning how to grocery shop is absolutely worth the effort.

The first thing to know is that the total amount of food in your shopping cart will likely increase dramatically. Remember, the calorie density of your food will decrease because you will be eating a larger amount of fiber- and water-rich foods. Luckily, fruits, vegetables, legumes, and intact whole grains are considerably less expensive than animal-based foods, so purchasing more of them may not increase the amount of money you spend (in fact your bill may even go down). As a general rule of thumb, when you have eyeballed your cart and believe that you have purchased enough fruits and vegetables, add about 50 percent more! We know that may seem wasteful, but we aren't kidding when we tell you that the amount of food you'll be eating will increase dramatically.

You can also save money by purchasing bulk items at stores such as Costco, Walmart, or Sam's Club. In addition to buying bulk items like beans and whole grains, you can purchase a wide variety of fresh produce and stock up on your favorite frozen fruits and vegetables. Other great options for sourcing tropical fruits are local farmers' markets, Asian markets, or Latino markets. We recommend looking for these markets in your area so that you can diversify your options and save money at the same time in many cases.

### Shopping Suggestions for Green Light Foods

- **Fresh and frozen fruit:** Remember, fruit is low in calorie density, so it will take a lot of fruit to fill you up. When buying fruit at the market, make sure to go *big*. If you were to visit our homes, you would find shelves stocked with large quantities of in-season fruit.

It's important to replenish your fresh fruit supply on a regular basis and stock fruit at varying stages of ripeness. That way you can eat some today, some tomorrow, and some a few days from now. Purchase your favorite fruits from the market, and try new ones that seem exciting, including bananas, kiwis, mangoes, nectarines, cantaloupes, papayas, oranges, apples, persimmons, figs, and pears. Also feel free to try new varieties of familiar fruit. Instead of getting Fuji apples every time, try Honey Crisp, Gala, or Braeburn—some are sweeter than others, and each has a different texture.

Unsweetened frozen fruit is a great option and can help you save money. Oftentimes frozen fruit is picked ripe before it's flash frozen, preserving many nutrients. Frozen berries are available year-round and don't spoil quickly like fresh berries. Try stocking your freezer with your favorite fruits including mangoes, cherries, peaches, pineapples, and frozen mixed berries. Just check the label to make sure no sugar has been added.

- **Fresh or frozen starchy vegetables:** Starchy vegetables are a staple in the Mastering Diabetes Method, and they can last for several weeks on your counter or in your fridge when raw. Oftentimes you can find precut starchy vegetables (fresh or frozen), which is a great way to save time. Examples include yams, potatoes, squashes, and pumpkin. Purchasing these vegetables in the freezer section of your grocery store will save you lots of time when preparing food in large quantities.
- **Dry or canned beans, lentils, and peas:** Legumes are another food group that we recommend buying in large quantities, especially because you can store them dried or canned for a long period of time. When you find them on sale, stock up! You can buy them in the bulk section of the grocery store, or you can buy them canned to save even more time. Consider selecting canned beans, lentils, and peas with no added salt for optimal heart health.
- **Intact whole grains (and pastas):** Intact whole grains are another great food group to buy in bulk. There are many options when it comes to buying intact whole grains, which store well in airtight

containers in your pantry or cupboards. Examples include buckwheat, spelt, farro, brown rice, millet, rye, sorghum, amaranth, teff, buckwheat, and bulgur. If you're looking for a time-saver, you can usually find precooked intact whole grains in the freezer section of the grocery store, and the most common options include brown rice and quinoa. Try a few different types of intact whole grains and see which ones you like best.

- **Fresh or frozen greens:** As we've discussed earlier, leafy greens are powerful additions to your meals because they slow the rate at which glucose is absorbed into your blood and contain tremendous nutrient density. Leafy greens store well in the refrigerator, but you can also find a great selection of greens in the frozen section of the grocery store. You can never have too many leafy greens in your diet, so stock up.

- **Fresh and frozen non-starchy vegetables:** Just like with frozen fruit, frozen vegetables are a terrific option. Frozen vegetables are usually flash frozen soon after harvest to preserve their nutritional value. Head to the produce section of the grocery store or your local farmers' market to find a wide variety of fresh non-starchy vegetables that you can use within the next week, or head to the freezer section to find frozen corn, broccoli, cauliflower, cauliflower rice, green beans, peas, and carrots.

- **Herbs and spices:** You can find a wide selection of herbs and spices at your local grocery store or farmers' market. Start by purchasing a few herbs and spices that you know you enjoy, then diversify your palate over the course of time. Fresh herbs will stay fresh on your countertop or refrigerator for only about one week, whereas dried herbs and spices can keep for months to years. Our favorites include cumin, paprika, curry powder, black pepper, red pepper, cayenne pepper, cinnamon, cardamom, and cloves. Experiment with new herbs and spices as the opportunities arise—they're a great way to add personality to any dish.

## Is It Important to Buy Organic Produce?

**We are often asked** if it's important to buy organic produce versus conventional. Choosing organic produce is almost always preferable, mainly because these plants have been grown using fewer chemicals, which translates to better health for you. One excellent online resource that we recommend consulting is the Dirty Dozen and the Clean Fifteen by the Environmental Working Group (EWG). Every year, the EWG does a comprehensive analysis of all fruits and vegetables in the United States to determine which foods have the highest and lowest pesticide residue. The Dirty Dozen is a list of twelve of the most contaminated fruits and vegetables, and the Clean Fifteen is a list of the fifteen least contaminated fruits and vegetables. When considering purchasing organic produce, first pay attention to these two lists, then branch out as your budget and mental capacity permit. Organic or not, though, when shopping at the grocery store, we recommend washing your produce first to remove any unhealthy substances that may have come into contact with your food during transit and handling.

At the beginning of your transition, we want you to focus more on eating plants and less on where they come from. The most important thing you can do is find a way to integrate as many green light foods into your diet as possible, regardless of whether they are organic or conventional. Over the course of time, as you become more comfortable with a plant-based lifestyle and shopping for produce, you can pay more attention to organic produce.

Once eating green light foods at every meal feels easy, natural, and enjoyable, then you can start considering adding more organic foods into the rotation. If you're buying organic foods at the grocery store, they will oftentimes be more expensive than conventional. (And for good reason—growing organically and responsibly requires more work!) As you begin to incorporate more of these foods, start with what works for your budget. Focus on buying organic versions of the fruits and vegetables that are most affected by pesticide use, as recommended by the EWG.

Eventually, you may want to explore buying your produce from a local farmers' market, where most of the fruits and vegetables have been grown without chemicals, using methods that not only improve the soil but also contribute to more nutritious food.

## Packaged Meals

If you are looking for premade meals made entirely from green light foods, unfortunately your options are quite limited. Plant-based packaged foods are becoming more widely available in the grocery store, although they often contain artificial sweeteners, vegetable oils, monosodium glutamate (MSG), artificial colors, texturizers, and preservatives, which can slow or stall your progress.

If you choose to incorporate more processed foods into your program, feel free to use some of the packaged meals that are available in the market, which may result in slower progress. We are not the food police. As coaches, we can help you understand the consequences of your choices on your insulin sensitivity and teach you how to make the most effective decisions to improve your metabolic health, one bite at a time. Your diligence and consistency in adopting lifestyle change is a personal decision, and we are here to support you to the best of our ability.

Think of your transition as an exercise in self-awareness rather than an exercise in self-judgment. Think about your life and figure out what level of commitment you choose to adopt. If cooking meals seems overwhelming or if eating at fast-food restaurants is familiar, then choosing packaged foods containing less than optimal ingredients may be a good way to transition to the full Mastering Diabetes Method. However, if you are fully committed to reversing insulin resistance and minimizing your risk for chronic disease, then we strongly suggest preparing your food yourself instead of relying on packaged meals.

To see a complete list of the packaged foods that we recommend in small proportions, visit www.masteringdiabetes.org/bookresources.

# Take-Home Message

Eating a nutrient-rich lunch can be easy, and we are very confident that you'll be surprised at how tasty and satisfying simple meals can be using only a few ingredients. Whether you choose a no-recipe lunch or use a recipe from our collection or elsewhere, the fundamental principle is the same: Build your lunch around a calorie-dense base, then garnish with less calorie-dense ingredients to add variety and flavor.

## How to Know When to Move On

As always, we suggest taking this process step by step. Work hard to construct lunch meals that you love before advancing to dinner. That way you will be sure to enjoy the process, experiment with new foods, and develop simple strategies to keep your blood glucose rock solid. We recommend moving on to dinner once you feel as though you have accomplished the following:

- You have eaten a low-fat plant-based whole-food lunch for a minimum of 7 consecutive days.
- You understand how much to eat in order to stay full for 3 to 4 hours throughout the middle of the afternoon.
- If you are insulin-dependent, you understand how much bolus insulin to inject in order to maintain a post-meal blood glucose between 80 and 140 mg/dL.

If you have accomplished these three tasks, then it's time to move on to dinner, the meal with the most variety.

To view the 10+ scientific references cited in this chapter, please visit us online at www.masteringdiabetes.org/bookinfo.

# Chapter 12

# Developing a Routine: Dinner

### Mastering Meal Prep: Tea

Tea loved to cook decadent meals for herself and her husband, but after years of indulging in rich meals, she was diagnosed with prediabetes in 2007. Five years later, she was diagnosed with type 2 diabetes and was able to keep her A1c at 7.2% with the use of metformin. However, even though her A1c approached a "safe" value, Tea began to experience nerve damage in her feet, chronic headaches, gallbladder inflammation, acid reflux, low energy, poor sleep, weight gain, and brain fog. She didn't fully understand why but reasoned that it had something to do with the typical approach to managing type 2 diabetes.

Dissatisfied with her worsening health, Tea began looking for alternative approaches to reverse type 2 diabetes altogether. One morning during her daily walk, Tea was having a difficult time feeling her feet due to peripheral neuropathy. In this moment, she decided to take her health into her own hands—and that's when a friend recommended the Mastering Diabetes Coaching Program. She joined the program immediately, intuitively knowing that eating a diet containing more fruits and vegetables could dramatically improve her overall health.

After only 2 weeks of following the Mastering Diabetes Method, Tea's headaches, brain fog, and acid reflux vanished. As she continued with the program, she watched her health continue to improve dramatically: Her lipid panel improved significantly, her blood pressure decreased, and her A1c fell by 1.7%. Over the course of just a few months, Tea learned how to replace her meals with delicious and satisfying green light foods. She quickly adopted the habit of batch cooking beans, vegetables, and rice along with oil-free dressings, which gave her great options for simple, tasty meals.

Over the course of nine months, Tea lost 75 pounds, reduced her A1c from 7.2% to 5.0%, decreased her LDL cholesterol from over 400 mg/dL to 127 mg/dL, lowered her triglycerides from 593 mg/dL to 136 mg/dL, and decreased her blood pressure from 122/80 mmHg to 112/72 mmHg. In addition to improved biomarkers, Tea's neuropathy has ceased getting worse and she can now walk long distances. Tea has reversed type 2 diabetes and peripheral neuropathy, no longer experiences acid reflux or brain fog, is free of food addiction, and was able to discontinue metformin completely. Her doctor was amazed, and she is so happy to be healthy again.

---

Now it's time to take another big leap forward and start eating a nutrient-dense low-fat plant-based whole-food dinner. In the typical Western diet, dinner is usually the largest meal of the day, containing high-calorie protein- and fat-rich foods like chicken, steak, fish, lamb, pork, and cheese. We, on the other hand, recommend eating lighter meals at the end of the day, especially if you are more sedentary in the evening hours, because you're preparing your body for sleep and have significantly lower energy requirements than in the beginning and middle of the day. You can still enjoy a large meal at dinner, but compared with your lunch, we recommend eating larger quantities of leafy greens and non-starchy vegetables instead of protein- and fat-rich foods.

You will notice that the perfect dinner is very similar to the perfect lunch with one small but important difference: At the center of your plate you'll find calorie-dense foods once again, but instead of eating non-starchy vegetables as garnishes, we recommend eating them in significantly larger proportions. Eating more leafy greens and non-starchy vegetables at dinner is a simple and very powerful addition to your evening meal because not only are they low in calorie density but they are also packed with anti-inflammatory micronutrients and will keep your blood glucose stable throughout the night. Legumes are also an excellent addition to your evening meal, because the second-meal effect helps keep your fasting blood glucose in range.

Using this dinner formula, you can make a virtually endless variety of dinner meals, including bean and whole-grain burgers, tacos, wraps, sushi, chili, soups, curries, pizza, stews, salads, and much more. Dinner is your opportunity to be as creative as you wish, and to help you get started, we have included a few dinner options in chapter 15. You can also find many more dinner recipes on our website by visiting www.masteringdiabetes.org/recipes.

## Understanding Decision Fatigue

Have you ever run into the following scenario? After a long day at work or school, you return home to find yourself extremely hungry. Even though you started the day with the best intentions, by the time you get home, you're exhausted and don't have the energy to prepare a home-cooked meal. You sit on the couch, take a deep breath, then reach for your computer or phone to order takeout from your favorite restaurant, knowing that the food you're about to eat is comforting but far from nutritious.

If you've ever experienced this situation, then join the club. After a day spent working or studying, most people experience *decision fatigue,* a mental and emotional state in which making decisions is incredibly challenging. Decision fatigue is an extremely common psychological state that often surfaces at the end of the day, when your brain is fatigued from having made a wide array of decisions. Research has shown that judges are more likely to make poor decisions at the end of a mentally draining day, drivers make riskier decisions in the evening than in the morning, and athletes are more likely to make a mistake at the end of a game than they are at the beginning. Food manufacturers take advantage of the decision fatigue that many shoppers experience in the grocery store by placing processed snack foods at the checkout line to entice consumers when they are tired and most likely to make poor decisions.

Because decision fatigue can affect your food choices, do your best to think about your dinner *in advance* of the evening hours. We recommend preparing either the majority of your dinner or your entire dinner before you return home from work or school to minimize the amount of mental energy you have to expend in the evening hours. That's exactly why we are such strong advocates of batch prepping on the weekend, because it is a simple way to shift important decisions to a time of the week when you're likely to make better choices.

## Eating at Restaurants and Cafés

In an ideal world, everyone would eat a home-cooked dinner so that they could have full control of the ingredients used in preparation. An ideal world would also include restaurants with menus including delicious meals containing green light foods. But in today's world, eating at a restaurant or café with few to no perfect options on the menu happens with increasing frequency, so it's smart to plan ahead to make sure that doing so doesn't break your insulin sensitivity strategy.

There is no doubt that participating in social situations with family, friends, and coworkers can be one of the most difficult aspects of following the Mastering Diabetes Method. The outside world presents serious challenges to following this lifestyle, which means that having a game plan is essential to asking for what you want as comfortably as possible. Don't worry, being insulin sensitive and being social are not mutually exclusive events. In fact, through our own personal experience, we have discovered several tricks that can help you succeed in social situations.

### Strategy 1: Pre-Eat Your Dinner

One of the most effective ways to socialize at a restaurant with family, friends, or coworkers and maintain your insulin sensitivity is to eat a meal *before* leaving your house. By enjoying a calorie-dense meal before you arrive at a restaurant or café, you'll be less preoccupied with what's on the menu because you won't be as hungry.

The most important thing to remember when pre-eating is to consume calorie-dense foods that make you feel full. When you're hungry or hypoglycemic, it can be hard to make good decisions because the thought of food overwhelms your logical decision-making process. By eating to satiation before you get to a restaurant, you're equipping yourself with the ability to make more logical and thoughtful decisions when you're at the restaurant or café. Then when it's time to order, you can take your time to identify meals that are prepared without excess salt, oil, sugar, or sauces that may contain hidden red light ingredients. Pre-eating is very effective (and is actually our preferred method) for several reasons:

- Pre-eating meals puts the power in your hands because you will likely have more confidence in selecting meals made with green light ingredients when your hunger is at a manageable level.
- Most restaurants do not provide sufficiently large dishes to satisfy a low-fat plant-based whole-food eater, and ordering seconds or thirds can become quite expensive. Pre-eating enables you to stay full for hours without spending so much money.
- Pre-eating makes you less likely to eat snack foods like bread and chips, which many restaurants serve before your meal. When you're less hungry, these nutrient-poor options are less appetizing and *much* easier to resist.

### Strategy 2: Order Green Light Foods at a Restaurant

While pre-eating can set you up for success, sometimes it may not be possible or practical. Either way, learning how to order a meal outside of the house is essential for your long-term success.

Most restaurants may not have meals on the menu containing only green light foods. Most restaurants have many green light *ingredients* interspersed throughout the menu—and this can be very helpful. In some cases, there might be dishes that contain predominantly green light foods and require only small modifications. Start by identifying foods that can serve as your calorie-dense base, then order side dishes like steamed vegetables or a salad. You can also bring your own sauce in a leakproof travel container (this may seem strange at first, but you might be surprised to find your friends and coworkers excited by what you're doing). Regardless of whether you're in a fine dining establishment that's accustomed to such requests or a fast casual restaurant that serves nachos and burgers, the two keys to your success at any restaurant or café are *planning* and *communication*.

## How to Plan When Eating at a Restaurant

The first thing you can plan when eating outside of your house is *where* to eat. Picking plant-friendly restaurants is very helpful and will provide you with more options on the menu—as well as a great-tasting meal. While you can successfully order a Mastering Diabetes–friendly meal just about any-where, we have found that Thai, Vietnamese, and Japanese restaurants gener-ally have many green light options to choose from. And if your city or neighborhood doesn't have any of those options, choose a restaurant with a salad bar. Ironically, steak houses often have all-you-can-eat salad bars and are also known to offer plain baked potatoes and steamed seasonal vegetables, so look for one in your area to eat a calorie-dense meal with plenty of vegetables.

The second thing to consider is *what* to eat. With only a few minutes of online research, you can easily figure out what to order before you walk into the restaurant. Look at the online menu before you get to the restaurant, or call ahead to speak with a host or manager and politely ask if they can serve you green light options without added oil or salt.

When choosing what to order, focus less on the prepared dishes and more on the ingredients available on the menu. By doing this, you can pick and choose various ingredients, then ask the waitstaff for a custom dish con-taining those ingredients. Look for options like potatoes, squash, corn, beans, lentils, quinoa, brown rice, oatmeal, or fruits, and then order side dishes containing leafy greens and non-starchy vegetables, with herbs and spices.

Start thinking of a menu as a "choose your own adventure" book and find ways to assemble insulin-sensitizing meals creatively, using ingredients from multiple prepared dishes. This strategy keeps you insulin sensitive and is actually quite fun!

- **How to locate starchy vegetables:** Starchy vegetables are quite easy to find on restaurant and café menus because many cuisines use potatoes, yams, squash, corn, and root vegetables as staples. Most restaurants offer these ingredients in various forms, so look out for them anywhere on the menu. If a dish has crispy potatoes offered as a side, ask your server if the kitchen can prepare those same potatoes steamed, baked, or broiled without cheese, cream, oil, or butter. You can do the same for foods like squash and yams because they're quite versatile and lend themselves to many cooking techniques. Be sure to communicate to your server that you would like your starchy vegetables prepared without oil, cheese, or butter—this single trick will keep you insulin sensitive and save you many days of frustration. The more you practice asking for foods you want at a restaurant, the easier it becomes to easily ask for a meal that works for you.

- **How to locate beans, peas, and lentils:** Legumes are another great calorie-dense option that you can oftentimes find on a menu, especially at restaurants and cafés that serve Mexican, Indian, Mediterranean, African, and Latin cuisine. As when ordering starchy vegetables, make sure to ask your server if they can be prepared without oil, butter, ghee, or lard. Legumes are used to make curries, soups, and dips, so look for chickpeas, lentils, beans, and peas in stews or chilis containing rice, roasted vegetables, and whole grains.

- **How to locate intact whole grains:** Brown rice, black rice, and quinoa are easy to find on Asian, Mexican, Mediterranean, and Middle Eastern menus. Make sure to ask your server if either oil or fish stock is used when preparing them in the kitchen. If they are, ask the waitstaff politely if they can make you an oil- and fish-stock-free version.

- **How to locate leafy greens:** Just about every menu is likely to have leafy greens, including romaine lettuce, iceberg lettuce, butter lettuce, spinach, arugula, kale, or Swiss chard, especially in the salad section of the menu. If a particular salad contains an oil-based dressing, cheese, bacon, or large quantities of seeds or nuts, ask that these ingredients be removed and replaced with additional vegetables like green beans, tomatoes, cucumbers, bell peppers, corn, peas, jicama, carrots, beets, cauliflower, or broccoli. Then ask for oil and vinegar on the side and just skip the oil. Or request a side of apple cider vinegar, balsamic vinegar, red wine vinegar, or slices of lemons or limes.

- **How to locate non-starchy vegetables:** It's generally also easy to find non-starchy vegetables like artichokes, carrots, cauliflower, broccoli, onions, mushrooms, eggplants, tomatoes, okra, asparagus, cucumber, zucchini, radishes, and jicama. They are usually offered as side dishes or used inside other dishes on the menu. Ask for these vegetables raw, lightly steamed, or baked without any added oil.

- **How to locate fruits:** Ordering fruit from a restaurant or café can be problematic because either it's usually served in small amounts or in an unripe state. Cafés that serve smoothies or fruit bowls are an exception to this rule, and are excellent choices for places to eat. If you do manage to find fruit-friendly cafés or restaurants, be sure to communicate that you are interested in large quantities so that they understand just how much to prepare in order to keep you full. If you are able to find a buffet that serves fruits like oranges, melons, grapes, or apples, this is a great way to eat a satisfying meal of fruit.

- **How to find herbs and spices:** One of Cyrus's favorite things to add to his dinner is a collection of spices, because they are very flavorful and can completely change the personality of a dish. Some of Cyrus's favorites include cumin, cayenne pepper, red pepper flakes, black pepper, thyme, oregano, curry powder, paprika, cinnamon, and cardamom. In addition, we both enjoy fresh herbs including cilantro, basil, mint, thyme, rosemary, and oregano. Do your best to avoid premade spice combinations because they often contain added salt. When you're at a restaurant, ask your server if the kitchen has herbs and spices available, and whether they can be added to your meal. Also consider bringing your own dried herbs and spices in a plastic bag—this is a simple trick that can make a huge difference in how much you enjoy your food.

## How to Communicate Politely . . . Without Being Awkward

As you can see, green light foods are widely available at many restaurants and cafés. It's your job to play detective and find them on the menu, then clearly communicate how you would like them prepared. In this section, we'll focus on simple, sometimes humorous, and always highly effective communication strategies that you can use to stay happy, healthy, and full. These techniques can take some getting used to, especially if you're nervous about feeling uncomfortable or "on the spot" in public places. We are pleasantly surprised at how helpful servers are in making sure that you get what you're looking for.

What we've found over the years is that the most effective way to communicate your desires in an unthreatening and polite way is to intercept your server *away* from the table and explain why you have special requests. This way you can speak with them in private about your preferences without the other people at the table overhearing the conversation, which could lead to unnecessary questions or make you feel uncomfortable when ordering. When you explain that you are living with diabetes and following a new diabetes protocol, you're increasing the likelihood that the server won't take your choices personally or as a knock against the food served at their restaurant. Most servers can relate to your efforts to improve your health and are likely to help you to the best of their ability. Here are the exact steps that you can take to eliminate awkwardness before it begins:

- **Step 1:** Before your server has taken your order, leave the table and pretend to go to the bathroom.

- **Step 2:** Find your server on the restaurant floor and say the following: "Excuse me, I eat differently than most people because I am living with diabetes. I am curious if you could help me create a custom dish from ingredients on the menu." When you explain that your choices stem from a health condition, their defense mechanisms will drop and their desire to help will likely escalate very quickly. Be sure to ask politely, and your server is bound to respond with an emphatic yes.

- **Step 3:** Next, explain that your preferences are focused on eating plants. Because eating a plant-based diet is becoming more common, your server may recognize this phrase. Then proceed to explain exactly what you *do* want to eat. By the time you are speaking to the waiter, you will have already identified what ingredients you have to work with. Restaurants want you to have a great dining experience, because it is a service industry and the employees are rewarded when customers have a great experience (in the form of a tip). We have found that servers actually enjoy a fun challenge because it keeps their job interesting and makes them feel good to know they could help you out. Feel free to also use the following statements or modify these as you see fit:

  - "I'm living with diabetes and I'm trying this new program to help me improve my diabetes health. If you can help me order a super simple meal, I would really, really appreciate it."
  - "I do not eat dairy products, so please do your best to keep the cheese, butter, and cream sauce away from my dish."
  - "I love to eat plainly steamed vegetables, and I see you have a lot of them on the menu. I'd like a dish with [insert exact list]. The bigger the bowl, the better!"
  - "Oil makes me feel terrible, so please keep the dressing on the side. I would really appreciate it."

- **Step 4:** Reiterate exactly what you do want. The clearer you can be, the better. Ask for dishes including a salad with steamed vegetables, beans, or potatoes on top; an oil-free vegetable or bean soup; or a heaping plate of potatoes and vegetables cooked without oil. Most of the time, your server or the chef will impress you with a fun, creative presentation of what you ordered. When it comes to condiments, we recommend bringing your own or adding lime juice, lemon juice, or vinegar on top of your meal.

- **Step 5:** Thank your server profusely for his or her help and personal attention. Giving your server a high five with a huge smile on your face can create a sense of camaraderie and reminds everyone to have fun.
- **Step 6:** When the server returns to the table and asks for everyone's order, you'll already be set and won't experience the anxiety of a potentially awkward public conversation.

### How to Add Humor to Lighten the Mood

One of the most important things you can do in social situations involving food is add humor. People enjoy interacting with others who don't take themselves too seriously and are willing to be lighthearted about their food preferences. Do your best to convey that you would like to customize your order while being comedic about why you choose to eat a plant-based diet. Try using some of the following statements the next time you're out at a restaurant and watch what happens.

- "I eat like a monkey. I love eating fruits and vegetables, so as long as you have those around, I'm all set!"
- "I'm trying to set the world record for maximizing insulin sensitivity, and eating fatty foods will crush my hopes and dreams. Do you think you can help?"
- "If I eat foods that contain fat, I get super angry and start breaking things. Trust me, you don't want to see that side of me!"

## How to Succeed at Dinner Parties

Let's say you are invited to a dinner party with some friends. In the past you may have just eaten whatever was served, but now that you're following the

Mastering Diabetes Method, you'll likely want to make some changes. It's normal to feel nervous about how to handle a dinner party or potluck, but don't worry, because there are simple ways to keep social gatherings at someone's house easy and fun.

As we've said previously, the most important thing you can do when enjoying a meal outside of your home is to plan ahead. In the same way that you can take matters into your own hands by pre-eating before going to a restaurant or asking your server for a custom meal, we recommend contributing a dish to a party and making enough of it to share with others. To do this, it's best to communicate with the host well in advance (usually between two and seven days) so that the host can plan his or her menu accordingly. Ask if it's okay for you to bring a dish to share, or if you can help prepare food that will work for you. You can also use the words *I'm living with diabetes* and *health* in this situation, just as you did before, or use one of the following statements:

- "I've been eating a plant-based diet recently and it's improving my diabetes health. I'd love to make a plant-based dish and contribute it to the party if that's okay with you."
- "This may sound completely bananas, but I'm following a program for my health and they guarantee that eating this way will improve my diabetes, so I'm giving it my best effort."
- "I feel as if I'm eating like an elephant these days! It's crazy, but the program creators guaranteed me it would work, and so far I'm seeing great results."

If you tell the host that you can't eat what he/she prepares for everyone else, he/she might become defensive, which can create tension that can become awkward very quickly. Do your best to avoid saying things like "Your food has too much oil/fat/salt." Instead, focus on communicating what you would like to eat, not what you would like to avoid. Communicating that you are living with diabetes and following a new diabetes program can help the host feel less defensive. Do your best to make it clear that you're coming from a place of love and appreciation rather than a competition about who makes healthier food. People are usually very accommodating, especially when you're asking for what you need and communicating authentically.

If your host is adamant about preparing everything, ask if he or she is willing to make a specific recipe that you provide. Communicate that it's super important not to deviate or improvise—even something as simple as using Parmesan cheese or making an oil-based vinaigrette will make the meal challenging for you to enjoy.

## How to Handle Being Interrogated

When you eat differently from others in social situations, you may begin to receive many questions about your food choices. These scenarios often begin when someone is genuinely curious about your habits, but it can sometimes turn into an uncomfortable interrogation session. Often these conversations can become intense, and without any preparation you may feel the need to defend your choices rather than talk about your new lifestyle from a place of curiosity and excitement. Some of the most common questions that many of our clients face include:

- Where do you get your protein if you don't eat meat?
- Carbs are bad for you. Isn't that too many carbohydrates?
- Fruit contains a lot of sugar. Isn't sugar bad for diabetes?
- What about calcium? Where is your calcium coming from if you don't drink milk?
- What about healthy fats? You must eat a lot of nuts and seeds.

If you find yourself unexpectedly involved in an interrogation session, take a deep breath. Start by saying something to the effect of "I'm happy to talk about my diet, but I may not have all the answers right now." Next, do your best to communicate your experience authentically by saying, "Please understand that I'm following this method to help me reverse insulin resistance and control my blood glucose." If you have already started to experience changes in the way you feel or in your blood glucose values, tell others exactly what you have experienced, whether positive, negative, or neutral. If you have not experienced any changes in the way you feel or in your blood glucose values, you can say, "I'm hopeful that this program will [state your goals]," and refer back to your *why* when you first started the program.

Also keep in mind that you're not obligated to answer anyone's questions (especially if they feel judgmental or threatening). Feel free to emphasize that you are trying something new as an experiment. Then refer people to this book to consult our more than 800 scientific references, or refer them to our website and tell them to read our evidence-based blog, listen to our podcast, attend our annual online summit, view our posts on Instagram and Facebook, or watch videos on our YouTube channel for more information. People may interrogate you without knowing that they are doing so, so do your best to thank others for their concern and gently communicate that you are following a program that is based on almost a hundred years of evidence-based science, even though it may seem contrary to popular opinion.

And always remember, if you are confident in the science backing the Mastering Diabetes Method, then it doesn't really matter what other people think. You are the master of your own decisions; your results will speak for themselves. Even though others may have the best intentions, maintaining your commitment to this program is a personal decision at all times regardless of what others may think.

## How to Know When to Move On

Now that you have the knowledge to make the best choices for the food you eat all day, every day, by constructing the perfect dinner in addition to the perfect breakfast and perfect lunch, it's time to begin experimenting with the final step in your daily meal plan: intermittent fasting. This addition to your new lifestyle routine can take your insulin sensitivity to the next level and dramatically improve your metabolic health. We recommend moving on to intermittent fasting once you feel as though you have accomplished the following:

- You have eaten a low-fat plant-based whole-food breakfast, lunch, and dinner for a minimum of 7 consecutive days.
- You understand how to order food at a restaurant or café and feel comfortable communicating your needs to others in an unthreatening and respectful manner.
- If you are insulin-dependent, you understand how much bolus insulin to inject in order to maintain a post-meal blood glucose between 80 and 140 mg/dL.

If you have accomplished these three tasks, then it's time to move on to intermittent fasting and begin to understand why *not eating* is one of the single most powerful tools for improving your metabolic health ever discovered.

# Chapter 13

# Intermittent Fasting for Increased Insulin Sensitivity and Weight Loss

## Life in the Fast Lane: Erica

Erica was diagnosed with type 1 diabetes at the age of 11 and did her best to control her blood glucose using basal and bolus insulin in addition to restricting her carbohydrate intake. Over the course of time, her energy levels dwindled significantly, she gained excess weight, and her blood glucose was difficult to control. In October of 2015, she injected 21 units of basal insulin and injected bolus insulin at a 6:1 carbohydrate-to-insulin ratio for meals, both of which indicated a high degree of insulin resistance. In addition, her A1c had climbed to 7.7%, and she grew increasingly frustrated that her blood glucose had become seemingly uncontrollable.

At first, Erica was apprehensive about adopting the Mastering Diabetes Method and didn't believe that it could help her gain better control of her blood glucose because it went against everything she had been taught. However, only one week after committing to the Mastering Diabetes Coaching Program her blood glucose values were much steadier. Within the first 30 days, Erica had lost 13 pounds, cut her basal insulin use by 50 percent, and increased her carbohydrate-to-insulin ratio from 6:1 to 11:1 at meals, and her energy levels were noticeably higher. Soon she began performing a once-per-week 24-hour fast to continue gaining insulin sensitivity. Within six months, Erica began experiencing regular menstrual cycles for the first time in six years, which made her hopeful that she could one day become pregnant. By May of 2017 she had lost 34 pounds, had increased her carbohydrate-to-insulin ratio at mealtime sixfold (from 6:1 to 36:1), and became pregnant for the first time.

During pregnancy, her doctor instructed her to decrease her carbohydrate intake to maintain excellent blood glucose control and expected that her basal rate would quadruple (from 11 units to 44 units per day). Instead, Erica continued eating a low-fat plant-based whole-food diet because she knew that it would maximize her insulin sensitivity, and as a result, her basal rate increased by only 3 units per day (from 11 units to 14 units per day).

At delivery, her mealtime carbohydrate-to-insulin ratio was 6:1, which greatly surprised her doctor because a typical carbohydrate-to-insulin ratio for a pregnant woman with type 1 diabetes is approximately 1:1. Throughout her pregnancy, Erica feasted on mangoes, papayas, pineapples, persimmons, tomatoes, beans, lentils, tempeh, tofu, potatoes, squash, and corn. Her baby boy, Eli, was born in February of 2018, and now eats just like his mom. At delivery, her A1c had dropped from 7.7% to 6.3%, and her nurse commented that she rarely sees women with a blood pressure of 100/70.

Now, more than four years since she began following the Mastering Diabetes Method, including a regular weekly intermittent fasting practice, Erica is in the best metabolic shape of her life and does her best to spread the message far and wide. "I'm a completely different person. I am laughing now because when my doctor looks at my continuous glucose monitor, it appears as though I don't have diabetes. This is the first thing that has worked well for me since I was eleven years old. It's been a while and I am very happy to have found this way of life."

---

When we ask our clients, "When was the last time you fasted for 24 hours?" Most people respond with "Never." Many of them then go on to say things like "I thought fasting was bad for me because it slows down my metabolism," or "I can't fast for 24 hours, that's too long." Here's the problem—neither of these statements is true.

For over 2 million years, our human ancestors were largely hunter-gatherers. They spent the bulk of their time gathering low-calorie foods, including wild grains, roots, and berries, and enjoyed the occasional high-calorie feast following a successful hunt. In truth, our human ancestors were actually *gatherer-hunters,* given that they spent the majority of their time gathering and a minority of their time hunting. In order to survive long periods of limited food availability, our human ancestors often fasted for extended periods of time, sometimes up to 10 days in a row.

This pattern of fasting and feasting—cycling between periods of high and low calorie intake—created a series of biochemical adaptations that naturally selected for those who could survive an uncertain food supply. Scientists believe that over the course of time, metabolic adaptations that allowed for regular intermittent fasting became ingrained in the genetic material of modern humans, and for this reason, modern-day humans are not only capable of fasting for extended periods of time but actually derive substantial metabolic benefit when fasting.

Fast-forward to the 1930s. Hard at work in a science lab at Cornell University, Clive McCay and his colleagues were the first to observe that restricting the calorie intake of laboratory rats allowed them to live longer than their *ad libitum* counterparts, who were given access to food 24 hours a day. McCay and his colleagues didn't realize it at the time, but what seemed like a simple observation would unlock an explosion of scientific research that would begin to explain biological mechanisms responsible for reducing the rate of aging, increasing longevity, improving memory, and stimulating weight loss, while simultaneously reducing the risk for chronic metabolic conditions such as heart disease, cancer, and type 2 diabetes. Even though their initial observations came from experiments with laboratory rodents, in almost every organism studied to date (including yeast, worms, flies, mice, rats, and most recently, monkeys), calorie restriction has been shown to increase longevity and prolong or delay the onset of many age-related diseases.

Thousands of research teams have since investigated the benefits of calorie restriction, attempting to explain why many species derive exceptional metabolic benefits from a reduced calorie intake. In graduate school, Cyrus and his colleagues took this research one step further by investigating the exact cellular mechanisms at play during calorie restriction that are responsible for a reduced risk for type 2 diabetes and cancer. What they confirmed was that restricting calorie intake by an average of 25 percent from *ad libitum* controls resulted in measurable decreases in insulin production, fasting blood glucose, postprandial blood glucose, and body weight. Even more incredibly, they found that only *a few days* of calorie restriction was enough to significantly increase insulin sensitivity. They discovered that calorie restriction dramatically increases fat oxidation and slows the rate at which mitochondrial proteins are synthesized and degraded.

Their research confirmed and advanced knowledge about calorie restriction that is also accepted by the larger scientific community—that calorie restriction is one of the most powerful methods of improving all aspects of glucose metabolism, including weight loss, reduced fasting blood glucose, reduced post-meal blood glucose, reduced insulin requirements, increased mitochondrial function, reduced oxidative stress, and dramatically increased insulin sensitivity. In fact, intermittent fasting is such a powerful insulin-sensitizing tool that it has become a cornerstone of our approach to reversing insulin resistance naturally.

## Why Intermittent Fasting Works

When you perform an intermittent fast, it provides you with an opportunity to enter *negative calorie balance,* a state in which your energy expenditure exceeds your energy needs. Operating in negative calorie balance for extended periods of time forces your muscles and liver to burn or off-load stored glucose and fatty acids, which in turn makes them more responsive to these fuels the next time they become available. This is great news for two main reasons.

First, oxidizing excess stored fat inside of your muscles and liver is a powerful way to increase their ability to communicate with insulin, as you learned in chapter 3. Reducing the burden that excess fatty acids place on your muscles and liver unlocks their ability to recognize and communicate with insulin effectively. Second, when your muscles and liver operate in negative calorie balance for extended periods of time, not only do they burn excess stored fatty acids but they also burn glycogen, the stored form of glucose. As the glycogen storage tank decreases in size, muscle and liver cells activate a series of intracellular mechanisms that make it easier to import glucose the next time it's available. In effect, negative calorie balance activates a few master enzymes in muscle and liver cells that create a state of cellular "hunger."

Calorie restriction is one of the most effective and reproducible ways to slow the speed at which organisms age and is the only known intervention to extend lifespan. A 20 to 50 percent reduction in calorie intake has been shown to increase lifespan by up to 50 percent and prevent or delay the onset of many chronic diseases including obesity, type 2 diabetes, cancer, nephropathy, cardiomyopathy, neurodegeneration, and multiple autoimmune diseases.

Because performing longevity experiments in humans presents ethical problems, it is difficult to know for certain whether inducing negative calorie balance in humans will extend lifespan. However, similar to animal studies, human experiments have demonstrated that calorie restriction delays the onset of many age-related diseases, which suggests that it is extremely likely that negative calorie balance increases longevity in humans.

Negative calorie balance also has tremendous benefits for cardiovascular health. It may seem illogical, but scientists have uncovered that reducing food intake for extended periods of time allows blood vessels everywhere to relax, which in turn reduces blood pressure. Studies have shown that calorie restriction improves the function of the endothelial cells that line the inside of blood vessels, improving their ability to manufacture nitric oxide (NO), a gas that allows blood vessels to dilate. And in addition to increased NO synthesis, negative calorie balance reduces cardiovascular inflammation, which increases blood flow to tissues. When it comes to the direct benefits of negative calorie balance on your risk for heart disease, studies show that calorie restriction substantially reduces LDL cholesterol and triglycerides and directly improves the function of your heart muscle.

In laboratory animals, negative calorie balance has been demonstrated to be a very effective strategy to prevent and reverse cancer. Research published in *Science* reported that in monkeys, restricting calorie intake by 50 percent significantly reduces the incidence of cancer. A large body of evidence suggests that negative calorie balance in humans shares many of the same molecular mechanisms found in other mammals, and researchers are very excited to learn more because calorie restriction is widely known to be the most reproducible way to increase lifespan and protect against cancer in mammals. Testing how calorie restriction affects cancer incidence in humans is significantly more challenging than it is in other mammals because it is difficult to conduct long-term survival studies due to compliance, cost, and ethical considerations. Despite this, data from studies of long-term calorie restriction in humans suggest that the molecular mechanisms are very similar to those found in rodents and monkeys.

There are many reasons that calorie restriction is very powerful at reducing cancer incidence, resulting from reduced body weight, reduced inflammatory cytokines, reduced growth factors, reduced oxidative stress, improved DNA repair processes, and reduced cell replication rates. As early as the 1940s, research published in *Cancer Research* identified that negative energy balance can decrease both tumor number and size, and since that publication the scientific evidence has grown substantially.

Research from Cyrus' laboratory at UC Berkeley showed that *negative calorie balance reduces the global cell proliferation rate,* which means that cells in all tissues reduce the speed at which they replicate, which in turn reduces the rate of formation of cancerous cells. Since being overweight dramatically increases your risk for the development of many cancers by increasing the global cell proliferation rate, weight loss that naturally occurs from being in negative calorie balance is one of the most powerful ways to prevent and reverse cancer.

No matter how you slice it, entering negative calorie balance isn't just good for you, it's *great* for you. So the question becomes . . . *how do you induce negative energy balance for optimal results?*

# Choose Your Fast Track

At this point, you may be thinking to yourself: "The effects of negative calorie balance sound great, but there's no way I can function in my everyday life without food." To that we say: True, in the real world, daily calorie restriction can be quite challenging. And continuous calorie restriction can place physical, emotional, and mental limitations on your daily life, as well as become quite limiting in the long term. To solve this problem, many research groups have developed lifestyle-friendly intermittent fasting strategies to mimic the metabolic effects of calorie restriction.

There are endless permutations of intermittent fasting regimens. Just do an online search for "intermittent fasting regimens" and you'll come across many different methods, each with its own set of benefits and limitations. The trick is to find an intermittent fasting regimen that works well in your lifestyle. The most common methods include:

- **The 16:8 Daily Intermittent Fast:** Fast for 16 hours a day, then eat for the next 8 hours. Repeat daily.
- **The 20:4 Daily Intermittent Fast:** Fast for 20 hours a day, then eat for the next 4 hours. Repeat daily.
- **25 Percent Daily Calorie Restriction:** Reduce your calorie intake by 25 percent every day.
- **Alternate-Day Fasting:** Alternate periods of 24 hours of eating with 24 hours of fasting.
- **Once-per-Week 24-Hour Intermittent Fast:** Fast for 24 hours once per week on the same day every week.

If you are living with insulin-dependent diabetes, please refer to chapter 9 for more details on how to use intermittent fasting to test your basal insulin strategy. If you are using oral or injectable medications (other than insulin), we strongly suggest talking with your physician about how to adjust or modify your medication schedule when you are fasting. Many oral medications are prescribed to be taken with food to minimize gastrointestinal side effects, including nausea, vomiting, diarrhea, gas, bloating, constipation, cramping, and abdominal pain. Discussing your fasting strategy and medication use with your physician will help you safely begin a regular fasting practice. If you inject bolus insulin at mealtime, then you will likely not need bolus insulin while fasting. We suggest making a plan with your physician to strategize your bolus insulin use in advance of your first intermittent fast.

We welcome you to experiment with any and all of the intermittent fasting regimens listed above. In our own experience and in that of our clients, the two most achievable and sustainable intermittent fasting regimens are the **Once-per-Week 24-Hour Intermittent Fast** and the **16:8 Daily Intermittent Fast**.

## The Once-per-Week 24-Hour Intermittent Fast

Just as the name implies, choose one day of the week that is the most convenient for you to fast for the majority of the day. We recommend a day when you're largely sedentary. We also recommend starting the fast after dinner the day before your fast, so that you're not ravenous when you wake up the next morning and can function well the next day. By doing so, you will start and end your fast in the evening time and count all sleeping hours toward your fasting period—meaning you're really only skipping two meals. Here's what a 24-hour fast would look like under these circumstances:

### Example Fasting Day: Thursday

**Wednesday at 6 P.M.:** Eat your last meal of the day. Drink 2 to 3 cups of water.

**Wednesday at 8 P.M.:** Start 24-hour intermittent fast.

**Wednesday at 10 P.M.:** Go to sleep.

**Thursday at 8 A.M.:** Drink 2 to 3 cups of water or 1 to 2 cups of green tea.

**Thursday at 12 P.M.:** Drink 2 to 3 cups of water or 1 to 2 cups of green tea.

**Thursday at 3 P.M.:** Drink 2 to 3 cups of water or 1 to 2 cups of green tea.

**Thursday at 6 P.M.:** Eat a reasonably sized dinner, complete with plenty of whole carbohydrate-rich food from fruits, starchy vegetables, beans, lentils, peas, or intact whole grains and plenty of non-starchy vegetables, mushrooms, and leafy greens. If you experience a high blood glucose reading after your dinner meal, increase your intake of non-starchy vegetables, mushrooms, and leafy greens the next time.

**Friday at 7 A.M.:** Return to eating green light foods.

### Tips and Strategies for Easing Through an Intermittent Fast

- Drink plenty of fluids. Doing this will help keep you hydrated and distend your stomach temporarily to mimic the feeling of being full. When your stomach distends, it sends a signal to your brain, which can curb your feelings of hunger. Feel free to drink as much water during your fast as you like, even if it's more than is included in the sample schedule.

- The green tea is not essential for fasting, but it can make the experience easier. Many people report that green tea is very effective at suppressing their appetite, in addition to having an exceptionally high antioxidant content.

- Be aware of your body cues. Are you feeling anxious, frustrated, or "upset" during your fast? This is very normal if you are not accustomed to being in a fasted state or skipping a meal. You can remind yourself that you're going to be OK and try to relax your mind. Take a few deep breaths and learn from this experience.

- Distract yourself with activities to keep your mind off your fasting or hunger. Read a book or magazine, watch a movie, take a walk, or perform some other activity that can help you stay focused on something other than your fast.

- Have low-fat plant-based whole-food options available in your house when you "break" your fast in the evening. This helps prevent the temptation to eat high-fat, high-protein, and refined foods.

## The Once-per-Week *Modified* 24-Hour Intermittent Fast

For some people, performing a full 24-hour fast can be particularly challenging. Especially for people with diabetes, fasting for extended periods of time can increase the risk for hypoglycemia, while others tend to get *hangry* (hungry + angry). If this is the case for you, a modified 24-hour intermittent fast is an effective way to get the benefits of intermittent fasting while keeping you safe. Consider performing a modified 24-hour intermittent fast if you fall into one of the categories below:

- You are living with type 1 diabetes and suspect that your basal insulin strategy may cause hypoglycemia.
- You are prone to frequent hypoglycemia.
- You have a very difficult time concentrating when fasting.
- You experience violent mood swings or get angry when hungry.

The main reason why it is difficult to perform a true 24-hour intermittent fast for some people is that consuming zero calories for an extended period of time can deprive your brain of glucose if the amount of glycogen stored in your liver is small, which can result in rapid mood swings, frustration, anger, inability to concentrate, shaky hands, sweating on the palms of your hands or forehead, and slurred speech.

The major differences between a true and a modified intermittent fast are the number of calories you consume in a 24-hour period and the period of time between snacks. In a true intermittent fast, you consume zero calories at mealtime, and in a modified intermittent fast, you consume a few snacks containing between 100 and 200 calories each. Even with a small intake of calories, you can still get some exceptional health benefits. Here is an example of a modified 24-hour intermittent fast:

## Example Fasting Day: Thursday

**Wednesday at 6 P.M.:** Eat your last meal of the day and drink 2 to 3 cups of water.

**Wednesday at 8 P.M.:** Start modified 24-hour intermittent fast.

**Wednesday at 10 P.M.:** Go to sleep. Nighty-night!

**Thursday at 8 A.M.:** Drink 2 to 3 cups of water, 1 to 2 cups of green tea, or 1 cup of non-starchy vegetable juice.

**Thursday at 12 P.M.:** Drink 2 to 3 cups of water or 1 to 2 cups of green tea.

**Thursday at 3 P.M.:** Drink 2 to 3 cups of water and have a small snack (see examples below).

**Thursday at 6 P.M.:** Eat a small dinner before bed, with plenty of whole carbohydrate-rich food from fruits, starchy vegetables, beans, lentils, peas, or intact whole grains and plenty of non-starchy vegetables, mushrooms, and leafy greens.

**Friday at 7 A.M.:** Return to your normal eating schedule.

### Snack Options During a Modified Intermittent Fast

Here are a few snack options to eat during your modified 24-hour intermittent fast. Do your best to eat small snacks and resist the temptation to eat large meals.

- 1 cup of non-starchy vegetable juice made from any combination of tomatoes, beets, celery, carrots, cucumbers, mint, parsley, arugula, or kale.
- 1 to 2 pieces of your favorite fruits (banana, apple, pear, persimmon, orange, a handful of berries, etc.).
- 1 to 2 handfuls of your favorite non-starchy vegetables (cauliflower, tomatoes, carrots, broccoli, Brussels sprouts, okra, etc.).
- A small salad containing 1 to 2 handfuls of non-starchy vegetables only.

## The 16:8 Daily Intermittent Fast

The second intermittent fasting option that is both effective and often-times less challenging than performing a 24-hour intermittent fast is the **16:8 Daily Intermittent Fast**. Many people find this option to be more achievable because it requires eliminating one meal per day, either breakfast or dinner. This is actually our preferred method of intermittent fasting, and we have found that a 16:8 daily fast helps many of our clients gain insulin sensitivity and lose weight at a faster pace. As opposed to the **Once-per-Week 24-Hour Intermittent Fast**, a daily 16:8 intermittent fast does require you to eliminate one meal every day, and it is important that you be very consistent in your daily activities. And most important, performing a 16:8 intermittent fast allows you to exercise during your 8-hour feeding window, which is always great news.

Below are two sample 16:8 intermittent fasts—the first does not include breakfast; the second does not include dinner.

### Example No-Breakfast Daily 16:8 Fasting Regimen

**Daily Fasting Window: 8:00 P.M. to 12:00 P.M.**
**Wednesday at 6 P.M.:** Eat a green light dinner.
**Wednesday at 8 P.M.:** Stop eating. *Begin fasting window.*
**Wednesday at 10 P.M.:** Go to sleep.
**Thursday at 8 A.M.:** Skip breakfast. Drink 2 to 3 cups of water or 1 to 2 cups of green tea.
**Thursday at 12 P.M.:** *Begin eating window.* Eat a green light lunch.
**Thursday at 3 P.M.:** Eat a snack if you feel hungry.
**Thursday at 4 P.M.:** Perform 30 to 60 minutes of exercise.
**Thursday at 6 P.M.:** Eat a green light dinner.
**Thursday at 8 P.M.:** Stop eating. *Begin fasting window.*
**Wednesday at 10 P.M.:** Go to sleep.
**Thursday at 8 A.M.:** Skip breakfast. Drink 2 to 3 cups of water or 1 to 2 cups of green tea.

Repeat the cycle for continuing benefits, or until you achieve your ideal body weight.

### Example No-Dinner Daily 16:8 Fasting Regimen

**Daily Fasting Window: 4:00 P.M to 8:00 A.M**

**Wednesday at 8 A.M.:** *Begin eating window.* Eat a green light breakfast.

**Wednesday at 11 A.M.:** Perform 30 to 60 minutes of exercise.

**Wednesday at 12 P.M.:** Eat a green light lunch.

**Wednesday at 3 P.M.:** Eat a snack if you feel hungry.

**Wednesday at 4 P.M.:** Stop eating. *Begin fasting window.*

**Wednesday at 10 P.M.:** Go to sleep.

**Thursday at 8 A.M.:** *Begin eating window.* Eat a green light breakfast.

Continue the cycle . . .

As you can see, whether you choose to skip your breakfast or your dinner, on a daily basis you have an 8-hour window of opportunity in which to eat 2 or 3 meals. It is often challenging to eat a day's worth of food in this 8-hour window, so resist the temptation to stuff yourself knowing that you'll be fasting for the next 16 hours, and instead finish your meals feeling full and comfortable. By doing so, you will likely accelerate the rate at which you lose weight, given that you'll reduce your calorie intake in this 24-hour period.

## How to Intermittent Fast If You Are Underweight

If you are hoping to gain weight in order to arrive at your ideal body weight, performing intermittent fasting will likely make it quite challenging. We recommend not performing intermittent fasting until you achieve your ideal body weight, at which point you can perform either a once-per-week 24-hour intermittent fast or a 16:8 daily intermittent fast and prevent against further weight loss. The way to do this is to eat enough calories during your feeding window to prevent against an overall reduction in total calories. Try the method of fasting that you prefer, then experiment with how much you have to eat during your feeding window in order to keep your weight stable. It's likely that a 16:8 intermittent fast will make it more challenging to keep your weight stable than will the once-per-week 24-hour intermittent fast.

## Hunger Comes in Many Flavors

Let's face it: We eat when we're feeling lonely. And sad. And frustrated. And angry. And happy. And confused. And excited. There is no denying the fact that humans are emotional creatures, and that it's common to eat in response to emotions. In the world of abundance in which we live, eating is a natural response to both favorable and unfavorable situations. But this direct connection between your emotional state and your food intake can often result in the overconsumption of calories.

Even though one of the biggest tenets—and benefits—of the Mastering Diabetes Method is that you can eat until you feel satisfied, we still want you to be mindful of *when* you eat in addition to *what* you eat. Knowing when to eat becomes easier when you understand what true hunger feels like, and it's an important step in increasing your insulin sensitivity over the course of time. Luckily, experiencing true hunger is something that you are likely to experience by performing a single intermittent fast. We have discovered that people eat in response to two types of hunger and often have a difficult time differentiating between the two.

*Physiological hunger* is the type of hunger you experience when your brain, muscles, and internal organs are in a true low-energy state. This is the type of hunger that you experience following a demanding workout or when you have exerted significant physical or mental energy and need high-quality fuel to replenish your energy needs. This is a type of hunger that you can feel not only in your stomach but also in your muscles and in your brain. Physiological hunger is your signal to eat low-fat plant-based whole foods to meet the energy requirements of repairing, growing, and energy-deprived tissues.

*Emotional hunger,* on the other hand, is the type of hunger you experience when a situation or thought process creates a desire to eat. As opposed to physiological hunger, emotional hunger creates a feeling of true hunger even though the biological requirement for fuel is low or nonexistent. If you've ever looked at someone else eating a plate of food and become instantly hungry, that's emotional hunger. Or perhaps you've experienced emotional hunger when you looked at the clock and thought to yourself, *It's six p.m. That's when I normally eat dinner.* Maybe you've been served a plate of appetizers at a friend's house and become hungry just because you saw other people eating. Once again, this is emotional hunger.

Understanding the difference between these two types of hunger can make a huge difference in your overall health, and performing regular intermittent fasting is a simple strategy that you can use to help you differentiate between the two. Think of intermittent fasting as an experiment in not eating that has tremendous benefits for your cardiovascular system, your muscles, your liver, your brain, and your digestive organs; it also helps you understand the difference between a true state of hunger and a hunger that's driven by situations around you. The combination of benefits to your physical and emotional health are well worth the experiment and are another tool to add to your insulin sensitivity toolbox that is guaranteed to improve your overall health.

## How to Know When to Move On

Once you've had a chance to experiment with intermittent fasting and observe the changes it makes to your appetite, your insulin use, your mood, your digestive function, your blood glucose, and your energy levels, it's time to add the final tool to your insulin sensitivity toolbox—exercise. In the next chapter, we'll describe the benefits of exercising and the effect that exercise has on your insulin sensitivity, and give you practical ways to begin or optimize an exercise regimen. We recommend moving on to the final step in the process once you have accomplished the following:

- You have performed either two 24-hour intermittent fasts, two modified 24-hour intermittent fasts, or seven consecutive days of

16:8 daily intermittent fasts, and understand how they affected your diabetes health.

- If you are living with insulin-dependent diabetes, you understand how much basal and bolus insulin you need to inject to prevent yourself from becoming hypoglycemic on a fasting day.

If you have accomplished these tasks, then it's time to start moving your body to take your insulin sensitivity to the next level. If you're ready to increase your hard-earned insulin sensitivity even more than you already have, exercise is your ticket!

To view the 50+ scientific references cited in this chapter, please visit us online at www.masteringdiabetes.org/bookinfo.

# Chapter 14

# Exercising for Maximum
# Insulin Sensitivity

## Running Strong: Paul

Paul is a competitive athlete and running coach who has been living with both type 1 diabetes and celiac disease since he was 6 years old. In his forties, Paul became concerned about an elevated A1c of 7.1%, weight gain, high cholesterol, and high blood pressure. In addition, Paul began experiencing pins and needles in his feet. Even with Paul's regimented half-marathon training schedule and seemingly meticulous low-carbohydrate diet, he found that exercising frequently did not prevent him from developing common diabetes complications. When he realized that it consistently took him nearly two months to feel fully recovered from running a half marathon, he knew that something had to change. That's when he joined and committed to the Mastering Diabetes Coaching Program.

Instead of limiting his carbohydrate intake to 50 grams per day and focusing on eating more protein, as he had been doing for many years, Paul began eating 400 grams of carbohydrate per day and quickly gave up meat, poultry, fish, milk, and eggs. Within only a few weeks, Paul began feeling noticeably more energy. His blood glucose control improved greatly as his total fat intake dropped and plant intake increased. In fact, Paul began feeling so vibrant that he decided to do something that few humans would even attempt—he decided to run forty half marathons in 365 days to celebrate his fortieth year living with type 1 diabetes. Between March of 2016 and March of 2017, Paul competed in forty half marathons around the world, an average of three half marathons per month.

Instead of worrying about his protein intake, Paul began concentrating on fueling his weary muscles with readily available carbohydrate energy from fruits, starchy vegetables, and legumes. For training and competition, Paul ate large bowls of fruit, which helped keep his muscle and liver glycogen stores full. In a short period of time, Paul's average fasting blood glucose decreased from 126 mg/dL to 94 mg/dL and his A1c decreased from 7.1% to 6.8%. His total cholesterol decreased from 201 mg/dL to 147 mg/dL, his blood pressure decreased from 140/80 mmHg to 126/80 mmHg, and he lost 15 pounds without even trying. He no longer experiences pins and needles in his feet or debilitating post-exercise fatigue. He enjoys running more than ever as a result of his dramatically improved metabolic health, and even successfully completed running forty half marathons in twelve months.

---

While it is true that eating a low-fat plant-based whole-food diet is your most powerful insulin sensitizer, this book would not be complete without an explanation of the incredible benefits of exercise, as well as a strategy to integrate daily movement into your regimen to further boost your insulin sensitivity and dramatically reduce your risk for long-term chronic disease. Because daily movement is such a powerful insulin sensitizer, we can all but guarantee that following these recommendations will further reduce your need for oral medication and insulin, reduce your fasting and post-meal blood glucose, reduce your total cholesterol, reduce your LDL cholesterol, increase your HDL cholesterol, and improve the condition of blood vessels in tissues all over your body.

# Mitochondria: The Powerhouses of the Cellular World

You've likely been told that moving your body is "good for you" and that moving your body daily will lead to better overall health, as in better blood glucose values, better sleep, improved mood, reduced depression, higher bone density, weight loss, better sex drive, and a betterment of your quality of life. And yet many people—regardless of whether they're living with diabetes— still don't take the necessary steps to incorporate movement into their lives. What we've found is that understanding *why* exercise positively impacts insulin sensitivity makes a big difference in the likelihood that you will adopt an exercise regimen.

So let's start by understanding the function of *mitochondria,* "mini organs" inside of cells that are essential for life. Mitochondria live in every cell of your body except for red blood cells, and they are the place where glucose, fatty acids, and amino acids get burned for energy. The number of mitochondria inside of a cell varies by type—skeletal muscle cells, heart muscle cells, skin cells, liver cells, sperm cells, neurons, and insulin-producing beta cells each contain a different mitochondrial density. Each cell can contain as few as 100 and as many as 5,000 copies of mitochondria. Inside each mitochondria, glucose, fatty acids, and amino acids are stripped of their energy- containing parts to produce a high-energy compound known as ATP, which is then used to power thousands of reactions inside the cell, including complex processes like protein synthesis, nutrient absorption, cell replication, and cell death.

As we discussed in chapter 6, your liver is one of the hardest-working and most underappreciated organs in your body and performs more metabolic processes than any other tissue. Think of your liver as a tireless supercomputer that runs your entire metabolic machine by coordinating, executing, and controlling thousands of simultaneous chemical reactions every second of every day. Maintaining top-notch liver health is essential for maximizing your long-term health.

Billions of mitochondria that exist in your liver fuel a vast number of critical metabolic functions. Specifically, the 1,000 to 2,000 mitochondria densely packed into each liver cell generate the large amounts of ATP required for deciding which glucose to keep, which glucose to export, which hormones to make, which fuels to break down, which fuels to store, which DNA to copy, which cells to destroy, which vitamins to store, which fatty acids to package, which proteins to degrade, which amino acids to convert, and which triglycerides to package into lipoprotein particles.

Mitochondria are densely packed in your muscle tissue as well. In non-obese people, muscle makes up between 40 and 50 percent of total body mass, and each muscle cell contains thousands of mitochondria. Muscle mitochondria are mainly responsible for generating ATP to control how nutrients get in and out of the cells and to contract and elongate muscle fibers when you exercise. When you engage in physical activity, mitochondria can increase the rate of ATP production by as much as 100 times.

Mitochondria are also crucial players in the insulin secretion game. Insulin-producing beta cells contain hundreds to thousands of mitochondria per cell, which are required to make split-second decisions about how much insulin to manufacture and release into circulation. Beta cells have a very difficult task at hand—not only do they produce insulin, but they are also responsible for producing the *right amount* of insulin. Releasing too much can result in life-threatening hypoglycemia, and releasing too little results in high blood glucose. So when this mitochondrial population is compromised, your chronic disease risk increases dramatically.

## Dysfunctional Mitochondria and Insulin Resistance: The Chicken-and-Egg Relationship

Because interconnected biological systems require that trillions of mitochondria function at peak performance, when mitochondria become *dysfunctional*, the effects are damaging and widespread, making it challenging for your brain, your muscles, your liver, your beta cells, and many other cell types to function properly. That said, the connection between insulin resistance and mitochondrial dysfunction is a classic chicken-and-egg story. Researchers know that mitochondrial dysfunction leads to insulin resistance, but they have also identified that insulin resistance can lead to mitochondrial dysfunction. And so there continues to be deliberation over *which came first?*

If insulin resistance causes mitochondrial dysfunction, then researchers could easily develop nutritional or exercise strategies to prevent mitochondria from becoming dysfunctional. On the other hand, if mitochondrial dysfunction causes insulin resistance, then promoting top-notch mitochondrial health could prevent insulin resistance from developing in the first place. It turns out that there is truth to both sides of this argument. Insulin resistance and mitochondrial dysfunction are inseparable processes, and because mitochondrial dysfunction plays an integral role in the development of insulin resistance (and vice versa), it is nearly impossible to separate one from the other. The beauty of this relationship is that regardless of which is the chicken and which is the egg, improving one improves the other.

**Making lifestyle changes that significantly improve mitochondrial function can dramatically increase your level of insulin sensitivity. Likewise, increasing your insulin sensitivity using your diet and exercise can indirectly improve mitochondrial function.**

Over the past fifteen years, studies have shown that people with type 2 diabetes also suffer from an insufficient number and quality of mitochondria in their muscle tissue. This presents a huge problem, because not only are there fewer mitochondria to begin with, the existing mitochondria don't burn fuel efficiently. The good news is that exercise is the single most effective way to make more mitochondria in muscle tissue. When you challenge your muscle to contract frequently (such as when you move your body during exercise), muscle fibers respond by increasing the number of mitochondria so that they can burn more fuel and process more oxygen the next time they are required to perform work. This results in improved endurance, increased strength, and an increased ability to perform work. The opposite is also true: Exercise physiologists have known for decades that a sedentary lifestyle can reduce the number of muscle mitochondria, leading to a decrease in muscular endurance, strength, and work output.

One of the main reasons mitochondria become dysfunctional is that they produce large quantities of free radicals, the unstable molecules that cause extensive cellular damage that you learned about in chapter 6. Large amounts of free radicals are formed in the mitochondria, and they damage cell membranes, protein, and DNA. Cells in your liver, muscle, and pancreas are notorious for accumulating free radical damage when you develop insulin resistance from a high-fat diet.

**When excess fatty acids accumulate inside muscle and liver cells from eating a high-fat diet, extensive scientific research has shown that mitochondria actually *increase* free radical production.**

But how is this possible? Low-carbohydrate diet advocates will tell you that eating a high-fat diet will improve mitochondrial efficiency and decrease inflammation in tissues all throughout your body, and that eating a high-fat diet turns you into a "fat-burning machine." While this sounds great, a closer look at rigorous science shows that even minor elevations in plasma lipids not only induce muscle insulin resistance but also alter the gene expression of key mitochondrial proteins, resulting in reduced mitochondrial function and a decreased rate of ATP synthesis. Research published in the journal *Diabetes* found that increasing dietary fat content from 35 to 50 percent (as is easily achieved on a low-carbohydrate diet) results in reduced expression of all genes involved in mitochondrial respiration—the very genes necessary for mitochondria to extract ATP from various intracellular fuels. This means that people who eat high-fat, low-carbohydrate diets often make more free radicals in their liver and muscle, dramatically increasing their level of cellular inflammation and silently crippling the function of trillions of muscle mitochondria.

## Exercise and Insulin

Aside from preventing and reversing chronic disease and promoting optimal mitochondrial health, the most powerful aspect of performing regular exercise when living with diabetes is that it acts as a *substitute* for insulin. Regardless of whether or not you inject insulin, performing daily exercise can significantly reduce the amount of insulin necessary to control your blood glucose.

When you contract and elongate your muscles hundreds or thousands of times during exercise, you force them to deplete the fuel in their internal storage tanks, including glycogen and triglycerides (the storage form of fatty acids). The type, duration, and intensity with which you exercise all have dramatic effects on how much glucose and how many fatty acids are burned for energy at any given moment in time.

All forms of exercise burn both glucose and fatty acids simultaneously, and your muscles always oxidize multiple fuels at the same time. Glucose is preferentially burned for energy during short-duration, higher-intensity bursts of energy, whereas fatty acids are preferentially burned for energy during longer-duration, lower-intensity exercise. Because of this complexity, the most important techniques to ensure that you are maximizing the opportunity to improve your insulin sensitivity using exercise are as follows:

- Move your body in ways that combine cardiovascular exercise and resistance exercise together.
- Exercise at a pace that makes it challenging to talk to someone else or sing your favorite song.
- Perform exercise that uses large muscle groups whenever possible, including muscles in your thighs (quadriceps), the back of your legs (hamstrings), your butt (gluteus), your core (rectus abdominis and obliques), your upper back (latissiumus dorsi), your chest (pectoralis), your biceps, and your shoulders (deltoids).

## Let's Get Moving!

You've now reached the crossroads. You've read the science of why exercise is so important for people living with insulin resistance. But the question still remains: How do I get started? It's a *great* question. We don't take the suggestion to exercise lightly; for many people, it's been years since they last had the habit of daily exercise. Or they've had to stop their exercise regimen owing to various diabetes-related aches, pains, and low energy levels. That's why we're going to take it slow, one step at a time—just like you're learning to add new foods into your diet one meal at a time. Here are our five easy steps for getting started.

## Step 1: Develop a Movement Goal

One of the easiest ways to stay motivated while getting the hang of a new exercise habit is to identify a goal. If you're new to exercise or just easing back in after some time away, a simple and highly effective goal is to move your body for a minimum of 180 minutes or 3 hours per week. That breaks down to 30 minutes a day, 6 days a week.

Chopping up your exercise into bite-sized chunks is a simple way to develop consistency and create an achievable habit. Remember that consistency is your best friend when it comes to building new habits, and this habit in particular can have a major impact on your insulin sensitivity and can maximize the health of your heart, blood vessels, liver, and muscles simultaneously. Consistency in your lifestyle habits is also highly beneficial in managing insulin-dependent diabetes because it helps keep your carbohydrate-to-insulin ratios predictable and repeatable.

To get maximum benefit from your time spent exercising, make sure that you're moving fast enough that you are unable to hold a conversation with someone and are unable to sing your favorite song. But contrary to popular belief, you don't have to exercise at high intensity to become more insulin sensitive. Working at a pace that makes it difficult to communicate is a simple way to ensure that you are working hard enough and will receive excellent metabolic benefit from each session.

If you hit this goal for one month—or if you are already active and consistently perform a minimum of 3 hours of exercise a week—you're doing great. Keep it up. You can always increase the amount of time you spend exercising or increase the intensity of your exercise sessions every few weeks, so that you can consistently increase the amount of work you perform. Exercising for 3 hours a week is sure to deliver exceptional results when you include both cardiovascular and resistance movements together, but if you're the type of person who really enjoys moving your body, then make sure that you're consistently challenging your musculature by diversifying your routine.

## Step 2: Define Your Exercise Preferences

The only exercise regimen that truly works is the one that *you will do*. Therefore, make sure that your exercise regimen is fun. Otherwise you're likely to abandon moving your body altogether. When it comes to choosing which activities to do, remember that there are two main types of exercise, each of which affects your body differently: cardiovascular exercise and resistance exercise.

**Cardiovascular exercise** is the most powerful insulin sensitizer and can reduce your blood glucose within 15 to 30 minutes of continuous movement. This effect can last for approximately 24 to 48 hours following your exercise session. Cardiovascular exercise includes movements that elevate your heart rate and can be maintained for extended periods of time without stopping. Examples of this type of exercise are walking, jogging, running, swimming, hiking, biking, jumping rope, cross-country skiing, snowshoeing, Zumba, dancing, soccer, basketball, rugby, racquetball, squash, water aerobics, and tennis.

**Resistance exercise** is a less powerful insulin sensitizer, but it has longer-lasting effects, reducing your body's need for insulin for approximately 24 to 72 hours following your exercise session. Examples include weight lifting, calisthenics, bodyweight resistance exercises (pull-ups, push-ups, lunges, air squats, plank holds), kettlebells, Pilates, and power yoga.

**Combination exercise** refers to any form of exercise that combines cardiovascular movements and resistance movements in the same exercise session. Combining cardiovascular movements and resistance movements together is the most powerful insulin sensitizer because it improves the ability of glucose and insulin to move in and out of your blood vessels and allows repairing muscle tissue to uptake large amounts of glucose. Examples of combination exercise include circuit training, CrossFit, boxing, kickboxing, gymnastics, and rowing. To capitalize on this difference between the two types of exercise, either perform exercise sessions involving both types of movements or aim for a 50:50 ratio of cardiovascular exercise and resistance exercise within a 7-day period. This way, you will derive the benefits of both types of exercise while building both muscular endurance and strength.

To become crystal clear on your exercise preferences, start by answering the following questions:

- What are your three favorite forms of exercise?
- What are your three least favorite forms of exercise?
- For each of your favorite forms of exercise, with how many people do you enjoy exercising (0, 1, 2, 3, or more)?
- For each of your favorite forms of exercise, what is your preferred time of day?

Once you have an answer to each of these questions, structure your exercise regimen the way that seems most exciting. Make sure that your preferences are very clear so that you maximize the chances of developing a routine that you truly enjoy.

A simple and powerful tool to use when you exercise is music, because it motivates you to work hard and distracts you from any discomfort that you may experience. Make a playlist of your favorite upbeat songs that lasts as long as your workout—we're confident that you'll feel the tremendous difference that it makes in keeping you motivated to move your body!

## Step 3: Find a Partner or Group to Exercise With

Accountability is another powerful motivator when it comes to starting a new exercise regimen. That's why we recommend developing your new routine with friends, coworkers, or family members—think of it as a built-in community that in turn provides support and accountability. If you enjoy exercising with one other person or with a small group, then build your exercise calendars together to capitalize on shared time.

If instead you prefer to exercise solo, you can still use this group to help you stay on track. Create a check-in system where you let one another know when you've completed a workout, or share your weekly workout schedule so that someone else knows what you plan to do. And don't forget to share your goals and accomplishments, too! Being able to get a big round of high fives as you hit those milestones (whether it's weight loss, decreased insulin requirements, or the fact that you can jog around the block without stopping) is a great way to keep you moving forward and feeling great.

Another great way to build in accountability is to join a class, a fitness group, or a club. If you enjoy a gym environment, ask for the gym's group class schedule and sample many different classes until you find one that you truly enjoy. You can also do an internet search for local walking or running clubs, swimming classes, hiking groups, dance classes, martial arts classes, boxing gyms, cycling teams, step aerobics classes, aqua jogging classes, yoga classes, or Pilates classes. Personal trainers are also excellent resources for learning how to move your body safely and effectively, while also providing lots of motivation, inspiration, and—that's right—accountability.

## Step 4: Schedule Your Exercise Routine and Make It Visible

The next step in this process is scheduling your exercise routine in a way that's *visible* to you. Do not rely on a mental calendar for keeping track of your workout regimen! Mental calendars are notoriously unreliable and are prone to overscheduling, excuses, or forgetting. Creating a visible calendar—whether it's digital, on a whiteboard, on a paper calendar, or elsewhere—is an essential part of creating a plan that sticks. Even though this may not seem important, trust us when we say that scheduling your exercise sessions is required for you to stay on track.

## Step 5: Start Slow and Be Consistent

What's most important when it comes to exercise is that you begin moving your body consistently. Only after you have that locked in place can you start thinking about increasing the intensity and duration of each exercise session. Give yourself permission to start slowly, then gradually do more over the course of time. If you are new to exercise, make sure that you talk with your doctor to choose the right type of exercise for your body.

For example, if you are initially performing 2 days of exercise per week, that's fine! Begin with 2 days the first week, then add a day a week until you arrive at 6 or 7 days of exercise in the fifth week. Once you are moving your body 6 or 7 days per week, keep that regimen steady for a few months and observe how different you feel physically, mentally, and emotionally. When you're feeling ready, slowly increase the intensity of each of your exercise sessions.

If you're an experienced athlete or already have a routine established, maintain a consistent regimen and increase intensity and volume as necessary to meet your specific goals in training for an endurance event, race, or competition.

# Controlling Your Blood Glucose Before, During, and After Exercise

It's very important that you approach exercise in a safe glucose range, do your best to stay in that range, and continue in that range after your workout is complete. We also want to make sure that you're able to maximize your performance during your workout. To help you achieve this, follow the strategies below to figure out what to do before, during, and after exercise.

## Before Exercise

### How to Control Your Blood Glucose

In general, your blood glucose is likely to decline during exercise, and because of that we recommend elevating your glucose prior to getting moving. In order to figure out your ideal pre-workout blood glucose range, you will have to experiment a bit so that it's tailored to your unique exercise regimen, as it is influenced by the type, duration, and intensity of the activity you perform.

**If You Inject Insulin:** If you are living with insulin-dependent diabetes, elevating your blood glucose before you begin exercising is a simple way to protect against unwanted hypoglycemia. To begin, we suggest an ideal pre-workout blood glucose range between 150 and 160 mg/dL, which you can adjust as you become more familiar with how your blood glucose changes during exercise. If you're worried that elevating your blood glucose before you exercise will increase your risk of developing diabetes complications, understand that the benefits your brain, heart, blood vessels, muscles, and digestive organs receive *far* outweigh the risks associated with temporarily elevated blood glucose.

You will likely have to work through a process of trial and error to get your pre-workout blood glucose values between 150 and 160 mg/dL and to prevent your blood glucose from dropping rapidly during your workout. Some people find that a 50 percent reduction in bolus insulin use in their pre-workout meal works well, while others using an insulin pump find that reducing their bolus insulin use by 30 percent and their basal insulin rate by 25 percent works well. Proper documentation for a period of about 2 weeks is the key to understanding exactly what to do.

If you choose to exercise in the morning, we highly recommend eating a small breakfast and injecting a small amount of bolus insulin prior to exercise. Attempting to exercise in the morning with zero bolus insulin in your blood creates a metabolic state that we call the *insulin drought*, and this state is notorious for causing high blood glucose in many people with insulin-dependent diabetes. Eating a small amount of food and injecting bolus insulin 30 to 60 minutes before exercise can make your blood glucose much more controllable during and after exercise.

**If You Do Not Inject Insulin:** If you are not insulin-dependent, then it is not necessary to elevate your blood glucose before exercise. Your liver and pancreas are finely tuned to maintain a safe blood glucose during exercise using insulin and glucagon, and therefore your risk for hypoglycemia is quite low. If you are concerned about hypoglycemia, start exercise with a blood glucose between 110 and 130 mg/dL as an added insurance policy against low blood glucose during exercise.

### What to Eat Before Exercise

Your muscle can store between 1,200 and 2,000 calories of glucose as glycogen, an easily accessible and quick-burning form of storage that contains glucose. When your muscles use glycogen as fuel, single glucose units are taken away on an on-demand basis. Once a glucose molecule is released from the glycogen granule, it undergoes a series of chemical reactions, ultimately gaining access to the mitochondria so that it can be burned completely for ATP.

The amount of glycogen you store in your muscles is a direct result of both your diet and your exercise patterns. Athletic trainers and coaches understand the importance of glycogen for athletic performance and instruct their athletes to carbo-load before a competition to temporarily increase the size of their muscle glycogen stores. While it is true that eating a carbohydrate-rich meal can temporarily increase the size of your glycogen stores, a single meal increases them only slightly.

Lucky for you, eating a diet high in whole carbohydrate-rich foods and low in both fat and protein allows you to carbo-load with every meal, providing your muscles with the impetus to regularly increase their glycogen stores. This in turn will give you the feeling of more energy during the day and during exercise. Not only does eating frequent meals high in whole carbohydrate energy increase the size of your glycogen stores, frequent meals low in carbohydrate energy also shrink your glycogen stores over time and cause your muscles to break down more protein during exercise. Ideal foods to eat before you begin exercising are carbohydrate-rich and include fruits like bananas, apples, oranges, pears, mangoes, or papayas, as well as starchy vegetables like potatoes, sweet potatoes, squash, or corn, or intact whole grains like quinoa or brown rice. Since fruits tend to move through your digestive system more quickly than whole grains and starchy vegetables, we recommend eating pre-workout meals containing a larger proportion of fruit.

Another extremely valuable type of food to add to your pre-workout meals are nitrate-rich vegetables, including beets, spinach, arugula, and Swiss chard. Recent compelling scientific research has shown that eating 1 to 2 servings of nitrate-rich vegetables 1 to 2 hours before your workout has a profound impact on blood vessels all over your body. The nitrate compounds undergo a complex series of reactions using enzymes in your small intestine and mouth, resulting in an increased production of nitric oxide (NO). This powerful gas helps relax the walls of your blood vessels and enhances the oxygen delivery to your muscles. This in turn allows you to perform more work with less perceived effort. In fact, many professional athletes are now "beet doping" to gain an advantage over their competitors.

Another option is to fast before exercising. Some people prefer to do this because they feel they can perform better with less material in their digestive system. We enjoy eating a small or medium-sized meal containing 2 to 5 servings of fruit about 1 to 2 hours before an exercise session, in conjunction with a 30 to 50 percent reduced bolus insulin dose. We encourage you to experiment so that you can find which strategy gives you energy while maintaining stable blood glucose values.

## During Exercise

### Controlling Your Blood Glucose

If you use an insulin pump to administer insulin electronically, it can be quite challenging to decide whether to stay connected to your insulin pump with a reduced basal rate or to disconnect from your insulin pump entirely. We have worked with many athletes with type 1 diabetes (and are athletes ourselves) and have found that the best insulin pump strategy depends on many factors. If you are consistently eating a low-fat plant-based whole-food diet, the two most important factors to take into consideration are (a) the length of time you perform exercise, and (b) the intensity of your exercise session.

**If you are performing exercise up to 1 hour in duration,** then you are likely not to require basal insulin while exercising. We suggest disconnecting your insulin pump altogether, because exercise will substitute for basal insulin while you exercise.

**If you are performing exercise between 1 and 2 hours in duration,** then it may be necessary to inject basal insulin after the 1-hour mark to prevent your blood glucose from rising unnecessarily. Even though exercise is a substitute for insulin, some people find that their blood glucose begins rising toward the end of an extended exercise session. If you have found this to be true, then connecting to your insulin pump toward the end of an extended exercise session to inject basal or bolus insulin may be necessary to prevent you from experiencing hyperglycemia after you have finished exercising.

The intensity of your exercise session is another large factor in determining whether you require basal insulin during exercise. In general, the higher your intensity level during exercise, the more likely it will be that you experience a high blood glucose during or after exercise. The reason for this is quite simple: Exercise that requires maximum effort stimulates your adrenal gland to produce the stress hormones cortisol and adrenaline, both of which signal your liver to dump glucose into your blood quickly. Think of cortisol and adrenaline as fast-acting and extremely powerful chemical signals that make sure your blood glucose stays high enough to perform movement at high intensity.

**If you choose to exercise at high intensity,** then consider observing how your blood glucose responds over the course of your exercise session. Some athletes find that they can manage their blood glucose well without the need for basal insulin, whereas others inject small amounts of basal insulin to prevent against an unwanted blood glucose high. As you gain more experience with high-intensity exercise, figure out which strategy makes the most sense for you.

**If you choose to exercise at a low- or medium-intensity level,** your adrenal gland will secrete small amounts of cortisol and adrenaline, which does not dramatically affect your blood glucose control. This makes your life significantly easier because these stress hormones are unlikely to affect your blood glucose profile.

### What to Eat During Exercise

Ideally, if you have taken steps to ensure that your glycogen stores are full before beginning a workout and have eaten a pre-workout meal 1 to 2 hours before beginning the session, chances are you will be able to exercise for as much as 60 to 90 minutes without eating any food and can get by with just drinking water to stay hydrated. However, if you find that you are getting light-headed, dizzy, or faint, or if your blood glucose is trending toward hypoglycemia, then it may be necessary to eat something small during your exercise session.

The best foods to eat during exercise are fruits because they are easily digestible, require zero preparation, and can help raise your blood glucose while exercising. We recommend having a few servings of fruit available in your gym bag or backpack, including bananas, plantains, dates, grapes, or oranges. These fruits work well to increase your blood glucose and keep your digestive system feeling light so that you can continue exercising. As you become more experienced with exercise, you're likely to find your favorite fruits and know exactly how much to eat to keep yourself feeling energized.

### How to Handle Hypoglycemia During Exercise

If you discover that your blood glucose is trending toward hypoglycemia during exercise, follow these steps:

1. Take a quick break and slow your heart rate temporarily.
2. Eat 1 to 2 pieces of fruit (bananas, dates, grapes, apples, peaches, and nectarines are good choices).
3. Wait 5 to 15 minutes.
4. Check your blood glucose and ensure that you are between 120 and 150 mg/dL.
5. Continue exercising until your session is complete (or stop exercising if you feel light-headed).

## After Exercise

### Controlling Your Blood Glucose After Exercise

As we discussed earlier, exercise and insulin do the same thing: They both shuttle glucose and fatty acids out of your blood and into tissues. (Insulin also shuttles amino acids out of your blood and into tissues, but because amino acids are seldom used for energy during exercise, we'll keep our comparison between insulin and exercise confined to glucose and fatty acids only.)

Exercise shuttles glucose and fatty acids out of your blood and into exercising muscles so that your muscles can use both fuels for immediate energy.

Insulin shuttles glucose and fatty acids into tissues all over your body, either to be burned for immediate energy or to be stored for later use. Both insulin and exercise stimulate glucose and fatty acids to leave your blood, resulting in lower blood glucose and triglyceride values. This is one of the advantages to using exercise as a substitute for insulin—in addition to hundreds of whole-body metabolic benefits, your muscles are hungry for glucose and small amounts of fatty acids for approximately 1 to 3 days after a single exercise session, reducing your insulin requirements dramatically.

**Phase 1 Afterburn:** Unlike insulin, however, exercise shuttles glucose and fatty acids into tissues not only during your exercise session, but for many hours afterward, resulting in an *afterburn* that can last for 24 to 72 hours, depending on the duration and intensity of your exercise session. In the immediate few hours after you exercise, muscles enter the *Phase 1 Afterburn,* in which they are at their most insulin-sensitive state. In stage 1, your muscles can absorb glucose from your blood either without the use of insulin or using only small amounts of insulin. In effect, your muscles are so hungry for glucose that they modify the action of some biochemical pathways to allow glucose to enter the cells of the tissue using very small amounts of insulin. Think of the Phase 1 Afterburn as your window of opportunity to eat carbohydrate-rich meals because your muscles are primed to absorb large amounts of glucose using small amounts of insulin.

**Phase 2 Afterburn:** In the *Phase 2 Afterburn,* your insulin sensitivity is higher than before you exercised, albeit slowly decreasing toward your pre-exercise level. Approximately 1 to 3 hours following your exercise session, your insulin needs will begin to increase once again as muscles readapt to their normal biochemical state. In comparison with the insulin sensitivity you experienced in phase 1, the Phase 2 Afterburn is not as powerful, but your insulin sensitivity will still be dramatically higher than it was before you began exercising. Your muscles are still capable of absorbing large amounts of glucose for smaller-than-normal amounts of insulin because your exercise session has increased their insulin sensitivity. Take a look at the graph on the next page to understand how the Phase 1 and Phase 2 afterburns affect your insulin sensitivity.

Your post-exercise insulin sensitivity is affected by many variables; however, time and diet composition are the two most important. As you can see

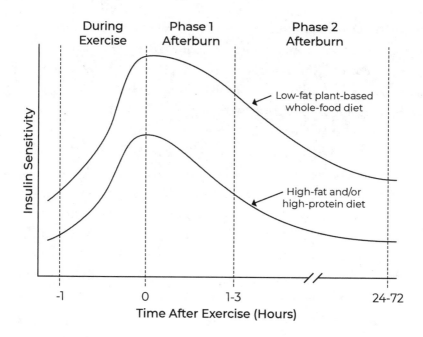

Your insulin sensitivity begins decreasing the moment you stop exercising, but eating a low-fat plant-based whole-food diet increases your baseline and peak insulin sensitivity.

in the graph, your insulin sensitivity begins decreasing from the moment you stop exercising and falls rapidly in phase 1, then less rapidly in phase 2. Eating a low-fat plant-based whole-food diet increases your baseline insulin sensitivity, your peak insulin sensitivity, and the speed at which your insulin sensitivity returns to its baseline value.

# You Can't Out-Exercise a Nutrient-Poor Diet

Even though exercising is a powerful tool at your disposal for increasing insulin sensitivity, it's very important to understand the following:

**Regardless of what you may have heard, performing frequent, long-duration, or high-intensity exercise is *less* powerful at improving your insulin sensitivity than eating a low-fat plant-based whole-food diet.**

Many people living with diabetes try to *out-exercise* a nutrient-poor diet by performing exercise frequently, for long periods of time, or at high intensity, thinking that the work performed during exercise cancels out the effects of poor nutrition. This could not be further from the truth. Even though exercise is an extremely effective insulin sensitizer, the quality of your diet is the most important indicator of your long-term metabolic health.

To illustrate this point, researchers at the University of Washington performed a study in which they compared the cardiovascular health of sedentary vegans eating a low-calorie, low-protein diet with highly competitive endurance runners eating the standard American diet to determine which group had better cardiovascular health. Most people would predict that competitive endurance runners would fare better, but what these researchers found was absolutely astonishing. Those in the low-calorie, low-protein group eating a 100 percent plant-based diet had lower total cholesterol, lower LDL cholesterol, lower triglycerides, and lower blood pressure than highly competitive endurance runners who ran an average of 2,500 miles per year for twenty-one years! The plant-based eaters were not exercising regularly, but they had measurably better cardiometabolic health than the endurance runners, despite the fact that the runners were 5 percent leaner.

### What to Eat After Exercise

Since the window of 1 to 3 hours after you finish exercising is your best opportunity to refill your liver and muscle glycogen tanks, it's important to eat a meal that is carbohydrate-rich and made from nutrient-dense plant material that is overflowing with micronutrients, especially antioxidants. Eating antioxidant-rich plant-based whole foods during this window of opportunity is tremendously beneficial because anti-inflammatory compounds will accelerate the rate of repairing muscle tissue, help reverse oxidative damage to blood vessels, and bathe all your tissues like your liver, brain, and kidneys in an "anti-inflammatory soup," thereby reducing inflammation all over your body.

The beauty of the Mastering Diabetes Method is that all green light foods are ideal options for eating after exercise. Of those foods, we suggest eating post-workout meals containing our favorite nutrient- and calorie-dense options, including fresh fruits, all varieties of beans, all varieties of lentils, green peas, quinoa, brown rice, millet, farro, sweet potatoes, purple potatoes, butternut squash, acorn squash, or corn. In addition to these options, feel free to add foods on the low-calorie density scale, such as including tomatoes, cucumbers, kale, spinach, arugula, onions, mushrooms, broccoli, or cauliflower. And don't forget to add spices like turmeric and ginger to your post-workout meals to increase their anti-inflammatory power. The options are seemingly endless, so take some time to find three or four nutrient-dense meals that maximize the inherent anti-inflammatory activity of these foods in the post-workout state. Your muscles will thank you for it. We guarantee it.

## How to Know When You've Optimized Your Insulin Sensitivity Toolbox

Once you've had a chance to integrate 3 hours of exercise into your weekly regimen in addition to periodic intermittent fasting and a low-fat plant-based whole-food diet, you're well on your way to implementing the most important tools in your insulin sensitivity toolbox. Because each of these habits can take time to develop, take your time to implement each one, experiment, and become as consistent as possible. Adding frequent movement into your regimen is an incredibly powerful tool that can take your insulin sensitivity to the next level, so be sure to develop a regimen that is truly fun and rewarding.

You'll know that you're implementing your insulin sensitivity toolbox to its fullest potential when the following is true:

- **Toolbox Strategy 1:** You are eating a green light breakfast, lunch, and dinner every day, and understand how much to eat at each meal to stay full for approximately 3 to 4 hours.
- **Toolbox Strategy 2:** If you are living with insulin-dependent diabetes, you understand how much bolus insulin to inject in order to maintain a postprandial blood glucose between 80 and 140 mg/dL after each meal.

- **Toolbox Strategy 3:** You have performed at least 10 intermittent fasts, and have a good idea of how your body responds to either a 16:8 intermittent fast (our preferred method) or a once-per-week 24-hour intermittent fast.
- **Toolbox Strategy 4:** You have integrated exercise into your daily schedule, and are consistently moving your body at a challenging pace for a minimum of 30 minutes per day, 6 to 7 days per week.
- **Toolbox Strategy 5:** You are working closely with your doctor or medical team to adjust your oral medication, insulin, and injectable medication needs as you gain insulin sensitivity.

If you are successfully integrating these tools in your daily life, we sincerely hope that you feel the difference that each tool can make, and benefit from the most powerful natural insulin-sensitizing method ever developed. If you want more education or guidance from our team of expert coaches, or are interested in joining a thriving online community of like-minded individuals who are reversing insulin resistance using their food as medicine, then visit www.masteringdiabetes.org/coaching/ and sign up today. Our members are excited to be part of a thriving online community that has changed the lives of thousands of people around the world. Get the guidance, accountability, and daily support required to make long-lasting lifestyle change that can truly transform your health from the inside out. We hope to see you inside!

To view the 65+ scientific references cited in this chapter, please visit us online at www.masteringdiabetes.org/bookinfo.

# Chapter 15

# Meal Plans and Recipes

And now for the most exciting part of the Mastering Diabetes Method: eating the world's most nutritious, disease-reversing, insulin-sensitizing food ever discovered. We know that some people are nervous to make the official leap to eating unprocessed whole-plant foods because they're worried that all they'll be able to eat is carrots and broccoli. Never fear, this is not the case with the Mastering Diabetes Method. We always look forward to our meals because they are not only nutrient-dense but also incredibly delicious, and they will keep you feeling satisfied. Very satisfied. In this section you will find thirty recipes for breakfast, lunch, and dinner, plus a 3-week meal plan to help you transition to the Mastering Diabetes Method smoothly.

We believe that it is *crucial* for you to fall in love with the food you eat in order to create a lifestyle that is enjoyable for years to come. We want you to look forward to each and every meal the way we do. As you're well aware by now, the recipes in this book are low in fat, and they're also salt-free. (High salt = increased appetite = weight gain = increased risk for type 2 diabetes.) So if you compare it to a double-bacon cheeseburger, our tasty Chickpea and Brown Rice Burger might not duplicate the flavors you know, although these flavors will be delicious in their own right. But as you begin to reduce or eliminate heavily salted, high-fat processed foods from your diet and increase the amount of nutrient-dense green light plants, your taste buds will begin to transform in ways that you can't predict right now. As your taste buds change, simple whole plant foods will begin to have more flavor and complexity, and before you know it, you're likely to begin craving them. Of course this can take time, depending on how consistent you are in limiting yellow light foods and completely eliminating red light foods. It's also okay to lightly salt your food, if that helps you during your transition. Be patient with yourself and know that as you become more consistent in your approach to the Mastering Diabetes Method, the food will come to life!

The recipes you'll find in this book are only a fraction of what can be created with green light foods. They're a great starting point, though, offering simple combinations and preparations. Over time, we encourage you to play around with these meals—swap out any ingredients you don't love or experiment with new ones. Our program is designed to be customizable and to accommodate your preferences, so many green light ingredients can be substituted for others. And as you feel more comfortable preparing meals with green light foods, branch out and get more adventurous—there's a whole world of nutrient-dense recipes that cater to those with a sweet tooth and to those who prefer eating savory dishes as well.

## Oil-Free Cooking Methods

The primary cooking methods called for in the Mastering Diabetes Method are **sautéing, stir-frying, steaming, boiling, roasting,** and **baking**—all without using oil. As you know, oils are a red light food that we recommend avoiding. You're probably thinking that aside from boiling and steaming that it's pretty difficult to get great flavor and texture without a pan full of hot oil. Not the case! By using a small amount of liquid instead (like broth or water), you can still achieve that tasty browned quality. In addition to being able to make our food without oil, we especially like cooking with liquid because it reduces the formation of the aforementioned AGE compounds. AGEs are formed when you cook at high temperatures in low-moisture environments (i.e., sautéing, stir-frying, and roasting), and they promote atherosclerosis, neuropathy, inflammation, endothelial damage, and kidney disease.

Luckily, it's completely possible to make dishes that are healthy, delicious, and satisfying. Here are our go-to techniques that have been perfected by our good friends at Forks Over Knives.

## No-Oil Sautéing and Stir-Frying

The key to building flavor and getting your food nice and browned in the pan is to cook over high heat, add a flavorful liquid, and frequently move the food in the pan to keep it from sticking.

Here's how:

1. Heat a dry pan over medium-high heat until it's smoking hot.
2. Add your vegetables, aromatics (garlic, ginger, onion), and anything else you're sautéing.
3. Let the ingredients begin to give up some of their moisture. You want them to stick to the pan just long enough to brown, but not so much that they burn.
4. When the moisture evaporates, start shaking the pan or using a spatula or spoon to move the ingredients in the pan to prevent burning.
5. When everything has started to brown, add a small splash of vegetable stock, juice, vinegar, or coconut water to the pan. This will loosen the ingredients from the pan and also help you scrape up all those delicious brown bits from the bottom of the pan.
6. Continue cooking until your ingredients are cooked to your liking.

## Baking and Roasting

Same deal as sautéing and stir-frying, but now you're using an oven. The biggest difference is that food dries out faster in the oven, so you'll add more liquid to the pan.

Here's how:

1. Preheat the oven to 400°F to 450°F. (Our recipes will give you specifics.)
2. Toss your vegetables with stock, juice, vinegar, coconut water, or any other flavored liquid so they're lightly coated.
3. Spread the vegetables in a single layer on a baking sheet lined with parchment paper or a silicone baking mat (for easier cleanup). Make sure there's at least an inch or two between the vegetables, which will encourage browning. Otherwise, the veggies will just steam.
4. Roast the vegetables until the bottoms begin to brown and can easily be loosened from the pan. Give everything a toss and continue roasting. If necessary, add a splash more liquid to help loosen any stuck vegetables. Continue until everything is tender and caramelized.

## Cooking Equipment

Because we want to set you up for long-term success, the recipes in the Mastering Diabetes Method are designed to be simple, quick, and easy. We want you to be able to create delicious meals that are high in nutrient density in a short period of time without complicated techniques or expensive cookware. While there are countless gadgets that you could purchase to simplify the process of preparing food—and you are welcome to buy them!—we'd rather you started with the basics. A sharp knife, an inexpensive blender and/or immersion blender, and a mixing bowl or two will get the job done.

## Time- and Health-Saving Cooking Strategies

We understand that cooking food without the use of salt, oil, and sugar can seem strange at first. But with some new, simple cooking techniques, you'll be making some delicious and satisfying meals in no time.

To start, here's a table you can refer to when adding extra flavor and texture to the dishes you're whipping up. Ingredients like vinegars, citrus juice, soy sauce or liquid aminos, and miso are great for adding brightness and saltiness; while vegetable broths and tomato juice help add body to sauces and stews (like adding a splash of cream); and broths and water are great stand-ins just about anywhere you'd use oil. Be mindful that the yellow light liquids can be somewhat problematic because of a high sodium or sugar content. Vegetable broth, miso products, liquid aminos, coconut aminos, and soy sauce are particularly high in sodium, so do your best to minimize your use of these flavorful liquids or use them in extremely small quantities. Many plant-based recipes ask you to use maple syrup to sweeten the flavor of the final dish, and for that reason we added it to our yellow light list. Even though pure maple syrup is technically a natural sweetener, even small amounts can elevate your blood glucose rapidly.

| Green Light Liquids | Yellow Light Liquids | Red Light Liquids |
| --- | --- | --- |
| Water | Low- or high-sodium vegetable broth | Vegetable or seed oils |
| Vinegars | | Butter and ghee |
| Tomato juice | Miso products | Milk |
| Lemon or lime juice | Liquid or coconut aminos | Animal-based broths |
| Homemade vegetable broth (no added salt) | Soy sauce (tamari) | Processed creamer (both dairy and nondairy) |
| | Maple syrup | Alcohol |

# Nutrient Profile

You'll notice that each of our recipes includes a nutrient profile, including energy (calories), fat, protein, total carbohydrates,* and fiber. That said, we assure you that every recipe in this book is more than adequate to meet your

---

* Please note that we have provided *total* carbohydrate, not *net* carbohydrate content for each recipe. If you are using bolus insulin, feel free to use either your total or net carbohydrate intake to calculate your carbohydrate-to-insulin ratio—both of them will work. Simply choose the one that works best for you, and do your best to be consistent for optimal results.

nutritional needs and that there's no need to micromanage individual nutrients. The foods that are part of the Mastering Diabetes Method are adequate for optimal human health, *but it's your job to ensure that you are eating enough to meet your energy needs and are not restricting your food intake as you may have done in the past.*

# A Meal Plan for Success

We consider ourselves compassionate and understanding coaches, but we also have a no-excuses methodology. Make sure that the goals you set for yourself match the level of commitment you make to the Mastering Diabetes Method. You may not want to go all the way and follow this method to a T, and that's okay. Just know that if you are not getting the results you are looking for, then it may be time to reevaluate your commitment to the four components of the Mastering Diabetes Method: low-fat plant-based whole-food nutrition, periodic intermittent fasting, daily movement, and completing decision trees.

The one thing we can absolutely guarantee is that if you follow one of the three-week plans outlined in this chapter, it is extremely likely that you will become more insulin sensitive. If you inject insulin, you are likely to need less insulin for a larger quantity of carbohydrate energy. If you do not inject insulin, you are likely to experience improved fasting and post-meal glucose values while eating larger amounts of carbohydrate-rich food. If you do choose to swap out ingredients, just make sure you're replacing them with other green light options (included in Appendix B).

In the following pages, you will find two different meal plans. If your level of baseline insulin resistance is low or medium (based on the Insulin Resistance Quiz in chapter 10), we suggest trying the first meal plan. If your level of baseline insulin resistance is instead high or very high, we suggest trying the second meal plan to help prevent against high blood glucose in the beginning stages of your transition. We want you to achieve excellent results, and following a time-tested and proven meal plan will hopefully simplify your life. Trust us when we say that you can do anything for three weeks, especially when your diabetes health noticeably improves.

# Meal Plan 1:
## For Low and Medium Baseline Insulin Resistance

## Week 1 (Breakfast Only)

|  | Breakfast Recipe | Lunch Recipe | Dinner Recipe |
|---|---|---|---|
| Day 1 | Robby's Antioxidant Delight | No change* | No change* |
| Day 2 | Refreshing Fruit Delight | No change* | No change* |
| Day 3 | Cyrus's Quinoa Special | No change* | No change* |
| Day 4 | Nature's Candy Bowl | No change* | No change* |
| Day 5 | Tropical Fruit Salad | No change* | No change* |
| Day 6 | Mexican Bean Breakfast Skillet | No change* | No change* |
| Day 7 | seasonal fruits | No change* | No change* |

*While we encourage you to make step-by-step changes and incorporate only one Mastering Diabetes–approved meal at a time, we also encourage you to modify other meals to include more green light foods in substitution for yellow and red light foods. During weeks 1 and 2 you might find opportunities where this is possible before you have actually changed all of your meals. Substituting as little as one green light food for a yellow or red light food can have a tremendous effect on your insulin sensitivity in the short and long term.

## Week 2 (Breakfast and Lunch)

|  | Breakfast Recipe | Lunch Recipe | Dinner Recipe |
|---|---|---|---|
| Day 8 | Nature's Candy Bowl | Curried Red Lentils over Fluffy Quinoa | No change* |
| Day 9 | Robby's Antioxidant Delight | Hearty Sweet Potato and Squash Soup | No change* |
| Day 10 | seasonal fruits | Curried Chickpeas and Potatoes | No change* |
| Day 11 | Refreshing Fruit Delight | Curried Chickpeas and Potatoes (leftovers) | No change* |

|  | Breakfast Recipe | Lunch Recipe | Dinner Recipe |
|---|---|---|---|
| Day 12 | Cyrus's Quinoa Special | Autumn Apple Salad | No change* |
| Day 13 | Tropical Fruit Salad | Marinara Zoodles with Chickpeas | No change* |
| Day 14 | Mexican Bean Breakfast Skillet | Mexican Kale Salad with Cilantro-Lime Dressing | No change* |

## Week 3 (Breakfast, Lunch, and Dinner)

|  | Breakfast Recipe | Lunch Recipe | Dinner Recipe |
|---|---|---|---|
| Day 15 | seasonal fruits | Curried Chickpeas and Potatoes | Lentil Dal over Cauliflower Rice |
| Day 16 | Refreshing Fruit Delight | Sweet Potato Bake | Chopped Power Salad with Mango Sauce |
| Day 17 | Robby's Antioxidant Delight | Sweet Potato Bake (leftovers) | Mushroom, Citrus, and Arugula Salad |
| Day 18 | Cyrus's Quinoa Special | Autumn Apple Salad | Roasted Root Vegetables with Portobello Mushrooms |
| Day 19 | Tropical Fruit Salad | Quick and Easy Brown Rice Pilaf with Mushrooms | Citrus Corn Carrot Salad |
| Day 20 | Mexican Bean Breakfast Skillet | Quick and Easy Brown Rice Pilaf with Mushrooms (leftovers) | Mandarin Sesame Salad |
| Day 21 | Nature's Candy Bowl | Mediterranean Lentil Tomato Salad | Pad Thai Zoodles with Ginger Sauce |

# Meal Plan 2:
## For High and Very High Baseline Insulin Resistance

### Week 1 (Breakfast Only)

|  | Breakfast Recipe | Lunch Recipe | Dinner Recipe |
|---|---|---|---|
| Day 1 | Chickpea Scramble | No change* | No change* |
| Day 2 | Kale and Lentil Breakfast Bowl | No change* | No change* |
| Day 3 | Mexican Bean Breakfast Skillet | No change* | No change* |
| Day 4 | Garden Breakfast Pan | No change* | No change* |
| Day 5 | Cauliflower Breakfast Scramble | No change* | No change* |
| Day 6 | Mexican Bean Breakfast Skillet | No change* | No change* |
| Day 7 | Cyrus's Quinoa Special | No change* | No change* |

### Week 2 (Breakfast and Lunch)

|  | Breakfast Recipe | Lunch Recipe | Dinner Recipe |
|---|---|---|---|
| Day 8 | Kale and Lentil Breakfast Bowl | Curried Red Lentils over Fluffy Quinoa | No change* |
| Day 9 | Cauliflower Breakfast Scramble | Hearty Sweet Potato and Squash Soup | No change* |
| Day 10 | Chickpea Scramble | Curried Chickpeas and Potatoes | No change* |
| Day 11 | Garden Breakfast Pan | Curried Chickpeas and Potatoes (leftovers) | No change* |
| Day 12 | Cyrus's Quinoa Special | Autumn Apple Salad | No change* |
| Day 13 | Mexican Bean Breakfast Skillet | Marinara Zoodles with Chickpeas | No change* |
| Day 14 | Mexican Bean Breakfast Skillet | Mexican Kale Salad with Cilantro-Lime Dressing | No change* |

## Week 3 (Breakfast, Lunch, and Dinner)

|  | Breakfast Recipe | Lunch Recipe | Dinner Recipe |
|---|---|---|---|
| Day 15 | Mexican Bean Breakfast Skillet | Colombian Black Bean Stew | Lentil Dal over Cauliflower Rice |
| Day 16 | Chickpea Scramble | Sweet Potato Bake | Chopped Power Salad with Mango Sauce |
| Day 17 | Mexican Bean Breakfast Skillet | Sweet Potato Bake (leftovers) | Mushroom, Citrus, and Arugula Salad |
| Day 18 | Cyrus's Quinoa Special | Autumn Apple Salad | Roasted Root Vegetables with Portobello Mushrooms |
| Day 19 | Cauliflower Breakfast Scramble | Quick and Easy Brown Rice Pilaf with Mushrooms | Citrus Corn Carrot Salad |
| Day 20 | Kale and Lentil Breakfast Bowl | Quick and Easy Brown Rice Pilaf with Mushrooms (leftovers) | Mandarin Sesame Salad |
| Day 21 | Garden Breakfast Pan | Mediterranean Lentil Tomato Salad | Pad Thai Zoodles with Ginger Sauce |

# Recipes

## BREAKFAST

### Refreshing Fruit Delight

YIELD: SERVES 1
Energy: 586 calories
Fat: 6 grams
Protein: 9 grams
Total carbohydrates: 141 grams
Fiber: 26 grams

1 papaya
1 mango
1 medium pear, cored and diced
1 medium cucumber, diced
½ cup blueberries
1 tablespoon freshly ground chia seeds
1 tablespoon fresh mint leaves, roughly chopped

Cut the papaya in half lengthways. Using a teaspoon, scoop out the black seeds and discard. Use a small sharp knife to cut the flesh away from the skin of each half. Discard the skin and slice the flesh into chunks. Toss them in a large bowl and set aside.

Use your small knife to carefully peel the skin from the mango and slice the flesh off the long, thin pit (discard the pit). Cut the mango into chunks and add to the bowl with the papaya. Add the pear, cucumber, blueberries, chia seeds, and mint and toss gently to combine.

## Robby's Antioxidant Delight

YIELD: SERVES 1
Energy: 582 calories
Fat: 7.5 grams
Protein: 11 grams
Total carbohydrates: 135 grams
Fiber: 34 grams

1 cup packed spinach
2 cups strawberries, hulled, halved, and rinsed
1 cup blueberries, rinsed
1 cup blackberries, rinsed
2 apples (any variety), cored and roughly chopped
1 large orange, peeled and roughly chopped
1 tablespoon freshly ground flaxseeds

In a large bowl, create a bed with the spinach. Top with the berries, apples, and orange and sprinkle with the flaxseeds.

# Nature's Candy Bowl

YIELD: SERVES 1
Energy: 632 calories
Fat: 4.6 grams
Protein: 7 grams
Total carbohydrates: 158 grams
Fiber: 25 grams

2 medium pears, rinsed, cored, and chopped
1 cup lettuce (any variety), rinsed and chopped
1 medium banana, mashed with a fork
½ cup chopped mango
3 Medjool dates
1 tablespoon freshly ground chia seeds

In a large bowl, combine the pears, lettuce, banana, and mango.

Slice the dates lengthwise until you hit a pit. Pull open the dates and remove and discard the pits. Add the dates to the bowl and toss everything with the chia seeds.

# Cyrus's Quinoa Special

YIELD: SERVES 1
Energy: 555 calories
Fat: 9.6 grams
Protein: 17 grams
Total carbohydrates: 107 grams
Fiber: 23 grams

½ cup dry quinoa (any variety)

1 medium apple (any variety), rinsed, cored, and diced

1 cup blackberries, rinsed

1 cup strawberries, rinsed, hulled, and quartered

1 tablespoon freshly ground flaxseeds

Ground cinnamon or cardamom, to taste

In a medium saucepan, combine the quinoa with 1 cup of water. Bring to a boil and reduce the heat to low. Simmer the quinoa, uncovered, until the liquid has evaporated, 10 to 15 minutes. Remove the pot from the heat, cover, and let the quinoa sit for 10 minutes. Fluff with a fork and set aside. (You can also do this up to 5 days in advance and store the cooked quinoa in the refrigerator.)

In a large bowl, create a bed with the quinoa and top with the fruit. Sprinkle with the flaxseeds and a pinch of the spices over the top.

## Tropical Fruit Salad

YIELD: SERVES 1

Energy: 517 calories

Fat: 9 grams

Protein: 16 grams

Total carbohydrates: 103 grams

Fiber: 22 grams

1 cup diced papaya

1 cup diced mango

1 cup cooked chickpeas, drained and rinsed

1 cup chopped romaine lettuce

1 tablespoon freshly ground chia seeds

Ground cumin, to taste

Curry powder, to taste

Fresh lemon juice, to taste

In a large bowl, assemble all the ingredients and sprinkle the spices over the top. Toss to combine and adjust the seasoning with lemon juice or more spices to taste.

## Mexican Bean Breakfast Skillet

YIELD: SERVES 1
Energy: 366 calories
Fat: 4.8 grams
Protein: 18 grams
Total carbohydrates: 67 grams
Fiber: 23 grams

1 medium yellow onion, diced
4 garlic cloves, minced
1 teaspoon ground cumin
Zest and juice of 1 lemon
1 cup low-sodium canned black beans, rinsed and drained
Freshly ground black pepper, to taste
5 grape tomatoes, halved
1 tablespoon chopped fresh cilantro
1 tablespoon freshly ground flaxseeds
I lemon, quartered

In a medium skillet over medium heat, sauté the onion with 2 tablespoons water until it starts to brown, 2 to 4 minutes. Add the garlic, cumin, and lemon zest and juice and cook until the garlic and cumin are fragrant, about 1 minute. Remove the pan from the heat.

Stir the beans into the pan, mixing well. Season the mixture with a pinch of black pepper and serve garnished with the grape tomatoes, cilantro, flaxseeds, and lemon wedges.

# Cauliflower Breakfast Scramble

YIELD: SERVES 1
Energy: 583 calories
Fat: 7 grams
Protein: 34 grams
Total carbohydrates: 109 grams
Fiber: 41 grams

1 red onion, diced
1 red bell pepper, cored, seeded, and diced
1 green bell pepper, cored, seeded, and diced
2 cups sliced mushrooms of your choice
1 large head cauliflower, cut into florets
1 cup low-sodium canned black beans, drained and rinsed
½ teaspoon freshly ground black pepper
1 teaspoon ground turmeric
¼ teaspoon cayenne pepper, or to taste
2 garlic cloves, minced
1 tablespoon chopped green onions
1 tablespoon freshly ground flaxseeds

In a large skillet over medium heat, sauté the diced onion, peppers, and mushrooms for 5 minutes, or until just beginning to soften. Add water as necessary to keep the vegetables from sticking to the pan (1 to 2 tablespoons at a time).

Add the cauliflower to the pan and cook for another 5 minutes or until tender. Stir in the beans until thoroughly mixed and season with black pepper, turmeric, cayenne, and garlic. Cook for 5 minutes more so the flavors can meld. Serve hot, garnished with green onions and flaxseeds.

# Garden Breakfast Pan

YIELD: SERVES 1
Energy: 553 calories
Fat: 5.9 grams
Protein: 33 grams
Total carbohydrates: 96 grams
Fiber: 32 grams

1 large shallot, minced
1 red bell pepper, cored, seeded, and diced
1 cup frozen green peas
5 cups packed baby spinach
1 cup low-sodium canned red beans, drained and rinsed
1 large carrot, peeled and grated
Freshly ground black pepper, to taste
1 tablespoon freshly ground flaxseeds

In a medium pan over medium heat, sauté the shallot and pepper with 1 tablespoon of water. Stir frequently for about 2 minutes, or until the shallot is translucent and the peppers are tender. Add the peas and 2 more tablespoons of water. Cook over low heat until the peas are just warmed through, about 2 minutes.

Stir in the spinach, beans, and carrots, tossing to combine. Cook for 1 to 2 minutes, just to lightly wilt the spinach and heat the mixture through. Season to taste with pepper and serve hot, garnished with flaxseeds.

# Kale and Lentil Breakfast Bowl

YIELD: SERVES 2
Energy: 420 calories
Fat: 4.3 grams
Protein: 29 grams
Total carbohydrates: 76 grams
Fiber: 22 grams

2 garlic cloves, minced

4 kale leaves, cut into ¼-inch-thin strips

1 cup cooked lentils (any type you prefer)

Freshly ground black pepper, to taste

2 medium tomatoes, diced

2 tablespoons chopped flat-leaf parsley

2 tablespoons chopped green onions (white and green parts)

1 tablespoon freshly ground flaxseeds

In a small nonstick skillet over medium heat, combine 2 tablespoons of water with the garlic and kale. Cook, stirring frequently, until the kale has wilted, about 2 minutes. Add the lentils and continue cooking until warmed through, about 2 more minutes. Divide the mixture between 2 bowls and season to taste with black pepper. Top with the tomatoes and sprinkle with the parsley, green onions, and flaxseeds.

## Chickpea Scramble

YIELD: SERVES 2

Energy: 338 calories

Fat: 7.5 grams

Protein: 17 grams

Total carbohydrates: 54 grams

Fiber: 16 grams

1 (15-ounce) can low-sodium chickpeas

½ teaspoon ground turmeric

½ teaspoon freshly ground black pepper

¼ white onion, diced

2 garlic cloves, minced

2 cups mixed greens

1 tablespoon freshly ground flaxseeds

Handful of minced fresh parsley

Handful of minced fresh cilantro

Fresh lemon juice, to taste

Drain the chickpeas over a bowl, reserving the liquid from the can. Add the chickpeas to another medium bowl and pour in about a tablespoon of the liquid. Use a fork to slightly mash the chickpeas, leaving some whole. Stir in the turmeric and pepper until well combined.

In a medium skillet over medium heat, add the onion and 2 tablespoons of water. Sauté until the onions are soft, about 3 minutes. Add the garlic and continue sautéing until the garlic is fragrant, a minute more. If the garlic cooks too quickly, adding a little more water to the pan will keep it from burning. Add the mashed chickpeas to the pan and sauté to warm through, 2 to 3 minutes more.

Assemble the breakfast bowls by arranging the mixed greens at the bottom and topping them with the chickpea scramble. Sprinkle with the flaxseeds and herbs and finish with a squeeze of lemon juice to taste.

# LUNCH

## Marinara Zoodles with Chickpeas

YIELD: SERVES 3
Energy: 436 calories
Fat: 4.5 grams
Protein: 16 grams
Total carbohydrates: 91 grams
Fiber: 17 grams

6 medium zucchini or 3 cups store-bought zoodles
20 cherry tomatoes
1 cup sun-dried tomatoes (not packed in oil)
6 Medjool dates, pitted
6 garlic cloves
1 small onion, roughly chopped
Juice of 1 lemon
1 teaspoon chopped fresh rosemary
2 cups low-sodium canned chickpeas, drained and rinsed

Create "noodles" from the zucchini using either a spiralizer or a vegetable peeler. Set aside.

In a blender, combine the tomatoes, dates, garlic, onion, lemon juice, and rosemary and blend until smooth, about 1 minute. You may need to pause to scrape down the sides of the blender, then continue blending.

In a large bowl, toss the noodles and chickpeas with the sauce.

## Curried Red Lentils over Fluffy Quinoa

YIELD: SERVES 3
Energy: 440 calories
Fat: 3.8 grams
Protein: 21 grams
Total carbohydrates: 84 grams
Fiber: 17 grams

2 cups uncooked quinoa, rinsed
2 cups cooked red lentils (drained and rinsed if canned)
4 cups homemade or low-sodium vegetable broth, or water
2 medium sweet potatoes, peeled and diced
1 large onion, chopped
½ cup chopped celery
½ cup chopped carrots
3 garlic cloves, minced
1 teaspoon minced fresh ginger
1 tablespoon curry powder
1 teaspoon ground cumin
¼ cup chopped fresh cilantro
1 tablespoon fresh lemon juice

In a medium saucepan, combine 2 cups of quinoa with 2 cups of water. Bring to a boil over high heat, then reduce to a simmer. Cook, uncovered, until the water has evaporated, 10 to 15 minutes. Remove the pot from the heat, cover, and let the quinoa sit for 10 minutes before fluffing it with a fork. Set aside.

In a large pot over medium-high heat, combine the lentils and broth or water. Bring to a boil, then reduce to a simmer. Add the sweet potatoes, onion, celery, carrots, garlic, ginger, and spices and stir until combined. Cover and cook for 15 to 20 minutes, until the lentils and potatoes are soft. Stir in cilantro and lemon juice and remove the pot from the heat.

Transfer half of the lentils to a blender and blend until smooth, then stir the blended lentils back into the pot. You could also use an immersion blender right in the pot; just leave some texture and chunkiness to the lentils. Spoon the lentils over quinoa and serve.

## Mexican Kale Salad with Cilantro-Lime Dressing

YIELD: SERVES 2
Energy: 529 calories
Fat: 4 grams
Protein: 26 grams
Total carbohydrates: 108 grams
Fiber: 32 grams

10 cups chopped curly kale
Juice of ½ large lemon
2 cups low-sodium canned black beans, drained
    and rinsed
2 cups corn kernels (fresh or frozen)
½ cup diced red onion
2 large red bell peppers, cored, seeded, and diced
2 jalapeño peppers, seeded and diced
    (scale back if you prefer less heat)
16 ounces cherry tomatoes, halved
Finely chopped fresh cilantro, for garnish
Cilantro-Lime Dressing (recipe follows)

In a large mixing bowl, sprinkle the kale with the lemon juice and give the kale a good massage until the leaves are tender and release bright green juice, about 2 minutes. Toss in the beans, corn, onion, peppers, and tomatoes. Sprinkle with cilantro and drizzle with the dressing.

### Cilantro-Lime Dressing
YIELD: MAKES 1½ CUPS (1 SERVING)
Energy: 28 calories
Fat: 0.2 grams
Protein: 1 gram
Carbohydrates: 6 grams
Fiber: 1 gram

1 cup loosely packed fresh cilantro
1 garlic clove
½ jalapeño, seeded
2 tablespoons fresh lime juice (about 1 lime)
2 tablespoons apple cider vinegar
Freshly ground black pepper, to taste

In a blender, combine the cilantro, garlic, jalapeño, lime juice, apple cider vinegar, and 1 tablespoon of water and blend until smooth. Season with pepper. This will keep in the refrigerator for up to 5 days.

# Mediterranean Lentil Tomato Salad

YIELD: SERVES 2
Energy: 501 calories
Fat: 3.9 grams
Protein: 27 grams
Total carbohydrates: 102 grams
Fiber: 22 grams

1 cup uncooked green lentils

2 garlic cloves

1 pint cherry tomatoes, quartered

1 cup sliced green onions (pale green and white parts only)

¼ cup chopped fresh basil

¼ cup chopped fresh dill

1 cup corn kernels (fresh or frozen and thawed)

2 teaspoons lemon zest

¼ cup freshly squeezed lemon juice

Freshly ground black pepper, to taste

In a large pot, combine the lentils and garlic with 4 cups of water. Bring to a boil and reduce to a simmer. Cook until the lentils are soft, about 15 minutes. Drain the lentils, discarding the garlic, and set aside to cool to room temperature.

In a large mixing bowl, combine the tomatoes, green onions, basil, dill, and corn with the cooled lentils. Add the lemon zest and juice, and toss to combine. Season with pepper. Serve at room temperature or chilled.

## Hearty Sweet Potato and Squash Soup

YIELD: SERVES 2

Energy: 428 calories

Fat: 3.2 grams

Protein: 11 grams

Total carbohydrates: 98 grams

Fiber: 23 grams

1 large butternut squash

2 large white onions, coarsely chopped

12 celery stalks, coarsely chopped

10 garlic cloves, finely chopped

6 medium sweet potatoes, peeled and diced

6 cups homemade or low-sodium vegetable broth

4 dried bay leaves

3 tablespoons cumin seeds

1 tablespoon crushed red pepper flakes

1 teaspoon ground cloves

Apple cider vinegar or champagne vinegar, to taste

Preheat the oven to 375°F.

Place the squash on a baking sheet and roast for 40 minutes, or until you can easily pierce the narrow end with a fork. Allow the squash to cool until you can comfortably handle. Remove the skin, halve lengthwise, remove the seeds and fibers, and dice. Set aside.

Heat 1 tablespoon of water in a large pot over medium heat. Add the onion, celery, and garlic and sauté until the onion is translucent and beginning to turn golden, about 10 minutes. If necessary, add more water to keep the vegetables from burning, about 1 tablespoon at a time.

Add the sweet potatoes and broth to the pot and bring to a low boil. Add the bay leaves, cumin, crushed red pepper, and cloves, and reduce to a simmer. Cover the pot and cook for 10 minutes.

Stir in the roasted squash and simmer over low heat until all the vegetables are tender, about 15 minutes.

Use a slotted spoon to scoop out 2 cups of the vegetables and transfer to a medium bowl. Use a fork to mash the vegetables well, then return them to the pot and stir to combine. Alternatively, you could use an immersion blender, or transfer the mixture to a blender and blend the soup until completely smooth. Taste the soup and adjust the seasoning with vinegar, if desired.

# Colombian Black Bean Stew

YIELD: SERVES 2
Energy: 634 calories
Fat: 3.7 grams
Protein: 34 grams
Total carbohydrates: 123 grams
Fiber: 46 grams

4 small yellow onions, finely chopped
7 garlic cloves, minced
2 (14-ounce) cans chopped tomatoes
4 cups low-sodium canned black beans, drained and rinsed
1 teaspoon ground cumin
2 cups homemade or low-sodium vegetable broth
1 teaspoon ground ginger
1 heaped teaspoon dried oregano
Pinch of freshly ground black pepper

In a large skillet over medium heat, sweat the onions until translucent, about 10 minutes. Add a couple tablespoons of water if necessary to prevent them from burning. Add the garlic and sauté for 2 minutes. Stir in the tomatoes, beans, and a scant ½ cup of water. Lower the heat to a simmer and add the cumin, broth, ginger, and oregano. Let the soup simmer for 15 to 20 minutes, so the mixture thickens and the flavors meld. Season with pepper and serve warm.

# Curried Chickpeas and Potatoes

YIELD: SERVES 2
Energy: 800 calories
Fat: 6 grams
Protein: 26 grams
Total carbohydrates: 171 grams
Fiber: 31 grams

2 medium onions, diced

5 garlic cloves, minced

1 tablespoon minced fresh ginger

½ teaspoon ground cumin

½ teaspoon ground coriander

1 teaspoon curry powder

1 cup tomato sauce (no salt added)

6 medium potatoes, peeled and diced

2 cups canned chickpeas, rinsed and drained

16 ounces cherry tomatoes, chopped

2 cups chopped cauliflower

½ cup chopped fresh cilantro, plus more for garnish

1 lemon, sliced into wedges

In a medium pot over medium heat, sauté the onion, garlic, ginger, and spices until the onions become translucent and begin to caramelize, 7 to 10 minutes. Add 1 tablespoon of water at a time, if necessary, to keep the ingredients from sticking to the pan.

Stir in the tomato sauce and potatoes. Cover and simmer until the potatoes are just tender, about 15 minutes. Add the chickpeas, cherry tomatoes, and cauliflower and simmer for another 5 minutes. Remove the pot from the heat and stir in the cilantro. Serve with a sprinkle more of cilantro and lemon wedges.

## Sweet Potato Bake

YIELD: SERVES 5
Energy: 466 calories
Fat: 3.3 grams
Protein: 17 grams
Total carbohydrates: 95 grams
Fiber: 19 grams

4 cups sweet potatoes, cut in ½-inch cubes

2 cups homemade or low-sodium vegetable broth

1 (15-ounce) can low-sodium black beans, drained and rinsed

1 cup uncooked quinoa, rinsed

1 cup frozen corn, thawed

2 teaspoons ground cumin

1 teaspoon chili powder

½ teaspoon dried thyme

½ cup chopped green onions (white and green parts)

Preheat the oven to 375°F.

In a large baking dish, combine the sweet potatoes, broth, beans, quinoa, corn, cumin, chili powder, and thyme. Stir until mixed well and cover with foil. Bake for 45 minutes. Remove the foil and bake for an additional 15 to 20 minutes, or until most of the liquid has been absorbed and the potatoes are tender. Let the dish sit for 5 minutes so any remaining liquid can be absorbed. Sprinkle with the green onions and serve.

## Quick and Easy Brown Rice Pilaf with Mushrooms

YIELD: SERVES 2

Energy: 424 calories

Fat: 3.4 grams

Protein: 12 grams

Total carbohydrates: 89 grams

Fiber: 6 grams

10 ounces sliced cremini mushrooms

1 cup diced yellow onion

2 garlic cloves, minced

2 cups homemade or low-sodium vegetable broth

1 cup brown rice, rinsed

¼ cup diced green onions (white and green parts)

In a medium pan over medium heat, sauté half of the mushrooms with 2 tablespoons of water. Cook the mushrooms until they brown, 2 to 3 minutes. Remove the mushrooms from the pan and set aside.

In a medium pot, combine 2 tablespoons of water with the onion and garlic. Sauté for 2 minutes. Add the other half of the mushrooms and sauté for another 3 to 4 minutes until they are brown.

Stir in the broth and rice, scraping up any browned bits from the bottom of the pot. Cover and simmer over very low heat until the broth is absorbed and the rice is al dente, 45 to 50 minutes. Mix in the reserved mushrooms, top with the green onions, and serve.

# Autumn Apple Salad

YIELD: SERVES 1
Energy: 478 calories
Fat: 1.7 grams
Protein: 14 grams
Total carbohydrates: 112 grams
Fiber: 23 grams

3 cups cherry tomatoes, halved
2 apples, grated
½ cup butternut squash, very thinly sliced (a vegetable peeler or mandoline works well here)
10 fresh basil leaves, thinly sliced
½ medium red onion, thinly sliced
1 head lacinato kale, thinly sliced
Juice of ½ large lemon, plus more to taste

In a large bowl, combine the tomatoes, apples, squash, basil, and red onion. Toss well, then set aside.

In another large bowl, combine the kale and lemon juice and give the kale a good massage with your hands until the leaves are soft and are starting to give up their green juice, 2 to 3 minutes. Mound the apple mixture over the kale and adjust the seasoning with more lemon juice, if desired.

# DINNER

## Pad Thai Zoodles with Ginger Sauce

YIELD: SERVES 2
Energy: 410 calories
Fat: 9.1 grams
Protein: 23 grams
Total carbohydrates: 72 grams
Fiber: 27 grams

8 large zucchini or 4 cups store-bought zoodles
4 cups chopped broccoli
2 cups shredded carrots
2 large red bell peppers, cored, seeded, and sliced
1 cup sugar snap peas
Ginger Sauce (recipe follows)
¼ cup chopped fresh cilantro
¼ cup chopped green onions (white and green parts)
2 tablespoons crushed peanuts

To make the zucchini noodles, use a spiralizer or a vegetable peeler to slice the zucchini into very thin strips. Set aside.

In a large skillet or wok over medium-high heat, combine the broccoli, carrots, pepper, and sugar snap peas. Sauté 5 to 6 minutes, until the vegetables are soft. Add the zucchini noodles and sauté for an additional 3 to 4 minutes, until the noodles are tender but not soft. Stir in the sauce. Remove the pan from the heat and top the noodles with the cilantro, green onions, and peanuts.

### Ginger Sauce
YIELD: MAKES ABOUT 2½ CUPS (1 SERVING)
Energy: 121 calories
Fat: 1.2 grams
Protein: 5 grams
Total carbohydrates: 27 grams
Fiber: 6 grams

2 cups roughly chopped zucchini
1 cup orange or tangerine segments
2 tablespoons sliced fresh ginger
Fresh basil, to taste
Curry powder, to taste

In the bowl of a food processor, combine the zucchini, oranges or tangerines, and ginger. Process until blended well. Adjust the seasoning to taste. Store in the fridge for up to 2 days.

## Roasted Root Vegetables with Portobello Mushrooms

YIELD: SERVES 2
Energy: 524 calories
Fat: 2.8 grams
Protein: 21 grams
Total carbohydrates: 117 grams
Fiber: 29 grams

10 portobello mushroom caps, sliced ½-inch thick
2 cups 1-inch cauliflower florets
2 cups diced sweet potato (about ½-inch cubes)
2 cups diced butternut squash (about ½-inch cubes)
1 cup diced beets (about ½-inch cubes)
1 medium red onion, diced
4 garlic cloves, minced
2 tablespoons fresh thyme leaves
1 tablespoon chopped fresh rosemary
1 tablespoon fresh lemon juice, or to taste

Preheat the oven to 425°F. Line 2 baking sheets with parchment paper and set aside.

In a large mixing bowl, combine all of the ingredients except the lemon juice and toss to mix well.

Spread vegetables evenly in a single layer over the baking sheets. Roast for 45 minutes, stirring once or twice, or until the vegetables are tender and easily pierced with a fork or knife.

Serve in a large bowl, dressed with lemon juice to taste

## Potato-Veggie Tian

YIELD: SERVES 2
Energy: 473 calories
Fat: 2.9 grams
Protein: 17 grams
Total carbohydrates: 107 grams
Fiber: 26 grams

8 medium tomatoes, sliced thin
1 red onion, sliced thin
3 medium zucchini, sliced thin
1 medium eggplant, peeled and sliced into ⅛-inch rounds
3 medium baking potatoes, peeled and sliced into ⅛-inch rounds
Freshly ground black pepper
2 teaspoons fresh rosemary, chopped, plus more for sprinkling
2 teaspoons fresh thyme, plus more for sprinkling
Juice of 1 lemon
1 tablespoon minced garlic

Preheat the oven to 375°F.

Combine the tomatoes, onion, zucchini, eggplant, and potatoes in a large bowl and season to taste with pepper. Sprinkle the vegetables with 1 to 2 tablespoons of water, enough to lightly and evenly coat them. Toss gently with the herbs, lemon juice, and garlic.

In a large baking dish, arrange the vegetable slices in rows in the following order: potato, tomato, eggplant, tomato, potato, zucchini, onion, tomato, eggplant, tomato. Layer them in such a way that they are stacked tightly on a diagonal.

Sprinkle the top with the extra herbs and pour any juice left in the bowl over the vegetables. Cover tightly with foil and bake for 1 hour. Remove the foil and continue baking for another 30 minutes, until the vegetables are completely tender and slightly browned around the edges.

## Lentil Dal over Cauliflower Rice

YIELD: SERVES 3
Energy: 548 calories
Fat: 2.6 grams
Protein: 36 grams
Total carbohydrates: 102 grams
Fiber: 32 grams

2 medium heads of cauliflower
2 medium yellow onions, diced
4 garlic cloves, minced
2 cups homemade or low-sodium vegetable broth
2 (6-ounce) cans tomato paste
1 tablespoon curry powder
4 cups cooked or canned brown lentils, drained and rinsed

Break up the cauliflower into individual florets and pulse them in a food processor until they reach a rice-like consistency. Be careful not to overprocess or it will become too watery. Transfer the rice to a large mixing bowl and set aside.

In a large skillet over medium heat, add the onion and cook until golden brown, about 10 minutes. Add a tablespoon of water, if necessary, to keep it from burning. Add the garlic and cook for 1 minute. Pour in ½ cup of the stock and cook for 2 minutes.

Stir in the tomato paste, curry powder, and remaining stock. Mix well and reduce the heat to medium-low. Add the lentils and cook until the mixture has heated through and thickened slightly, about 10 minutes.

Serve the dal over cauliflower rice.

## Hot and Spicy Broccoli-Cauliflower Rice

YIELD: SERVES 3
Energy: 471 calories
Fat: 3.4 grams
Protein: 28 grams
Total carbohydrates: 92 grams
Fiber: 34 grams

2 medium heads of cauliflower
2 medium heads of broccoli
1 cup homemade or low-sodium vegetable stock
4 large carrots, diced
2 large yellow onions, chopped
2 cups chopped kale leaves
2 cups low-sodium canned black beans, drained and rinsed
2 cups frozen green peas
4 large celery stalks, diced
2 teaspoons ground turmeric
Cayenne pepper, to taste

Break up the cauliflower into individual florets and pulse in a food processor until it reaches a rice-like consistency. Be careful not to overprocess or it will become watery. Transfer the cauliflower rice to a large mixing bowl.

Break up the broccoli into individual florets and pulse in a food processor until it reaches a rice-like consistency, also taking care to not overprocess. Add the broccoli rice to the bowl with the cauliflower rice.

In a deep saucepan over medium-high heat, combine the stock and carrots and cook until they are semi-soft, about 5 minutes.

Add the onion, kale, beans, peas, and celery and cook, stirring often, until all of the vegetables are soft and any excess liquid in the pan has cooked off, about 5 minutes. Add a splash more stock to the pan if it gets too dry and the vegetables need to cook longer.

Season the mixture with the turmeric and a pinch of the cayenne. Stir in the broccoli/cauliflower rice and season with more cayenne to taste, if desired.

## Chopped Power Salad with Mango Sauce

YIELD: SERVES 1
Energy: 690 calories
Fat: 7.6 grams
Protein: 31 grams
Total carbohydrates: 139 grams
Fiber: 31 grams

**For the Mango Sauce**

1 cup diced mango
2 cups diced tomato
2 tablespoons nutritional yeast

**For the Salad**

1 medium sweet potato, peeled and diced
1 bunch of curly kale, washed, stems removed, and chopped
Juice of ½ large lemon
¼ teaspoon freshly ground black pepper
1 cup low-sodium canned garbanzo beans, drained and rinsed
1 yellow bell pepper, cored, seeded, and chopped
½ cup fresh or frozen cranberries, roughly chopped
¼ cup chopped red onion

Make the sauce: Combine all of the ingredients in a blender and process until smooth. Set aside.

In a small pot, combine the sweet potato with enough water to cover and boil until fork-tender, 15 to 20 minutes. Drain and set aside.

In a large bowl, combine the kale, lemon juice, and black pepper. Use your hands to massage the kale until the leaves are tender and start to give up their dark green juices, about 2 minutes. Fold in the cooked sweet potato, beans, bell pepper, cranberries, and red onion. Drizzle with the mango sauce and serve.

## Greens and Beans

YIELD: SERVES 2
Energy: 423 calories
Fat: 1.8 grams
Protein: 25 grams
Total carbohydrates: 84 grams
Fiber: 19 grams

2 small yellow onions, diced
4 garlic cloves, minced
2 cups low-sodium canned white beans, drained and rinsed
6 cups de-stemmed and chopped kale
4 cups de-stemmed and chopped Swiss chard
2 medium green bell peppers, cored, seeded, and chopped
Juice of 2 lemons
Pinch crushed red pepper flakes (optional)

In a large skillet over medium heat, sauté the onion and garlic until translucent, about 7 minutes. Add 1 tablespoon of water to the pan if needed to prevent burning.

Add the white beans, kale, chard, bell pepper, and the juice. Stir and cover. Cook, stirring frequently, until the greens are wilted, 2 to 5 minutes. Add 1 tablespoon of water if needed to prevent the greens from sticking to the pan. Sprinkle with the red pepper flakes, if desired, and serve.

## Citrus Corn Carrot Salad

YIELD: SERVES 1
Energy: 438 calories
Fat: 3.1 grams
Protein: 18 grams
Total carbohydrates: 77 grams
Fiber: 26 grams

2 medium oranges, peeled and segmented or sliced into rounds
2 medium carrots, shredded
2 medium tomatoes, sliced
1 cup frozen corn, thawed
½ red onion, chopped
2 tablespoons chopped fresh cilantro
1 tablespoon fennel seeds
6 cups of mixed greens

In a large bowl, combine the oranges, carrots, tomatoes, corn, onion, cilantro, and fennel seeds and mix well, ensuring that the juice from the oranges and tomatoes coats the mixture, creating a dressing. Serve over a bed of the greens.

## Mandarin Sesame Salad

YIELD: SERVES 2
Energy: 344 calories
Fat: 3.9 grams
Protein: 13 grams
Total carbohydrates: 75 grams
Fiber: 19 grams

1 head of Napa cabbage, shredded

6 small mandarin oranges, peeled and segmented

1 cup snow peas, halved

6 green onions (white and green parts), cut into 1-inch
    pieces

1 large carrot, grated

½ cup bean sprouts

2 tablespoons rice wine vinegar

1 tablespoon black sesame seeds

In a large bowl, combine the cabbage, oranges, snow peas, onions, carrot, sprouts, and vinegar and toss well. Sprinkle the salad with the sesame seeds and serve.

## Mushroom, Citrus, and Arugula Salad

YIELD: SERVES 1

Energy: 362 calories

Fat: 3.3 grams

Protein: 17.4 grams

Total carbohydrates: 79 grams

Fiber: 19 grams

3 medium oranges, peeled and segmented or
    sliced

2 cups cremini mushrooms, sliced

½ cup cherry tomatoes, halved

2 zucchini, sliced lengthwise into long strips

½ tablespoon fennel seeds

5 cups arugula

½ tablespoon balsamic vinegar

Fresh lemon juice, to taste

In a large bowl, toss together the oranges, mushrooms, tomatoes, zucchini, and fennel seeds.

Arrange the mixture over the top of the arugula and serve sprinkled lightly with balsamic vinegar for added flavor. Adjust the seasoning with lemon juice to taste, if desired.

# Appendix A:
# C-Peptide Testing

## How to Get Your C-Peptide Tested

It's actually very easy to get your C-peptide level tested. This entails an inexpensive blood test that you can request from your doctor, or you can order the test for yourself online and schedule to have your blood drawn at a local LabCorp or Quest Diagnostics facility. Sometimes paying out of pocket is more convenient than waiting to see your primary care physician or endocrinologist. If you are going to use the latter method, we suggest ordering from one of the following online laboratories:

- **Option 1:** Request a Test—$59.00 online order
- **Option 2:** Direct Labs—$69.00 online order
- **Option 3:** Personalabs—$106.00 online order

Select where you would like to get your blood drawn, enter your credit card information, and then take the order form to your local facility. The results are quick and often ready in 1 to 3 days.

# Interpreting Your C-Peptide Test Results

We recommend using the following guidelines to interpret your C-peptide test results. As you can see, your C-peptide results are best read in conjunction with an islet antibody test—interpreting the results of both tests together provides the most accurate information.

## Your fasting C-peptide is less than 1.0 ng/mL:

Your endogenous insulin production is very low, which means that you fall into one of the three categories below:

- **If you test positive for one diabetes antibody** (and are over the age of 30), you are likely living with type 1.5 diabetes and may require both basal and bolus insulin to control your blood glucose.
- **If you test positive for multiple diabetes antibodies** (irrespective of your age), you are likely living with type 1 diabetes, and may require both basal and bolus insulin to control your blood glucose.
- **If you test negative for diabetes antibodies,** you are likely living with insulin-dependent type 2 diabetes (low insulin production). You are likely to require both basal and bolus insulin in order to control your blood glucose.

## Your fasting C-peptide is 1.0–2.0 ng/mL:

Your endogenous insulin production is medium, which means that you fall into one of the following three categories:

- **If you test positive for one diabetes antibody** (and are over the age of 30), you are likely living with type 1.5 diabetes and may experience a decline in your insulin production with an increased need for exogenous basal and bolus insulin over time.
- **If you test positive for multiple diabetes antibodies** (irrespective of your age), you are likely living with type 1

diabetes and are currently in the "honeymoon" phase, during which your endogenous insulin production is declining quickly. You will likely experience an increased need for exogenous basal and bolus insulin over time.

- **If you test negative for diabetes antibodies,** you are likely living with type 2 diabetes (impaired insulin production). Adopting the Mastering Diabetes Method to maximize your insulin sensitivity is your best chance at remaining free of exogenous insulin.

### Your fasting C-peptide is 2.0 ng/mL or above:

Your endogenous insulin production is medium to high, which means that you fall into one of the following three categories:

- **If you test positive for one diabetes antibody** (and are over the age of 30), you are likely living with type 1.5 diabetes and may experience a decline in your insulin production with an increased need for exogenous basal and bolus insulin over time even though your endogenous insulin production is sufficient now.
- **If you test positive for multiple diabetes antibodies** (irrespective of your age), you are likely living with type 1 diabetes and are currently in the "honeymoon" phase, during which your endogenous insulin production is declining quickly, even though your endogenous insulin production is sufficient now. You will likely experience an increased need for exogenous basal and bolus insulin over time.
- **If you test negative for diabetes antibodies,** you are likely living with type 2 diabetes (high insulin production). You are likely to remain free of exogenous insulin as long as you continually improve your insulin sensitivity.

The following table summarizes our C-peptide guidelines.

| | Low C-Peptide (<1.0 ng/mL) | Medium C-Peptide (1.0–2.0 ng/mL) | High C-Peptide (2.0 ng/mL+) |
|---|---|---|---|
| **Negative Antibody Test** | Type 2 diabetes with low insulin production (insulin likely) | Type 2 diabetes with impaired insulin production (insulin unlikely) | Type 2 diabetes with high insulin production (insulin unlikely) |
| **Positive (1 diabetes Antibody)** | Type 1.5 diabetes (insulin necessary) | Type 1.5 diabetes (insulin necessary) | Type 1.5 diabetes (insulin necessary over time) |
| **Positive (2+ diabetes Antibodies)** | Type 1 diabetes (insulin necessary) | Type 1 diabetes (insulin necessary) | Type 1 diabetes (insulin necessary over time) |

# Appendix B:
# A Complete List of Green Light Foods

Since green light ingredients will now account for the majority of your meals, we figured it would be helpful to include a one-stop reference for many of the fantastic options you have. And this is only the beginning—many of these foods have many varieties that change throughout the course of the year.

For example, you can likely find at least eight varieties of potatoes easily: russet, sweet, red, white, purple, fingerling, Yukon gold, and Japanese. For mangoes, look for Haden, Kent, Ataulfo, Manila, Champagne, and Keitt. The same rules apply to tomatoes, persimmons, pears, grapes, apricots, citrus, plums, nectarines, peaches, squashes, beans, and intact whole grains.

With this much variety to choose from, you can see how it's very difficult to get bored with eating the same foods over and over! You may even be surprised at how many tasty foods are easily accessible in your local area. We highly suggest referencing this list any time you want to add diversity to your menu.

As you may remember from chapter 9, it's important to focus on green light foods that provide substantial calorie density. The four green light categories that provide the most are fruits, starchy vegetables, legumes, and intact whole grains. For simplicity's sake, we've listed these foods in order of descending calorie density. So if you are feeling hungry between meals, make sure to focus on eating more calorie-dense green light foods at the beginning of your meal. This will help ensure that you don't fill up on low-calorie items, then get hungry one to two hours after your meal.

## Master List of Green Light Foods

For each category, the foods below are listed from highest to lowest calorie density.

### FRUITS

Mamey sapote
Plantains
Persimmons
Breadfruit
Custard apple
Passion fruit
Jackfruit
Sugar apple
Bananas
Pomegranate
Sapodilla
Jujube
Crab apples
Cherimoya
Figs
Elderberries
Kumquats
Grapes
Guavas
Lychees

Soursop
Cherries
Currants
Oranges
Kiwifruit
Longans
Mangoes
Pears
Blueberries
Muscadine grapes
Quinces
Apples
Tangerines
Raspberries
Pineapple
Apricots
Loquats
Clementines
Cranberries
Plums

Gooseberries
Nectarines
Horned
    melon
Blackberries
Mulberries
Papayas
Grapefruit
Asian pears
Prickly pears
Peaches
Pomelo
Honeydew
    melons
Cantaloupe
Strawberries
Carambola
    (star fruit)
Watermelons
Casaba melons

## STARCHY VEGETABLES

| | | |
|---|---|---|
| Taro | Cassava (yuca) | Carrots |
| Yams | Red potatoes | Butternut squash |
| Corn | Parsnips | Spaghetti |
| White potatoes | Acorn squash | squash |
| Sweet potato | Hubbard squash | Pumpkin |

## BEANS, PEAS, LENTILS

| | | |
|---|---|---|
| Chickpeas | Adzuki beans | Lentils |
| Pink beans | Kidney beans | Lima beans |
| Pinto beans | Fava beans | Broad beans |
| White beans | Pigeon peas | Mung beans |
| Navy beans | Great Northern | Green peas |
| Cranberry beans | beans | Yard-long beans |
| Black beans | Split peas | Yellow beans |
| French beans | Moth beans | Green beans |

## INTACT WHOLE GRAINS

| | | |
|---|---|---|
| Khorasan wheat | Millet | Amaranth |
| (kamut) | Rye | Wild rice |
| Spelt | Sorghum | Teff |
| Barley (hulled | Quinoa | Buckwheat |
| only, no pearl) | Wheat, hard red | Bulgur |
| Brown rice | winter | |

## NON-STARCHY VEGETABLES

| | | |
|---|---|---|
| Mountain yam | Shallots | Tomatillos |
| Artichokes | Broccoli | Rutabagas |
| Beets | Eggplant | Kohlrabi |
| Onions | Brussels sprouts | Chayote |

| | | |
|---|---|---|
| Cabbage | Turnips | Celery |
| Bok choy | Rhubarb | Radishes |
| Cauliflower | Asparagus | Cucumber |
| Radicchio | Tomatoes | Zucchini |
| Okra | Summer squash | |

## LEAFY GREENS

| | | |
|---|---|---|
| Dandelion greens | Arugula | Pokeberry |
| Seaweed | Spinach | Purslane |
| Parsley | Beet greens | Endive |
| Collards | Turnip greens | Romaine lettuce |
| Lamb's-quarters | Fennel | Red leaf lettuce |
| Leeks | Green onions | Green leaf lettuce |
| Chives | Swiss chard | Iceberg lettuce |
| Kale | Watercress | Butter lettuce |
| Mustard greens | Chard | Nopales |

## HERBS AND SPICES

All herbs and spices, fresh or dry, excluding spice mixtures containing salt

## MUSHROOMS

All culinary mushrooms, fresh or dry

## SPROUTS

All sprouts

# Appendix C:
# Sample Decision Trees

## Sample Decision Tree: Insulin-Dependent Diabetes

Below you will find sample decision trees for a person living with type 1 diabetes and a person living with type 2 diabetes. These are basic examples to illustrate the fundamentals of how to use a decision tree. Your initial decision trees may be more complex and you may have more data to document, which will require a second page to complete a full day. The more detailed you are in this process, the more you will benefit.

Let's walk through a sample for an insulin-dependent person living with type 1 diabetes and evaluate each decision together. Jim uses Lantus as a long-acting insulin and Humalog as a fast-acting insulin.

- Jim wakes up.
    - 5:30 A.M.—Jim wakes up with a fasting blood glucose of 105 mg/dL. He injects 1 unit to treat the dawn phenomenon.
- Jim prepares for exercise.
    - 6:15 A.M.—Jim tests his blood glucose before a cycling class, and he is at 110 mg/dL. He eats 1 medium banana, which has 30 grams of carbohydrate, and injects 0.5 unit

of Humalog insulin. He chooses to under-inject insulin given that he is about to exercise and he predicts that his pre-exercise carbohydrate-to-insulin ratio is 60:1.

- 6:30 A.M.—Jim starts a 45-minute cycling class.
- Jim is finished with exercise.
  - 7:30 A.M.—While talking with friends and stretching, Jim measures his post-exercise blood glucose to be 115 mg/dL. It's time to prepare for eating breakfast.
- Jim prepares to eat breakfast.
  - 8:45 A.M—Seated at his desk to start the workday, Jim calculates his breakfast meal to contain approximately 175 grams of carbohydrate from bananas, mangoes, and apples. He predicts that a 25:1 carbohydrate-to-insulin ratio is the correct insulin sensitivity after exercise, and injects 7 units of fast-acting insulin 15 minutes before he eats (following our insulin timing strategies, pages 200–202).
  - 9:00 A.M.—Jim measures his blood glucose and it is 130 mg/dL. He is confused why his blood glucose is on an upward trend. He patiently waits for the insulin he injected 15 minutes ago to start working.
  - 9:15 A.M.—Jim measures his blood glucose again at 118 mg/dL. Given that he is under 120 mg/dL and trending down, he begins eating his breakfast.
- Jim checks his blood glucose two hours after breakfast.
  - 11:30 A.M.—Two hours after he is done eating, Jim measures his blood glucose at 126 mg/dL. He is excited because his predicted breakfast carbohydrate-to-insulin ratio of 25:1 worked well.
- Jim prepares to eat lunch.
  - 12:30 P.M.—Jim is ready to eat lunch, which he brought from home, so he knows it contains 150 grams of carbohydrate. His blood glucose is 120 mg/dL. His predicted carbohydrate-to-insulin ratio is 25:1 at lunch, so he injects 6 units of fast-acting insulin.

- 12:45 P.M.—Jim's blood glucose is 105 mg/dL. Since he is under 120 mg/dL and trending downward, he begins eating immediately.
- Jim checks his blood glucose two hours after lunch.
  - 3:30 P.M.—Jim measures his blood glucose at 200 mg/dL. He suspects it's high because of an adrenaline rush owing to a very important presentation he'll be delivering to his boss and colleagues. Jim takes a 1 unit fast-acting insulin correction bolus.
- Jim prepares to eat dinner.
  - 6:00 P.M.—Jim is home and ready to eat dinner. His blood glucose is 111 mg/dL and his dinner contains 115 grams of carbohydrate energy. Jim knows that he tends to be more insulin sensitive in the evening, so he injects with a predicted carbohydrate-to-insulin ratio of 32:1 and injects 3.5 units of fast-acting insulin.
  - 6:15 P.M.—Jim starts to enjoy his delicious dinner after waiting for 15 minutes to allow insulin to start working.
- Jim corrects hypoglycemia.
  - 7:45 P.M.—90 minutes after Jim started eating his dinner, he feels shaky. He measures his blood glucose at 65 mg/dL and eats 1 Medjool date to recover. He writes down that he consumed 15 grams of carbohydrate energy. In 15 minutes he feels great. Now Jim can calculate his actual carbohydrate-to-insulin ratio, which is 115 + 15 / 3.5 = 37. Tomorrow when he injects bolus insulin for his dinner meal, he will inject at a 37:1 ratio rather than the 32:1, which led to hypoglycemia today.
- Jim prepares for bed.
  - 10:00 P.M.—Before going to bed, Jim injects 14 units of long-acting insulin. He also measures his blood glucose at 98 mg/dL and is confident that his blood glucose will remain steady throughout the night.

Name ___Jim___     Insulin Dependent 24-Hour Decision Tree     Date _6_/_18_

| A Time | B BG (mg/dL) | C Activity | D Carbs (g) | E Fat (g) | F Predicted Carb:Insulin Ratio | G Injected Insulin (U) | H Actual Carb:Insulin Ratio | I Detailed Information About the Food You Ate (Elaborate on Back) | J Notes |
|---|---|---|---|---|---|---|---|---|---|
| 5:30 am | 105 | Fasting BG | | | | 1 u | | | Dawn phenomenon |
| 6:15 am | 110 | Pre Workout | 30 g | 0.4 g | 60:1 | 0.5 u | | Banana before workout | |
| 6:30 am | | Workout | | | | | | | Cycling class |
| 7:30 am | 115 | BG Check | | | | | | | |
| 8:45 am | | Injection | 175 g | 3.1 g | 25:1 | 7 u | 25:1 | Banana, mangoes, apples | |
| 9:00 am | 130 | BG Check | | | | | | | Wait 15 minutes to eat |
| 9:15 am | 118 | Begin Breakfast | | | | | | | |
| 11:30 am | 126 | BG Check | | | | | | | |
| 12:30 pm | 120 | Lunch Injection | 150 g | 4.5 g | 25:1 | 6 u | | Sweet potatoes, broccoli, green onion, lettuce, chickpeas | |
| 12:45 pm | 105 | Begin Lunch | | | | | | | |
| 3:30 pm | 200 | Correction | | | | 1 u | | | Adrenaline high from presentation |
| 6:00 pm | 111 | Dinner Injection | 115 g | 7 g | 32:1 | 3.5 u | 37:1 | Quinoa, black beans, carrots, garlic, onion, arugula, 1/4 avocado | Actual CI adjusted to 37:1 |
| 6:15 pm | | Begin Dinner | | | | | | | |
| 7:45 pm | 65 | Feeling Shaky | 15 g | | | | | 1 medical date | |
| 10:00 pm | 98 | Basal Injection | | | | 14 units | | | |
| TOTALS | -- | -- | 485 g | 15 g | | 33 u | | | |

# Sample Decision Tree:
# Non-Insulin-Dependent Diabetes

Veronica is living with type 2 diabetes and uses oral medications to manage her blood glucose, cholesterol, and blood pressure. She tests her blood glucose only twice per day, as we suggested in chapter 9. She does not monitor her calorie intake; instead she pays attention to her hunger signals for guidance about how much and how often to eat. She eats delicious nutrient-dense meals and documents her total carbohydrate and total fat intake on her decision tree to ensure that the food she is eating does not exceed our recommendations for maximum insulin sensitivity.

- Veronica wakes up.
  - 6:30 A.M.—Veronica wakes up with a fasting blood glucose of 173 mg/dL and is happy that it is lower than yesterday's fasting blood glucose of 205 mg/dL.
- Veronica exercises.
  - 7:30 A.M.—Veronica starts a 45-minute group fitness class.
- Veronica eats breakfast.
  - 9:00 A.M.—Veronica eats a Refreshing Fruit Delight (page 321), ensuring that her total fat intake is less than 10 grams at any given meal. She takes 1,000 mg of metformin (oral diabetes medication), 10 mg of lisinopril (an oral high blood pressure medication), and 25 mg of Crestor (an oral cholesterol-lowering statin medication).
- Veronica eats lunch.
  - 12:30 P.M.—Veronica eats the Sweet Potato Bake (page 336).
  - 3:30 P.M.—Veronica eats a snack of 2 apples at the office.
- Veronica eats dinner.
  - 6:00 P.M.—Veronica returns home and eats one of her favorite dinners, the Pad Thai Zoodles with Ginger Sauce (page 339), which has 9 grams of fat. She also takes 1,000 mg of metformin with her dinner.

- Veronica goes for a walk.
  - 7:00 P.M.—About 30 minutes after she has finished eating, Veronica goes for a walk with her kids to get her heart rate up for 15 minutes.
- Veronica prepares for bed.
  - 10:00 P.M.—Before going to bed, Veronica measures her blood glucose at 122 mg/dL.

Name _Veronica_    Non-Insulin Dependent 24-Hour Decision Tree    Date _2/18_

| Time | BG (mg/dL) | Activity | Carbs (g) | Fat (g) | Foods Eaten | Notes |
|---|---|---|---|---|---|---|
| 6:30 am | 173 | Fasting BG | | | | BG lower than yesterday!!! :) |
| 7:30 am | | Exercise | | | | Group fitness class 45 minutes |
| 9:00 am | | Breakfast | 141 g | 6 g | Refreshing Fruit Delight | Medications - 1000 mg Metformin, 10mg lisinopril, 25 mg Crestor |
| 12:30 pm | | Lunch | 95 g | 3.3 g | Sweet Potato Bake | |
| 3:30 pm | | Snack | 50 g | 0.6 g | 2 Sliced Apples | Feeling hungry |
| 6:00 pm | | Dinner | 72 g | 9 g | Pad Thai Zoodles with Ginger Sauce | 1000 mg Metformin |
| 10:00 pm | 122 | BG check before bed | | | | |
| | | | | | | |
| | | | | | | |
| | | | | | | |
| TOTALS | -- | | 358 g | 18.9 g | | Total fat less than 20 for the day :) |

# Acknowledgments

**Cyrus:** I would like to acknowledge my wife, Kylie Buckner, for her relentless dedication to improving the lives of thousands of people around the world, for the brilliance that she brings to my life, and for helping to improve the quality of information in this book. I would also like to thank my mom for preparing a home-cooked lunch for me every day from the first day of kindergarten through the last day of high school, with *zero* exceptions. Her dedication to grocery shopping, meal planning, and feeding me real food did not go unnoticed for even one day, and many of my habits today are a result of her unending desire to eat real food. I would also like to thank my dad for getting me addicted to mangoes from the Indian market at a young age, and for always encouraging me to higher education.

I'd like to thank my sister Persis for opening my eyes to being a vegetarian from a young age, for starting my addiction to green peas, and for always encouraging me to challenge the status quo. I'd like to thank my sister Shanaz for being the first person to figure out that I had type 1 diabetes, and for setting the example of what it means to work hard and always strive for excellence in the medical profession. And last but certainly not least, I'd like to thank my adorable and silly kittens, Mew and Blu, for always keeping me company, for making me laugh, and for allowing me to be your dad. I would be nothing without my family, so thank you for all that you've done to make me who I am today.

**Robby:** I would like to acknowledge my parents, Paul and Peggie Barbaro. Thank you for your unconditional love and unwavering support. My upbringing has set me up for success and true fulfillment. I am eternally grateful for your encouragement to pursue whatever is in my heart.

The encouragement and support I have received from family and dear friends throughout the book-writing process have meant the world to me. My sincere thanks to Adam Sud, Ally Ertel, Ashley and Britton Foster, Casey and Phil McCluskey, John Pierre, Melissa Pampanin, PJ Barbaro, Setareh Khatibi, Steve and Sara Cunning, Sterling Phillips, and Tara Kemp.

Brian Wendel, my respect for you is immense. Your true friendship and mentorship have shaped who I am and influenced me in immeasurable ways.

Taylor Call, your wisdom, guidance, and faith mean everything. Thank you.

Last but certainly not least, I want to express my gratitude for Cyrus. You are the best partner I could ever ask for, in a million ways and more. Your commitment to excellence and scientific rigor inspire me daily. Plus, you're the most fun and brilliant human I've ever met!

**We would both like to acknowledge** our agent, Janis Donnaud, for believing in us, and our editor, Caroline Sutton, for giving us an opportunity of a lifetime.

**Additionally, we would both like to acknowledge** the incredible team of talented people who have supported *Mastering Diabetes* from the time it began. Without their efforts, this book would simply not exist, and because of that we feel indebted to them for their hard work and dedication to changing the lives of thousands of people around the world. This list of exceptional individuals includes Adam Sud; Alex MacDowell; Chelsea Morrisey; Clay Crenshaw; Dave Rogenmoser; Heather Brock; Heather Harden; Ioana Pasarin; Jamie Marie Koonce; Jessica Stidham; Jewels Christine; Jonny Morelli; Jose Roman; Jose Tejero; Kylie Buckner, RN, MSN; Sam and Josh Ovett; Shelly Nason, PhD; Laurie Masters; Lindsay Garcia; Mariela Artega; Marc Ramirez; Navin Gupta; Rachel Kersten; and Tara Kemp.

**We would also like to acknowledge** the doctors, experts, pioneers and health professionals whose contributions have set a strong foundation for our work:

Alona Pulde, MD; Alan Goldhamer, DC; Angie Sadeghi, MD; Anthony Lim, MD; Brenda Davis, RD; Caldwell B. Esselstyn Jr., MD; Caroline Trapp, DNP; Chef AJ; Chris Wark; Clint Paddison; Columbus Batiste, MD; David Katz, MD, MPH; Dan Buettner; Danielle Belardo, MD; Dean Ornish, MD; Dean and Ayesha Sherzai, MD; Doug Lisle, PhD; Doug Graham, DC; Dustyn Williams, MD; Garth David, MD; Gemma Newman, MRCGP; Hans Diehl, DrHSc, MPH; Jane Esselstyn, RN; Julieanna Hever, RD; Laurie Marbas, MD; Marc Hellerstein, MD, PhD; Matthew Lederman, MD; Mauricio González, MD; Michael Greger, MD; Michael Klaper, MD; Michelle McMacken, MD; Monica Aggarwal, MD; Nancy Bohannon, MD; Neal Barnard, MD; Jay Sutliffe, PhD; Jeff Novick, MS, RDN; Jim Loomis, MD; John McDougall MD; Joel Fuhrman, MD; Joel Kahn, MD; Ray Cronise; Rick Dina, DC; Rip Esselstyn; Robert Ostfeld, MD; Ron Weiss, MD; Rosane Oliveira, PhD; Scott Stoll, MD; Steve Lawenda, MD; Susan Peirce Thompson, PhD; Susan Levin, MS, RD; T. Colin Campbell, PhD; Thomas Campbell, MD; Ocean Robbins; Valter Longo, PhD; Will Bulsiewicz, MD; and William Gibson, MD.

# Index

and diabetic ketoacidosis, 191
effect of plant-based diet on blood glucose,
    x, 5, 6
and exercise, 21–22, 149, 294–95,
    300–307, *307*
fasting, 147–48, *188*
and fat in diet, 45, 69, *70*, 168–69
fiber's effect on blood glucose, 113
and first 30 days of MDM, 147–48
fluctuations in blood glucose, 192
and glycemic index versus glycemic load,
    220–21
and heme iron, 87–88
and intermittent fasting, 21, 276, 281
and Kempner's rice-fruit diet, 135
and ketogenic diets, 121, 122, 123–24, 144
and legumes, 260
and low-carbohydrate dogma, 150
and low-carbohydrate plant-based diets, 131
and low-fat diets, 134–35
and medicinal plants, 222–24
and metabolizing of glucose, 48
monitoring, 4, *188*, 193
and oils, 159
and red light foods, 238
and refined carbohydrates, 113
and spikes following consumption of
    carbohydrates, 41, *42*
and sweeteners, 104, 219
time required for change in blood glucose
    level, 148–49
and trans fats, 68
and transitioning to MDM diet, 192
and yellow light foods, 154
blood pressure
    adjusting medications, 4
    and consumption of sodium, 89
    effect of plant-based diets, x, 4, 5, 10, 43
    and insulin resistance, 11
    and intermittent fasting, 277
    and ketogenic diets, 122
    and low-fat plant-based diets, 138, 140
    monitoring, *188*
body fat, conversion of glucose to, 114. *See
    also* adipose tissue
body weight
    and consumption of sugar, 102

conventional views on weight gain, 41
and insulin sensitivity/resistance, 61
monitoring, *188*
and plant-based diets, 3, 5, 10, 43, 139
*See also* weight loss
bolus insulin, 203–4
bone fracture risk, 156
brain
    and excess glucose, 114
    glucose and insulin required by brain, 48,
        117, 118
    and glycogen stores in liver, 116–17
    and ketone bodies manufactured by
        liver, 117
bread, 90, 153
breakfast, 212–32
    and caffeinated beverages, 227–29
    hunger soon after, 231
    importance of eating breakfast, 214
    and medicinal plants, 222–24
    options, 218–19, 221–22
    recipes, 321–29
    reexamining approach to, 19
    smoothies, 229–30
    and troubleshooting high blood glucose
        levels, 230–31
breastfeeding, xi
brewer's yeast, 182
*British Medical Journal*, 88
brown rice, *168*
Buettner, Dan, 143
bulk in foods, 240
butternut squash, *168*

caffeinated beverages, 227–29
caffeine, 161
calorie counting, x, 164–65, 235–36
calorie density, 235–38, 252
calorie restriction, 21, 275–76. *See also*
    intermittent fasting
cancer
    and consumption of animal-sourced
        foods, 85, 126
    and consumption of sugar, 102
    and green tea, 161
    and insulin resistance, 11, *12*

In the process of writing this book, we read thousands of scientific papers and referenced more than eight hundred peer-reviewed articles. Even though there are too many references to print in this book, we are passionate about empowering you to make informed decisions for your health. Visit www.masteringdiabetes.org/bookinfo to explore every scientific reference in this book.